Caring for the Elderly

The Johns Hopkins Series in Contemporary Medicine and Public Health

Consulting Editors:

Martin D. Abeloff, M.D.
Samuel H. Boyer IV, M.D.
Gareth M. Green, M.D.
Richard T. Johnson, M.D.
Paul R. McHugh, M.D.
Edmond A. Murphy, M.D.
Edyth H. Schoenrich, M.D., M.P.H.
Jerry L. Spivak, M.D.
Barbara H. Starfield, M.D., M.P.H.

———

Also of Interest in This Series:

Adding Life to Years: Organized Geriatrics Services in Great Britain and Implications for the United States,
William Halsey Barker
The Hospice Experiment,
edited by Vincent Mor, David S. Greer, and Robert Kastenbaum

Caring for the Elderly

Reshaping Health Policy

362.6
Ei 81

WITHDRAWN

EDITED BY

Carl Eisdorfer, PH.D., M.D.
Professor and Chairman, Department of Psychiatry
Director, Center on Adult Development and Aging
University of Miami School of Medicine

David A. Kessler, M.D., J.D.
Medical Director, The Jack D. Weiler Hospital of the
Albert Einstein College of Medicine
Montefiore Medical Center

Abby N. Spector, M.M.H.S.
Project Director, Philadelphia Geriatric Center

The Johns Hopkins University Press
Baltimore & London

LIBRARY ST. MARY'S COLLEGE

183413

© 1989 The Johns Hopkins University Press.
Copyright does not include
the separate content of chapter 27,
which was written as a work of
the United States government.
All rights reserved
Printed in the United States of America

The Johns Hopkins University Press
701 West 40th Street
Baltimore, Maryland 21211
The Johns Hopkins Press Ltd., London

The paper used in this publication meets the minimum requirements of
American National Standard for Information Sciences—Permanence of Paper
for Printed Library Materials, ANSI Z39.48-1984.

Library of Congress Cataloging-in-Publication Data

Caring for the elderly: reshaping health policy/edited by Carl Eisdorfer, David
A. Kessler, and Abby Spector.
    p.   cm.   (The Johns Hopkins series in contemporary medicine and
public health)
    Includes bibliographies and index.
    ISBN 0-8018-3810-X (alk. paper)
    1. Aged—Medical care—United States.   2. Aged—Long term care—
United States. [1. Medical care, Cost of—United States.] I. Eisdorfer,
Carl. II. Kessler, David A. III. Spector, Abby. IV. Series.
    [DNLM: 1. Health Insurance for Aged and Disabled, Title 18.
2. Health Policy—United States. 3. Health Services for the Aged—
United States. WT 30 C277]
RA564.8.C38   1989
362.1'9897'00973—dc20
DNLM/DLC
for Library of Congress   89-2199
                                                    CIP

$51.15 ᕼᕮᑎ 5-7-91 (ᐯ.ᐯ.)

LIBRARY ST. MARY'S COLLEGE

For Susan, Erica, Marc, Jason, Seth, and Noah Eisdorfer
For Paulette, Elise, and Benjamin Kessler
For Gerald Skillings

Contents

Five. Ethical and Political Dimensions of Reform

Six. Reconceptualizing the Problem

Contributors

Linda H. Aiken, Ph.D., Trustee Professor of Nursing and Sociology, School of Nursing and Department of Sociology, and Associate Director, Leonard Davis Institute for Health Economics, University of Pennsylvania

Stuart H. Altman, Ph.D., Dean and Professor, Florence Heller Graduate School for Advanced Studies in Social Welfare, Brandeis University

Lisa F. Berkman, Ph.D., Associate Professor of Epidemiology, Department of Epidemiology, School of Medicine, Yale University

Robert H. Binstock, Ph.D., Henry R. Luce Professor of Aging, Health, and Society, Department of Epidemiology and Biostatistics, School of Medicine, Case Western Reserve University

Philip W. Brickner, M.D., Director, Department of Community Medicine, St. Vincent's Hospital and Medical Center of New York

Elaine M. Brody, M.S.W., Sc. D. (Hon.), Associate Director of Research, Philadelphia Geriatric Center

Stanley J. Brody, J.D., M.S.W., Professor of Physical Medicine and Rehabilitation in Psychiatry Emeritus, University of Pennsylvania

Francis G. Caro, Ph.D., Professor of Gerontology and Director of Research, Gerontology Institute, University of Massachusetts, Boston (formerly Director of Research, Community Service Society, New York, N.Y.)

Donna Cohen, Ph.D., Professor of Public Health, and Director, Gerontology Center, Department of Community Health Sciences, University of Illinois, Chicago

Cynthia A. Coombs, M.S., Associate Director, The Robert Wood Johnson Foundation Program for Hospital Initiatives in Long-Term Care, New York, N.Y.

Karen Davis, Ph.D., Professor and Chairman, Department of Health Policy and Management, School of Hygiene and Public Health, Johns Hopkins University

Paul M. Densen, D.Sc., Professor of Community Health and Medical Care Emeritus, School of Medicine, Harvard University (formerly Director, Harvard Center for Community Health and Medical Care, School of Public Health and Medical School, Harvard University)

Carroll L. Estes, Ph.D., Professor and Chairman, Department of Social and Behavioral Sciences, and Director, Institute for Health and Aging, School of Nursing, University of California, San Francisco

Msgr. Charles J. Fahey, M.S.W., M.Div., Marie Ward Doty Professor of Aging Studies, and Director, Third Age Center, Fordham University at Lincoln Center

Judith Feder, Ph.D., Co-Director, Center for Health Policy Studies, and Research Associate Professor, Department of Community and Family Medicine, School of Medicine, Georgetown University

Karyn L. Feiden, B.A., Consultant, The Robert Wood Johnson Foundation Program for Hospital Initiatives in Long-Term Care, New York, N.Y.

James P. Firman, M.B.A., Ed.D., President, United Seniors Health Cooperative, Washington, D.C.

Iris C. Freeman, M.S.W., Executive Director, Minnesota Alliance for Health Care Consumers, Minneapolis

Eli Ginzberg, Ph.D., Director, Conservation of Human Resources, Columbia University

Jay N. Greenberg, D.Sc,. Executive Vice President, LifePlans, Inc., Waltham, Mass.

Charlene A. Harrington, Ph.D., R.N., Professor, Institute for Health and Aging, Department of Social and Behavioral Sciences, School of Nursing, University of California, San Francisco

Margaret M. Hastings, Ph.D., Associate Professor, Health Resources Management, School of Public Health, University of Illinois, Chicago

William R. Hazzard, M.D., Professor and Chairman, Director, J. Paul Sticht Center on Aging, Department of Internal Medicine, Bowman Gray School of Medicine, Wake Forest University, Winston-Salem, N.C.

Tom Joe, Director, Center for the Study of Social Policy, Washington, D.C.

Ellen W. Jones, M.P.H., Associate Professor of Community Health Emerita, Preventive Medicine and Clinical Epidemiology, Harvard Medical School (formerly, Assistant Director, Harvard Center for Community Health and Medical Care, School of Public Health and Medical School, Harvard University)

Robert L. Kane, M.D., Dean, School of Public Health, University of Minnesota

Rosalie A. Kane, D.S.W., Professor, Schools of Social Work and Public Health, University of Minnesota

Mary C. Kapp, M.Phil., Epidemiologist, Health Department, Hartford, Conn. (formerly Senior Project Director, Center for Gerontology and Health Care Research, Brown University)

Sidney Katz, M.D., M.A. Professor of Bio-Architectonics and Medicine, Bio-Architectonics Center and Department of Medicine, Case Western Reserve University (formerly Professor of Community Health, School of Medicine, Brown University)

Lambert N. King, M.D., Ph.D., Medical Director and Vice President for Professional Affairs, St. Vincent's Hospital and Medical Center of New York

Philip R. Lee, M.D., Professor of Social Medicine and Director, Institute for Health Policy Studies, School of Medicine, University of California, San Francisco

Walter N. Leutz, Ph.D., M.S.W., Senior Research Associate, Florence Heller Graduate School for Advanced Studies in Social Welfare, Brandeis University

Barbara Lyons, M.H.S., Research Associate, Department of Health Policy and Management, School of Hygiene and Public Health, Johns Hopkins University

George L. Maddox, Ph.D., Chairman, University Council on Aging and Human Development and Professor of Sociology and Medical Sociology, Departments of Sociology and Psychiatry, Duke University

Judith S. Magel, M.C.P., M.B.A., Senior Policy Analyst in Long-Term Care, Department of Health Care Delivery, American Medical Association

Kenneth G. Manton, Ph.D., Research Professor, Demographic Studies, Duke University

James L. O'Brien, Jr., M.A., Assistant Director, Quality Measurement and Management Project, The Hospital Research and Educational Trust, Chicago

William A. Read, Ph.D., Associate Director, The Flinn Foundation, Phoenix (formerly President, Hospital Research and Educational Trust, Chicago)

Dorothy P. Rice, B.A., D. Sc. (Hon.), Professor in Residence, Institute for Health and Aging, Department of Social and Behavioral Sciences, School of Nursing, University of California, San Francisco

Diane Rowland, Sc.D., Assistant Professor, Department of Health Policy and Management, School of Hygiene and Public Health, Johns Hopkins University

William J. Scanlon, Ph.D., Co-Director, Center for Health Policy Studies, and Research Associate Professor, Department of Community and Family Medicine, School of Medicine, Georgetown University

Linda K. Scharer, M.U.P., Assistant Director, Department of Community Medicine, St. Vincent's Hospital and Medical Center of New York

Helen L. Smits, M.D., Director, John Dempsey Hospital, Professor of Community Medicine, School of Medicine, University of Connecticut Health Center

Anne R. Somers, B. A., Sc.D. (Hon.), Adjunct Professor, Department of Environmental and Community Medicine, Robert Wood Johnson Medical School, University of Medicine and Dentistry of New Jersey

Bruce C. Vladeck, Ph.D., President, United Hospital Fund of New York

Terrie Wetle, Ph.D., Director of Research, Braceland Center for Mental Health and Aging, Institute of Living, Hartford, Conn; Associate Professor, Department of Community Medicine and Health Care, University of Connecticut; and Lecturer, Division on Aging, School of Medicine, Harvard University

T. Franklin Williams, M.D., Director, National Institute on Aging, National Institutes of Health

James Williamson, CBE, M.B., Ch.B., FRCPE, Sc.D. (Hon.), Professor Emeritus, Department of Geriatric Medicine, University of Edinburgh

Acknowledgments

In expressing our appreciation to those who participated in this project, we must begin by acknowledging the contributing authors. We are grateful for what we believe to be their very significant contributions to a much-needed effort to reshape health-care policy for the elderly, and thereby to improve health-care policy for the nation.

The United Hospital Fund of New York also has our deep appreciation for helping to underwrite the expense in organizing the volume. We are especially grateful to its president, Bruce Vladeck, not only for his support of the book from the start but also for his willingness to serve as one of the contributing authors. He offered many thoughtful recommendations as we formulated our ideas for the book, and helped us to move the project from conception to reality. Few individuals bring his breadth of perspective and depth of insight to the field of health policy. His studies of nursing home care and hospital payment systems, areas addressed in this book, have been instrumental in shaping national debate on these important issues.

We also wish to acknowledge the important assistance of The Robert Wood Johnson Foundation, whose Program for Hospital Initiatives in Long-Term Care provided the stimulus and partial support for this book. As we observed hospitals in the program changing their service delivery practices, it became clear that effective new strategies were being developed to improve the care of the elderly. We are indebted to Cynthia Coombs, who administered the program. She reviewed the manuscript at each stage of its development and contributed valuable ideas and criticisms throughout.

We would like to acknowledge the contributions of several individuals who were instrumental in giving the volume its final form. We are indebted to Maria Coughlin for her indispensable work in shaping and bringing clarity to the manuscript. She is responsible for reducing redundancy among the chapters and copyediting the full text. We are also deeply grateful to Karyn Feiden, whose thoughtful and creative editorial work and writing gave the manuscript its cohesion. Credit for the section introductions rests largely with her. We would also like to thank Susan Aldrich for her critical review of the entire book. Her many useful suggestions sharpened specific portions of the manuscript as well as its overall organization.

Our very special gratitude goes to Lorraine White for her exceptional assistance in preparing this volume. Throughout this process, she kept careful track of us, the contributors, and the chapters; organized the extensive correspondence, coordinated communications, and answered myriad questions; and typed (and re-typed) portions of the manuscript. We are immensely grateful for the precision, patience, perseverance, and humor with which she approached this project. We also wish to thank Patricia Kenneally and Helen Surita for their assistance with typing.

Finally, we would like to acknowledge our appreciation to our editor, Wendy Harris, at the Johns Hopkins University Press. She has been a continual source of support, encouragement, and expert advice throughout the lengthy process of producing this volume.

Introduction

Meeting the needs of an aging population is one of the country's most critical policy challenges. Traditional societal values have held that older people are entitled to access to health care that will enable them to live out their years with dignity. But, faced with a burgeoning elderly population and rising federal budget deficits, can we fulfill this broad promise?

To answer this question, we must confront a multitude of vexing pragmatic concerns: How much is society willing and able to spend on the health care of older people? Can access to health care be ensured both equitably and affordably? What are the appropriate responsibilities of the public and private sectors, and how can responsibility best be shared between the formal and informal systems of care? With the availability of life-sustaining technologies, what are the rights of individuals to mediate their own care, and what happens when individual rights conflict with societal needs? Will medical care be rationed, and if so, how will this be accomplished?

The imperative of addressing these difficult issues can be illustrated with a single statistic: Within the next 40 years the number of older persons in the United States will more than double. Currently, 29 million people are age 65 or older. By 2030, that number will climb to 64 million, or one in five Americans. Advanced age is associated with an increased risk of physical and psychiatric disability. Today, more than 80% of elderly persons have at least one chronic health problem, and many have multiple conditions. Older persons are already the leading consumers of health-care services; currently, they obtain approximately 40% more care in outpatient settings than the general population, they are admitted to hospitals twice as often, their hospital stays extend 50% longer, and they account for more than 90% of the long-term care bed occupancy in the United States. As we succeed in lengthening the life span, will we be prepared to meet the increased demand for services required by an aging population with multiple and chronic health problems?

In this volume, national experts address the complex demographic, financial, organizational, ethical, and political issues involved in planning health care for an aging society. The contributors to this volume are scholars, clinicians, and scientists of extraordinary repute who have devoted many years to examination of the issues described in their chapters. They include epidemiologists and ethicists, physicians and political scientists, empiricists and philosophers, economists and social workers. In assembling the volume, we asked each of these leading experts to define what they thought were the most important aspects of health care for the elderly, to look to the future, and to develop, from their own vantage points, strategies for improving existing systems of care. What has emerged from their work is a collection of essays examining a comprehensive range of issues in health care for the elderly.

The book is divided into six major sections. The first one, "Setting the Stage," presents a summary of the demographic, socioeconomic, and health characteristics of the elderly population. These objective data are an essential basis for any discussion or debate about our policy options for addressing the needs of the elderly.

The second section, "Paying for Services," begins by describing and evaluating our current systems of health-care financing and then turns to analyzing recent and proposed reforms. This section examines the questions of what quality health care for the elderly will cost and who will pay for it.

The third section, "Available and Emerging Sources of Care," points out the major strengths and weaknesses of our current health-care systems— although an impressive and varied range of services is available for the elderly, the services are so fragmented that access to and coordination of them prove difficult. This section focuses on the changing roles of hospitals, long-term care facilities, families, and consumer organizations in their attempts to provide integrated acute and long-term care for the elderly.

The fourth section, "Special Problems of Geriatric Health Care," brings a clinical perspective to the discussion of the health-care needs of the aged. Because their medical conditions are frequently multiple and chronic, the elderly have a distinct set of health-care needs that must be taken into account when developing health-care policy. This section drives home this point through discussions of lens implants, hip replacements, alcoholism, mental health, and preventive health care.

Some of the most difficult issues that policymakers must face are addressed in the fifth section, "Ethical and Political Dimensions of Reform." Essays in this section grapple with the allocation of scarce medical care, the use of life-sustaining technology, ageism, and equitable access to care.

The final section of the book, "Reconceptualizing the Problem," argues that a transformation of health care for the elderly is inevitable, and that reconceptualizing the way we think about health care for the elderly will help to ensure that this change is productive. Essays in this section challenge traditional perspectives on such topics as health maintenance, medical education, and the artificial separation of acute and long-term care and of medical and social services.

We developed this book for a broad audience of individuals concerned with health care for the elderly. It is intended to serve as a resource for health-care policymakers, planners, practitioners, and researchers as well as for students of health policy, administration, and research. Our goals in producing the volume were to provide important background about the elderly population and the problems in existing systems of care, as well as to offer a variety of proposed solutions to improve the care of older people.

Part One

Setting the Stage

Today's over-65 population has been slotted into three categories—the old, the old-old, and the oldest-old, a linguistic testimony to the graying of America. The highly subjective process of reshaping health policy to meet the demands of this aging segment of society, which is the mandate of this volume, is best begun with a compilation of facts. Therefore, we open with Dorothy P. Rice's stage-setting overview of the demographic, socioeconomic, and health characteristics of the elderly population. Her statistical data on the numbers of old people, the extent to which they require health services, and their access to care establish the heterogeneity of our target group. Building upon this factual baseline, she then dissects the strengths and weaknesses of the current health system. To meet the special needs of the elderly effectively and efficiently, the organization, delivery, costs, and financing of medical, social, and long-term care services must be restructured, writes Rice.

Among the signal changes of shifting demographic realities is an escalating need for particular medical services—the incidences of Alzheimer's disease and hip fractures, for example, are expected to jump, and with them the demand for appropriate care. Similarly, as the percentage of the elderly older than 85 spirals upward, the pressure to expand long-term care facilities will intensify.

However, much is still unknown about the demands that an aging population will place on the health-care system: Will more people grow increasingly frail and dependent over longer periods of time or will lifestyle improvements delay the onset of disability, reduce the prevalence of chronic disease, and compress morbidity at older ages? As the burgeoning elderly population stretches limited resources to the breaking point, will interest in primary care be rekindled, or will the elderly be forced to postpone medical treatment until they are in crisis?

Whatever the answers are, the growth of the aging population clearly challenges the nation's health-care delivery system in ways that elude the grasp of patchwork solutions. The changing circumstances highlighted here point up systemic cracks, but they also create a mood of uncertainty receptive to innovation. By arming policymakers with facts about the elderly population, this section provides the tools necessary to substitute coherent national health-care planning for short-term, piecemeal solutions.

One

The Characteristics and Health of the Elderly

Dorothy P. Rice

Americans are living longer today than ever before. Improvements in living conditions and lifestyles, as well as advances in science, medical technology, and pharmaceutical therapies, have meant tremendous reductions in the number of deaths from formerly fatal infectious diseases, dramatic gains in life expectancy, and a rapid growth of the number of older Americans. This demographic change has important implications for the nation's health, social, and economic institutions.

Contrary to popular belief, the elderly are generally healthy. However, they are more likely than younger people to suffer from chronic illnesses that cause limited or total disability. The probability of increasing disability and the need for medical care are greater for aged persons with multiple chronic conditions. Thus, the effect of increased longevity on health status and the quality of life has become a focal issue.

This chapter defines the elderly population, describes the changing demographic structure of the population, and focuses on the socioeconomic and health characteristics of the elderly. The health of the elderly is examined in terms of their health status, their use of medical care services, and their future morbidity and mortality patterns.

3

Definitions of the Elderly

Most geriatric literature seems to accept age 65 as the beginning of old age, although there are no precise biological reasons to do so. The operational definition of old age required to administer public programs is determined by custom and by the legal definition of retirement age, rather than by objective criteria.

In 1982, the World Health Organization selected age 65 as the beginning of old age. This was recognized as an arbitrary threshold for statistical purposes and corresponded with the generally agreed upon age of retirement and completion of professional activity in most countries.[1] In the United States, full Social Security retirement benefits, Medicare, and many private retirement plans now take effect at age 65, although eligibility criteria are beginning to change in response to social and economic pressures.

Public Law 98-21, the Social Security Amendments of 1983, legislated an increase in the age of eligibility for unreduced monthly benefits from 65 to 67 years on a gradual phase-in schedule beginning in the year 2000, with full implementation occurring in the year 2027.[2] Similarly, the 1982 Advisory Council on Social Security recommended a gradual increase in the age of eligibility for Medicare benefits from age 65 to 67, beginning in 1985, with full implementation by 1990,[3] but no enabling legislation has been passed.

It is clear that many factors have challenged the sanctity of age 65 as the age of retirement, including increased life expectancy, improved health, the growth of private and public pensions, increased service jobs, and changing social attitudes. Furthermore, as the number of elderly has grown, differences among them have become apparent. Subgroups of the elderly have been identified: those fit and active, and those 75 and older— the old-old, who have a much higher prevalence of illness and disability.[4] More recently, the latter population group has been further subdivided, with those age 85 and older identified as the oldest-old.[5]

The Changing Demographic Structure of the Population

The rapid growth of the elderly population in the United States is expected to continue well into the next century. In the period from 1930 to 1980, the elderly population grew four times as fast as the under-65 population. Projections made by the United States Bureau of the Census indicate that this differential rate of growth will continue for another 50-year period, 1980–2030.

At the turn of the century, the nation's 3.1 million elderly people comprised 4.0% of the total population (Table 1.1). Forty years later, the

Table 1.1. Number and Distribution of the Population, All Ages and 65 and Over, United States, 1900–2050

| Year | Population All Ages | Population 65 Years and Older | | | |
		Total	65–74	75–84	85 and Over
		Number (in thousands)			
1900	76,303	3,084	2,189	772	123
1910	91,972	3,950	2,793	989	167
1920	105,711	4,933	3,464	1,259	210
1930	122,775	6,634	4,721	1,641	272
1940	131,669	9,019	6,375	2,278	365
1950	150,697	12,270	8,415	3,278	577
1960	179,979	16,675	11,053	4,681	940
1970	204,879	20,085	12,486	6,166	1,432
1980	227,704	25,714	15,652	7,791	2,271
Projections[a]					
1990	249,657	31,697	18,035	10,349	3,313
2000	267,955	34,921	17,677	12,318	4,926
2010	283,238	39,196	20,318	12,326	6,551
2020	296,597	51,422	29,855	14,486	7,081
2030	304,807	64,580	34,535	21,434	8,611
2040	308,559	66,988	29,272	24,882	12,834
2050	309,488	67,412	30,114	21,263	16,034
		Percentage Distribution			
1900	100.0	4.0	2.9	1.0	0.2
1910	100.0	4.3	3.0	1.1	0.2
1920	100.0	4.7	3.3	1.2	0.2
1930	100.0	5.4	3.8	1.3	0.2
1940	100.0	6.8	4.8	1.7	0.3
1950	100.0	8.1	5.6	2.2	0.4
1960	100.0	9.3	6.1	2.6	0.5
1970	100.0	9.8	6.1	3.0	0.7
1980	100.0	11.3	6.9	3.4	1.0
Projections[a]					
1990	100.0	12.7	7.2	4.1	1.3
2000	100.0	13.0	6.6	4.6	1.8
2010	100.0	13.8	7.2	4.4	2.3
2020	100.0	17.3	10.1	4.9	2.3
2030	100.0	21.2	11.3	7.0	2.4
2040	100.0	21.7	9.5	8.1	4.2
2050	100.0	21.8	9.7	6.9	5.2

Source: Ref. 6.
[a]Middle series.

number of elderly had tripled to 9 million and constituted 6.8% of the nation's total. By 1980, the elderly population almost tripled again, to 25.7 million persons, representing 11.3% of the total population. By the year 2030 it is likely that one out of five Americans will be 65 years old or older, and the total number of elderly is projected to be 64.6 million.

Furthermore, the number and proportion of the very old have also increased rapidly. In 1900, fewer than 125,000 persons were 85 years old and older, comprising 4% of the population over 65 years old; by 1980, there were 2.3 million persons in this age group, or 9% of the elderly. In the period from 1980 to 2030, the very old population is projected to quadruple, comprising 13% of the elderly by 2030.

A child born in 1985 will be 65 in the year 2050. The total population under age 65 will number 242 million in 2050, a one-seventh increase in the 65-year period from 1985 to 2050. During the same period, the elderly population will multiply 1⅓ times, while the number of very old (age 85 and older) will increase by almost five times. Thus, the group age 85 and older is projected to be the fastest growing part of the population. This growth in the number of persons who survive into their eighties and nineties also makes it increasingly likely that many elderly persons will have a surviving parent. These projections are the "middle series" projections of the U.S. Bureau of the Census, based on the assumption of slightly increasing fertility rates and increasing life expectancy—for females, from 77.4 years in 1980 to 83.6 years in 2050, and for males, from 70 years to 75.5 years during the same period. Net immigration is assumed to be constant, at 450,000 persons each year.[6] How closely these population projections will correspond to future demographic changes is clearly uncertain, but they reflect expert opinion that is generally molded by the events of the recent past.

Socioeconomic Characteristics of the Elderly Population

The elderly of the United States are predominantly female (in 1985, there were 68 elderly men for every 100 elderly women), and the sex differential increases significantly with age. In 1985 there were 78 men 65–74 years old for every 100 women in the same age group, and only 54 men age 75 and older for every 100 women of the same age. This differential in the ratio of elderly men to women is projected to remain approximately the same in the future.

Not only do women live longer than men, they tend to marry men older than themselves, so they are often widowed, and they are unlikely to remarry once widowed. In 1985, two-fifths of all noninstitutionalized women age 65 to 74 and two-thirds of those age 75 and over were widowed. In contrast, less than one-tenth of the men age 65 to 74 and one-fourth of those age 75 and over were widowed.[7] An increasing number of older persons live alone rather than in family settings. In 1950, 14% of all elderly persons lived alone; by 1985 this proportion increased to 30%. The disparity in the marital status of older men and women results in significant differences in their living arrangements. In 1985, three out of four elderly men were married and living with their wives, but only two-fifths of all elderly women were married and living with their husbands.

As people age, they tend to leave the labor force or to work fewer hours. When they retire, their pensions are generally lower than their prior earnings. Thus there is a pattern of declining income for older persons. The lower incomes of the elderly are associated with factors over which they have little control: their sex and race, the health and survival of their spouses, their health, their ability to work, their educational attainment (which is strongly associated with lifetime earnings), their investments, and their assets.[8] For men, income tends to increase with age until about age 55, when significant numbers of individuals retire and income levels begin to decline steadily. Median income for women begins at lower levels than for men and starts to decline at age 50. In 1984, the median income of men 65 years old and older was $10,450, about 74% higher than that for elderly women ($6,020).[9]

In 1986, 67% of the 55- to 64-year-old men and 42% of the women in the same age group were in the labor force. For persons age 65 and over, however, these figures dropped to 15% for men and 7% for women.[10]

Social Security benefits are the largest source of income for the elderly; 91% of the elderly population receive benefits. More than half of the population age 65 and over depend on Social Security for over half their income, and a fifth receive 90% or more of their income from this source.[11]

In 1983, 3.7 million persons, or 14.1% of elderly persons, lived in poverty.[12] (This rate represents a significant improvement from 1967, when the poverty rate was 29.5%.) Poverty among the elderly is explained partly by the substantial reduction in income occurring at retirement and by the likelihood of major expenditures for health care. Poverty is disproportionately high among elderly women (17%) and blacks (36%). The current government definition of poverty does not include the value of in-kind transfers. If the value of in-kind food, housing, and medical care transfers received by the low-income elderly population were regarded as income, the poverty rate figure would be reduced.[13] There is serious disagreement, however, about whether payments for medical care, especially institutional care, should be counted when measuring poverty.

The demographic and socioeconomic characteristics of the elderly affect their health status and use of health-care services. Therefore, these statistics serve as a basis for understanding the magnitude of the problem of providing medical and other long-term services to the increasing number of persons who live to an age at which they are vulnerable to chronic illnesses that can cause limited or total disability.

Mortality

The rapid increase in the elderly population is attributable partly to declining mortality rates across the entire life span. Early in the century, the decline in mortality rates was greatest at younger ages, so that the proportion of babies surviving to adulthood increased. An individual born in 1900 could expect to live an average of 47.3 years, whereas by 1985, life expectancy reached 74.7 years (Table 1.2). Declining mortality rates for the elderly are also reflected in their improved life expectancy. In 1900, a 65-year-old person would expect to live 11.9 additional years, to age 77; by 1985, life expectancy at age 65 increased to 16.8 years, to about age 82.[14]

Mortality rates have dropped for males and females and for white and black persons, but women and white persons have shown the most rapid decreases. Between 1960 and 1985, women age 65 and over gained 2.8 years of life expectancy, compared with only 1.8 years for men. Elderly white persons gained 2.4 years, compared with only 1.6 years for blacks.

The leading causes of death for the elderly are heart disease, cancer, stroke, influenza, pneumonia, and arteriosclerosis. Death rates for all these causes except cancer have been declining. From 1950 to 1982, the death rate for people 65 years old and over decreased 19%, and the decline for females was nearly twice as great as that for males. Of the leading causes of death among the elderly, cancer has the most pronounced sex differences. Lung cancer exhibits the greatest disparity, with male mortality nearly five times greater than female mortality.

About half of the overall decline in mortality among the elderly during the period 1950–1982 was a result of the decline in heart disease mortality, the leading cause of death; another third is associated with the fall in death rates for stroke, the third leading cause of death. Cancer, the second leading cause, increased 14% and is the only major cause of death for the elderly to have increased in the 32-year period. A variety of factors are responsible for the substantial declines in mortality from heart disease and stroke during the past three decades. These include improved medical care and interventions, greater availability of coronary care units, advanced surgical and medical treatment of coronary heart disease, improved control of blood pressure, decreased smoking, modified eating habits, increased exercise, and more healthy lifestyles in general. A recent study estimated that more than half the decline in ischemic heart disease mortality between 1968 and 1976 was related to reductions in serum cholesterol levels and decreased cigarette smoking, and another 40% of the decline was attributed to specific medical interventions, such as coronary care units,

Table 1.2. Life Expectancy at Birth and at 65 Years of Age, by Sex and Race, United States, Selected Years 1900–1985

Specified Age and Year	Remaining Life Expectancy (in years)				
	Total	Males	Females	Whites	Blacks
At Birth					
1900	47.3	46.3	48.3	47.6	33.0
1950	68.2	65.6	71.1	69.1	60.7
1960	69.7	66.6	73.1	70.6	63.2
1970	70.9	67.1	74.8	71.7	64.1
1980	73.7	70.0	77.4	74.4	68.1
1985[a]	74.7	71.2	78.2	75.3	69.5
At Age 65					
1900	11.9	11.5	12.2	na	na
1950	13.9	12.8	15.0	na	13.9
1960	14.3	12.8	15.8	14.4	13.9
1970	15.2	13.1	17.0	15.2	14.2
1980	16.4	14.1	18.3	16.5	15.1
1985[a]	16.8	14.6	18.6	16.8	15.5

Source: Ref. 14.
[a]Provisional data.

arrhythmia prophylaxis, prehospital resuscitation, coronary artery bypass surgery, and treatment of blood pressure and clinical ischemic heart disease.[15] However, other interventions, such as pacemakers, may also have contributed to the decline.

Health Status

The health of the elderly can be measured several ways: their own perception of their health, limitations in their usual activities, and restricted-activity and bed-disability days. Table 1.3 summarizes these health-status measures by age. In 1985, 31% of the noninstitutionalized elderly reported that their health was fair or poor compared with other people their age. Approximately 33 million persons, 14% of the noninstitutionalized population, reported limitations of activity due to chronic diseases. Not surprisingly, the percentage of the population suffering limitation of activity increases with age: it is 5% of the total population under 18, 8% of those age 18–44 years, 23% of those 45–64, and 40% of those 65 and over.[16]

Health status data for the Medicare population are available from the National Medical Care Utilization and Expenditure Survey.[17] As shown in Table 1.4 and as expected, restricted-activity days and activity limitation increase with age. For example, of persons 64–69 years old, 31% reported some limitation in activity, compared with 52% of those 80 years old and over. Interestingly, the number of illnesses reported during the year and

Table 1.3.   Health Status and Utilization Measures by Age, United States, 1985

					65 and Over		
Measure	All Ages	Under 18	18–44	45–64	Total	65–74	75+
Percent Feeling Fair or Poor	10.3	2.6	5.6	18.5	31.4	na	na
Percent Limited in Activity	14.0	5.1	8.4	23.4	39.6	39.2[a]	39.8[b]
Percent Unable to Carry on Major Activity	3.9	0.5	2.1	8.7	10.4	17.0[a]	6.9[b]
Restricted Activity Days (per person)	14.8	8.5	11.2	20.3	33.1	na	na
Bed-Disability Days (per person)	6.1	4.0	4.5	8.3	13.7	na	na
Physician Visits (per person)	5.3	4.2	4.7	6.1	8.3	7.7	9.3
Percent Seeing Doctor in Last Year	75.4	77.9	70.2	74.4	83.8	83.8	86.9
Short-Stay Hospital Discharges[c] (per 100 persons)	12.4	5.0	11.0	16.2	28.1	24.7	33.6
Days of Care (per 100 persons)	83.4	25.7	55.3	129.2	245.5	207.2	307.1
Average Length of Stay	6.7	5.1	5.0	8.0	8.7	8.4	9.1
Needs Help in One or More Basic Activities (per 1,000 persons)	22.5[d]	—	5.1	20.6	90.2	52.6	157.0

Source: Refs. 16 and 19.
[a]Rates are for the 65–69 age group.
[b]Rates are for the 70 and over age group.
[c]Including deliveries.
[d]Includes adults age 18 and over.

perceived poor health status increased to age 80, but those 80 years of age and over averaged slightly fewer conditions and a smaller proportion of them reported poor health status than those in the 75–79 age group. The very old also perceived their health as somewhat better than that of those at younger ages. It is likely that at 80 years and over, the very sick and functionally disabled persons are institutionalized.

Table 1.4. Health Status Measures for Medicare Population by Age, 1980

Measure	Age				
	65 and Over	64–69	70–74	75–79	80 and Over
Restricted-Activity Days					
Average for all persons	31	26	32	37	39
Average for persons with at least one	50	42	51	55	61
Illness Conditions					
Average for all persons	4.4	4.0	4.4	5.1	4.9
Average for persons with at least one	4.8	4.4	4.7	5.5	5.2
Percent Limited in Activity	40	31	39	47	52
Percent with Conditions Unattended	95	94	95	96	98
Perceived Health Status (percent)					
Excellent	26	27	26	21	28
Good	37	38	37	36	37
Fair	25	26	24	26	24
Poor	12	9	13	15	12

Source: Ref. 17.

Although men and women differ little in the proportion reporting fair or poor health, there are substantial differences in the ability they report to carry on with their usual (major) activity because of health. Forty-five percent of elderly men, but only 35% of elderly women, report that they cannot carry on with their usual activity because of health problems. The men may actually be in poorer health—certainly death and hospital utilization rates are higher for men than for women—or their reports of poorer health may be a reaction to mandatory retirement because of age. [18]

Since need for help increases sharply with age, the very old require more assistance than the younger old. For instance, in 1979, 5% of the non-institutionalized people 65–74 years of age needed help in one or more basic physical activities, such as walking, going outside, bathing, dressing, using the toilet, getting in and out of bed or a chair, or eating, compared with 35% of those 85 years old and over. Similar patterns of need are also reported for other types of assistance. [19]

Chronic Illness

The incidence of chronic illness increases with age and becomes a major cause of disability requiring medical care. The cost of care for those suffering from chronic illness accounts for a large proportion of national expenditures for health care. Health trends of middle-aged and older persons since the late 1950s paradoxically include both longer life and worsening health.[20] The apparent worsening health, as reflected in the increasing prevalence of many chronic conditions, is attributed to greater awareness of diseases due to earlier diagnosis and earlier accommodations to disease. Longer life, as reflected in decreased mortality rates, may be attributed to earlier and better medical care of diagnosed cases, earlier and better self-care after diagnosis, and possibly lower incidence of some chronic diseases. Data from the longitudinal study of Du Pont Company male employees show that the incidence of first major coronary events declined steadily from 1957 to 1983.[21] This finding is in accord with the view that improvements in lifestyles plus better control of hypertension have been important to the declining rates of mortality from coronary heart disease.

Severe effects of chronic illness may prevent people from functioning independently. Almost nine out of ten aged persons whose activity is limited because of chronic conditions are limited in the amount or kind of major activity engaged in (e.g., working or keeping house). In 1985, elderly persons with acute and chronic conditions experienced almost one billion days of restricted activities; of this total, 41% were bed-disability days. Among the elderly with restricted activity, 33 days per year were restricted-activity days, 14 days of which were days of being confined to bed (Table 1.3).[16]

The prevalence of specific chronic conditions causing limitations of activity among the noninstitutionalized elderly is high. In 1985, 47% had arthritis, 41% had hypertensive disease, and 30% had heart conditions. Many elderly persons suffered from impairments: 29% had hearing impairments, 10% had visual impairments, and 17% had orthopedic impairments.[16]

It is generally recognized that many people, especially the elderly, suffer from multiple chronic conditions and disabilities. Table 1.5 shows the relationship to age of multiple chronic conditions and the various burdens they create. The data on multiple chronic conditions are tabulated for one, two, and three or more conditions causing limitation of activity.[22] Multiple chronic conditions causing limitation of activity increase with age. For example, only 3% of persons under age 17 report three or more chronic conditions causing limited activity, but 16% of those age 75 and over report the same.

The numbers of restricted-activity and bed-disability days are also significantly affected by the number of conditions. Persons with only one chronic condition report 57 restricted-activity days and 18 bed days per person per year. Persons with two conditions causing limitation of activity report about 50% higher rates; those with three or more conditions have more than twice the rates of those with only one condition. Although the number of restricted-activity days increases with age and the number of conditions, the highest rates are for those age 45–64 years. Bed-disability

Table 1.5. Health Status and Medical Care Use of Persons With Chronic Conditions Causing Limitation of Activity, by Age and Number of Conditions, 1979–1981

Number of Conditions	Total	Age				
		Under 17	17–44	45–64	65–74	75 and Over
Number of Persons (in thousands)[a]	31,738	2,243	8,045	10,479	6,292	4,678
One condition	21,575	1,897	6,412	6,680	3,765	2,821
Two conditions	6,650	275	1,243	2,434	1,598	1,099
Three or more conditions	3,513	72	390	1,365	929	758
Restricted-activity Days (per person)	68.7	37.3	60.2	77.6	72.3	73.4
One condition	56.8	35.3	54.4	62.4	58.4	61.1
Two conditions	83.5	45.4	73.0	92.9	84.7	82.3
Three or more conditions	113.6	61.3	114.2	124.4	107.4	106.4
Bed-Disability Days (per person)	22.3	13.8	18.9	24.0	22.8	27.5
One condition	18.3	13.1	16.3	19.6	19.1	22.6
Two conditions	26.7	16.3	25.4	27.4	26.0	30.6
Three or more conditions	38.1	23.0[b]	42.0	39.8	32.6	41.0
Physician Visits (per person)	9.6	10.3	10.0	10.1	9.2	8.1
One condition	9.0	10.0	9.2	9.3	8.7	7.9
Two conditions	10.3	11.1	11.5	10.7	9.7	8.5
Three or more conditions	12.1	12.9	18.6	13.5	10.3	8.6
Hospital Days (per 100 persons)	369	200	311	385	402	466
One condition	313	175	281	333	347	388
Two conditions	441	301	398	441	451	513
Three or more conditions	570	462[b]	541	538	539	689

Source: Computed from the 1979, 1980, and 1981 National Health Interview Survey micro data tapes.
[a]Total may not add due to rounding.
[b]Greater than 30% relative standard error.

13

days, however, gradually increase with more advanced age and the number of conditions.

Medical care use—measured in physician visits per person and hospital days per 100 persons—is also shown in Table 1.5 according to age. Although multiple chronic conditions affect the number of physician visits, the effect is small—physician visits per person rise from 9.0 for those reporting only one cause of limitation of activity to 10.3 for two causes and 12.1 for three or more causes; a similar pattern is seen among the elderly.

The number of hospital days varies more than the number of physician visits according to the number of conditions. The number of days per 100 persons rises from 313 for those with only one cause of limitation of activity to 441 for those with two causes and 570 for those with three or more causes. As expected, the rate per 100 persons also increases with age. All these patterns combined support the hypothesis that multiple chronic conditions create a significantly greater burden than having only one chronic condition, and that the burden increases with age.

Use of Health-Care Services

Use of health-care services increases with age. For example, elderly people visit physicians more frequently than younger people. In 1985, noninstitutionalized elderly people (other than hospital inpatients) saw physicians on an average of 8.3 times per year, in contrast to an average of 6.1 times for persons age 45–64. About 84% had contact with a physician during the preceding year. Nine out of ten elderly people had a regular source of care and eight out of ten saw a single doctor for their care.

Elderly people are hospitalized more frequently and stay in the hospital longer than younger persons. There were 7.6 million elderly discharges from nonfederal short-stay hospitals in 1985, with a total of 66 million days of care.[16] More than one-fourth (26%) of all people discharged were elderly and two-fifths (34%) of all days spent in hospitals were spent by elderly people. Less than 5% of the civilian noninstitutionalized population were 75 years of age or older in 1985, yet they accounted for 12% of all discharges and 16.3% of all days of care.

Although life expectancy for women is higher than for men, elderly women are more limited in activities of daily living, visit physicians more frequently, and use more days of hospital and nursing home care than men do.[23,24]

Not surprisingly, older persons who suffer from chronic and disabling conditions heavily utilize medical resources. The elderly with chronic activity limitation had 8.7 visits to physicians per year, in contrast to 4.3 visits for persons with no activity limitation. They had 41.2 hospitalizations per 100 persons per year, in contrast to 14.8 for those with no limitation of activity. The 46% of elderly people who were limited in activity because of a chronic condition accounted for 63% of physician contacts, 71% of hospitalizations, and 82% of all the days that older people spent in bed because of health conditions.[25]

According to the 1985 National Nursing Home Survey, about 5% of the elderly (compared with 22% of the old-old) are in nursing homes.[26] In 1985, a total of 1.5 million persons were in nursing and related care homes, of which 88% were 65 years and over. Other chronically ill elderly persons are in psychiatric or other chronic disease hospitals, Veterans Administration hospitals, and other long-term care facilities. In general, elderly residents of nursing homes suffer from multiple chronic conditions and functional impairments. Almost two-thirds (63%) are senile, 36% have heart trouble, and 14% have diabetes. Using the life-table method, it has been estimated that the elderly individual's risk of institutionalization approaches and may exceed 50%.[27]

Access to Medical Care

In the two decades since the establishment of Medicare and Medicaid, impressive strides have been made in ensuring that more Americans have access to the benefits of the health-care system. More people have attained regular access to health services, and a backlog of long-neglected needs, especially of the elderly and the poor, has been specifically addressed. For example, cataract operations, which improve vision, increased significantly after the introduction of Medicare. In 1985, the rate for this operation for both elderly men and women was three times that for 1965.[28,14]

Although the elderly have increased their use of health services during the past two decades, significant gaps still exist between subgroups of the elderly defined by income, race, and place of residence.[29] The poor tend to be sicker than the nonpoor, so that the higher medical care use rates among the poor do not necessarily indicate that they get more care given similar health status. After adjustment for health status, poor elderly persons who report their health as fair or poor make 25% fewer visits than those in the highest income groups. The use–disability rate, a measure of the number of physician visits per 1000 disability days, shows a wider differential among income classes.[30]

Other measures of access to care are identification of a regular source of care, characteristics of physical access to the regular source (transportation mode, travel time, waiting room time), insurance coverage, and the existence of medically unattended conditions. Data from the 1980 National Medical Care Utilization and Expenditure Survey show that from these measures of entry into the system, access to health care among elderly Medicare participants is judged to be good.[31] About 10% of elderly Medicare participants reported no regular source of care, compared with 14% of those under 65 years of age. In contrast to the white elderly population, however, a higher proportion of blacks have no regular source of care (9% versus 14%). In addition, black elderly were more likely than white elderly to have a clinic as their source of care (16% versus 9%). These findings are consistent with the findings from the 1977 National Medical Care Expenditure Survey.[32]

Another perspective on equity of and access to care by the elderly is offered by the provision of Medicare benefits. Medicare was clearly intended to provide equal access to medical care regardless of race, income, or location of residence. However, research has shown that Medicare benefits have been provided disproportionately to whites as compared to nonwhites. In 1969, payments per beneficiary were 40% higher for whites than for nonwhites.[33] Disparities in use and reimbursement of services by race decreased between 1967 and 1977, but relatively more whites than nonwhites still received reimbursement. Lower access to physicians and hospitals by nonwhites persists, especially in the South. However, once nonwhites exceeded the deductible, their reimbursements per person using reimbursed services were generally comparable to or higher than reimbursements to whites.[34] Clearly, differences between the elderly poor and nonpoor and between white and nonwhite persons in use of health-care services have diminished since Medicare and Medicaid began, but gaps persist.

Long-Term Care Needs

In addition to medical care, many elderly persons who have lost some capacity for self-care require a wide range of social, personal, and supportive services. Long-term care (LTC) is defined as physical care over a prolonged period for those persons incapable of sustaining themselves without this care.[35] LTC is viewed as a spectrum of services responding to different needs across a range of chronic illness and disability. To address the multiple and varied LTC needs of the aged population, services must cross the boundaries between income maintenance and health, social, and housing programs.[36]

Data from the Home Care Supplement[19] of the 1979 and 1980 National Health Interview Survey showed that an estimated 2.7 million elderly persons in the civilian noninstitutionalized population needed functional assistance from another person for selected personal care or home-management activities. The proportion of the population needing help increased with age among those 65 years of age and older. About 7% of those 65–74 years of age needed help, compared with about 16% of those 75–84 years old and 39% of those 85 and older. The need for personal care assistance results in a dependency that is reflected in the living arrangement of these individuals. About 3% of those 75–84 years of age and living alone required personal care, while 6% of those living with a spouse and 11% of those living with other relatives required this kind of assistance—and these rates are higher for those 85 years old and older. In contrast to adults needing personal care, the elderly who lived alone were twice as likely as those living with a spouse to need assistance in home-management activities, a finding suggesting that older people are more likely to be able to maintain independent living when home-management assistance is involved than when personal care is needed.

Expenditures for Medical Care

The elderly represented only 11% of the population in 1980, but they accounted for 31% of expenditures for personal health care. Per capita spending for elderly persons was 3½ times that for persons under 65 years of age. The level of per capita spending is directly related to the prevalence of disease, the number of services used by each patient, and the average cost of each service. The very large differences in per capita spending between the elderly and younger persons are chiefly the result of the higher prevalence of heart disease among the elderly. Both younger and elderly women used more medical services and incurred disproportionately higher expenditures relative to their numbers than did men. Women represented 59% of the aged population and they incurred 63% of the expenditures.[37]

The economic burden imposed by a disease type varied with the age and sex of the population. Table 1.6 shows 1980 expenditures for the costliest medical conditions according to age and sex. For the elderly, diseases of the circulatory system were the leading cause of health-care expenditures, accounting for about 30% of the total for older males and females and requiring $674 and $848 per capita, respectively. Also among the five most expensive conditions for both sexes were diseases of the digestive system and mental disorders. Injury, poisoning, and diseases of the musculoskeletal system and connective tissue completed the top five most expensive conditions for older women but ranked eighth and ninth for older men. Neoplasms were the second most expensive category among elderly males but ranked sixth for women 65 years of age and over. Similarly, diseases of the respiratory system were relatively important for older males, ranking fourth, but they ranked ninth among females.

Elderly people approaching death or institutionalization incur very high expenses for medical care. In 1978, the 1.1 million Medicare enrollees in their last year of life represented 5.9% of all enrollees, but they accounted for 28.2% of program expenditures. Medicare users who died in 1978 were reimbursed an average of $4909 for all covered services in their last year,

Table 1.6. Total and Per Capita Personal Health-Care Expenditures for Leading Medical Conditions, by Age and Sex, United States, 1980

Medical Condition	Total Expenditure (in millions)	Per Capita Expenditure				
		All Ages	Under 65 Years		65 Years and Over	
			Males	Females	Males	Females
All Conditions	$219,400	$947	$627	$791	$2,278	$2,667
Circulatory Diseases	33,184	143	67	61	674	848
Digestive Diseases	31,755	137	110	143	213	223
Mental Disorders	20,301	88	73	69	181	246
Injury and Poisoning	19,248	83	86	61	105	203
Nervous System and Sense Organ Diseases	17,499	76	57	69	168	176
Respiratory Diseases	17,305	75	60	68	192	137
Musculoskeletal System Diseases	13,645	59	40	55	91	187
Neoplasms	13,623	59	30	50	244	178
Genitourinary System Diseases	13,162	57	21	82	128	70
Endocrine, Nutritional, and Metabolic Diseases	7,656	33	15	31	82	138
All Other Diseases	32,022	138	67	104	200	261

Source: Ref. 37.

about four times the amount reimbursed for services provided to survivors. Average reimbursement per decedent for hospital care was 7.3 times higher in the last year of life than for survivors, 3.9 times higher for physician and other medical services, and 12.7 times higher for nursing home care.[38]

Data from the 1980 National Medical Care Utilization and Expenditure Survey confirm these findings—elderly persons approaching death or institutionalization have very high expenditures for medical care.[39] High medical costs at the end of life are not a new phenomenon and available data do not support the assumption that high medical expenses at the end of life are due largely to aggressive, intensive treatment of patients who are moribund. The data suggest that most sick people who die are given the medical care generally provided to the sick, and such care is expensive.[40]

Future Morbidity Patterns

Changing morbidity and mortality play an important part in estimating future illness patterns and in developing population projections, and considerable conjecture and controversy have arisen about future morbidity patterns. One theory holds that improvements in lifestyle will delay the onset of disability, reducing the prevalence of morbidity from chronic disease and compressing morbidity at older ages. A continuing decline in premature death is foreseen, along with the emergence of a pattern of natural death at the end of a natural life span.[41] Another theory argues that the prevalence of chronic disease and disability will increase as life expectancy increases, leading to a "pandemic" of mental disorders and chronic diseases.[42] Thus, the extension of life will bring on an extension of disease and disability. This increase in the prevalence of chronic conditions due to medical technology is seen as "the failure of success."[43]

A review of the evidence concludes that the number of old-old is increasing rapidly, the average period of diminished vigor will probably rise, chronic diseases will probably occupy a larger proportion of our life span, and the needs for medical care in later life are likely to increase substantially.[44] It is, of course, possible that both phenomena will be taking place simultaneously: there may be an increasing number of individuals in good health nearly up to the point of death and an increasing number with prolonged severe functional limitation, with a decline in the duration of infirmity. The effect on the prevalence of morbidity would, of course, depend on the relative magnitude of the various changes. Models linking morbidity and mortality can be developed to predict how healthy or ill cohorts of the older population will be in the future.[45]

Both the Bureau of the Census and the Social Security Administration have assumed continued reductions in mortality and improved life expectancy to the year 2050, resulting in a rapidly aging population. Based on

Table 1.7. Current and Projected Population, Limitations in ADL, Medical Care Utilization and Expenditures, United States, By Age, 1980–2040

Characteristic and Year	All Ages	Under 65	Age		
			Total	65 and Over	
				65–74	75 and Over
Population (thousands)					
1980	232,669	206,777	25,892	15,627	10,265
2000	273,949	237,697	36,252	18,334	17,918
2020	306,931	254,278	52,653	30,093	22,560
2040	328,503	261,247	67,256	29,425	37,831
Persons with Limitation in Activities of Daily Living (thousands)					
1980	3,142	1,362	1,780	648	1,132
2000	4,509	1,734	2,775	784	1,991
2020	5,952	1,998	3,954	1,309	2,645
2040	7,922	2,002	5,920	1,288	4,632
Physician Visits (millions)					
1980	1,102	936	166	100	66

2000	1,314	1,083	231	116	115
2020	1,499	1,164	335	191	144
2040	1,621	1,193	428	187	241
Days of Hospital Care (millions)					
1980	274	169	105	49	56
2000	371	211	160	58	102
2020	459	234	225	95	130
2040	549	236	312	93	219
Nursing Home Residents (thousands)					
1980	1,511	196	1,315	227	1,088
2000	2,542	226	2,316	265	2,051
2020	3,371	242	3,129	434	2,695
2040	5,227	248	4,979	425	4,554
Personal Health Expenditures (in constant 1980 billions of dollars)					
1980	$ 219.4	$ 154.9	$ 64.5	na	na
2000	273.4	183.1	90.3	na	na
2020	328.3	197.1	131.2	na	na
2040	369.0	201.5	167.5	na	na

Source: Ref. 46.

population projections made by the Social Security Administration, estimates have been made of the national effect of these demographic changes on health status, health services utilization, and expenditures for health care to the year 2040.[46] The projections were based on current age- and sex-specific rates of health status and utilization patterns, although it is expected that additional changes in levels of morbidity, in therapies and technologies and their availability, in the cost of care, and in social and economic conditions will also contribute to altered patterns and levels of utilization of services. Whatever else happens, the projected changes in the size and age distribution of the population alone would have a significant effect on utilization, and consequently on expenditures. Table 1.7 presents the results of these projections for the period 1980–2040. The total population is projected to increase 41%, while the group age 65 and older will increase 160%. The total number of persons limited in activities of daily living is projected to more than double; the elderly with limitations will more than triple. The effect of the aging of the population on physician visits and hospitalizations will be great. In 2040, 40% of the days of care are projected to be used by those age 75 and older, compared with 20% in 1980. The effect on the number of nursing home residents will be greatest: it is projected to more than triple, increasing from 1.5 million to 5.2 million in 2040—to meet the needs of the aging population. In 1980, 11% of the population age 65 and older accounted for 29% of the total health expenditures; by 2040 the elderly are projected to comprise 21% of the population, and almost half of the expenditures will be made on their behalf.

Short-term Bureau of Census population projections to the year 2000 show significantly different rates of changes in the population of the four regions of the United States. The West and South will be the fastest growing regions, with their populations increasing 45% and 31%, respectively, from 1980 to 2000. The North Central population is projected to rise only 1.5% while the Northeast is projected to lose population during the same period. The elderly population in all regions, however, is projected to rise, ranging from a 12% increase in the Northeast to a 60% increase in the South and West.[47]

These changing demographics will have different effects by region on medical care services. Applying current age- and sex-specific utilization rates to these projected population estimates shows significant regional variations in days of hospital care, physician visits, and nursing home care by the year 2000 to meet the needs of an aging population. The days of hospital care are projected to increase from only 6% in the Northeast to 57% in the West, reflecting regional population shifts as well as the aging of the population. A 5% decrease in physician visits is indicated for the Northeast; the West and South, however, with their large projected population growth, will need to increase physician visits 46% and 33%, respectively, to meet the medical care needs of the growing number of elderly persons in their regions. Lastly, the aging effect is much greater for nursing home care. The total number of nursing home residents in the United States is projected to increase 69%, almost four times the growth in the population. In the Northeast and North Central regions, the number of nursing home residents will increase 44%. In the South and West, where the elderly population will increase 60%, the number of nursing home beds will have to more than double to meet the needs of the projected elderly population.[48]

Conclusions

The socioeconomic characteristics and health status of the elderly, changes in the size and demographic structure of the population, use of medical and LTC services, and the effect of the aging of the population on the health-care system are reviewed here. It is difficult to accurately forecast changes in the medical care system and in patterns of medical treatment, government regulations and legislation, inflation, insurance coverage, education, income, and other important parameters of health care; however, continuing rapid growth in the number and proportion of aged in the population is certain.

The burden of an increasingly larger number and percentage of elderly persons will greatly affect Social Security, welfare, and Medicare benefit payments. An aging population raises many important policy issues.[49] Included are the integration of medical, social, and LTC systems and their financing, political and ethical concerns, geriatric medical care needs versus supply, alternative delivery systems, and the roles of health-care providers, all of which are discussed in subsequent chapters. The heterogeneity of the aged population and its special health and LTC needs present challenges for policymakers who are concerned with equity, effectiveness, and the quality of life. The organization, delivery, costs, and financing of medical, social, and LTC services will need to be restructured and reshaped to effectively and efficiently meet the special needs of the elderly.

References

1. Davies, A. M. 1985. Epidemiology and the challenge of ageing. *Int J Epidemiol* 14(1):9–21.
2. Svahn, J. A., Ross, M. 1982. Social Security amendments of 1983: Legislative

history and summary of provisions. *Soc Secur Bull* 46(7):3–48.
3. Bowen, O. R. (Chairperson) 1984. *Report of the 1982 Advisory Council on Social Security. Medicare Benefits and Financing.* Washington, D.C.: Government Printing Office.
4. Ouslander, J. G., Beck, J. C. 1982. Defining the health problems of the elderly. *Annu Rev Public Health* 3:55–83.
5. Suzman, R., Riley, M. W. 1985. Introducing the "oldest old." *Milbank Memorial Fund Q* (2):177–186.
6. United States Bureau of the Census. 1984. Projections of the population of the United States, 1983 to 2080. *Current Population Reports,* Series P-25, No. 952. Washington, D.C.: Government Printing Office.
7. United States Bureau of the Census. 1985. Household, families, marital status and living arrangements: March 1985 (advance report). *Current Population Reports,* Series P-20, No. 402. Washington, D.C.: Government Printing Office.
8. United States Bureau of the Census. 1983. America in transition: An aging society. *Current Population Reports,* Series P-23, No. 128. Washington, D.C.: Government Printing Office.
9. United States Bureau of the Census. 1985. Characteristics of the population below poverty level: 1983. *Current Population Reports,* Series P-60, No. 147. Washington, D.C.: Government Printing Office.
10. United States Bureau of Census. 1987. Statistical Abstract of the United States: 1988 (108th Edition). Washington, D.C.: Government Printing Office.
11. United States Senate, Special Committee on Aging and the American Association of Retired Persons. 1984. *Aging America: Trends and Projections,* PL 3377(584). Washington, D.C.: Government Printing Office.
12. United States Bureau of the Census, 1984. Money income and poverty status of families and persons in the United States: 1983. *Current Population Reports,* Series P-60, No. 147. Washington, D.C.: Government Printing Office.
13. United States Bureau of the Census. 1984. Estimates of poverty including the value of noncash benefits: 1979 to 1982. Technical Paper 51. Washington, D.C.: Government Printing Office.
14. National Center for Health Statistics. 1986. *Health, United States, 1985.* DHHS Pub. No. (PHS) 87-1232. Washington, D.C.: Government Printing Office.
15. Goldman, L., Cook, E. F. 1984. The decline in ischemic heart disease mortality rates: An analysis of the comparative effects of medical interventions and changes in lifestyle. *Ann Intern Med* 101(6):825–836.
16. National Center for Health Statistics. 1986. Current estimates from the National Health Interview Survey: United States 1985. *Vital and Health Statistics,* Series 10, No. 160, DHHS Pub. No. (PHS) 86-1588. Washington, D.C.: Government Printing Office.
17. United States Health Care Financing Administration. 1983. Health status of aged Medicare beneficiaries. *National Medical Care Utilization and Expenditure Survey,* Series B, Descriptive Report No. 2, DHHS Pub. No. 83-20202. Washington, D.C.: Government Printing Office.
18. Kovar, M. G. 1977. Health of the elderly and use of health services. *Public Health Rep* 42(1):9–19.

19. National Center for Health Statistics. 1983. Americans needing help to function at home. *Advance Data From Vital and Health Statistics*, No. 92, DHHS Pub. No. (PHS) 83-1250. Hyattsville, Md.: National Center for Health Statistics.

20. Verbrugge, L. M. 1984. Longer life but worsening health? Trends in health and mortality of middle-aged and older persons. *Milbank Memorial Fund Q* 62(3):475–519.

21. Pell, S., Fayerweather, W. 1985. Trends in the incidence of myocardial infarction and in associated mortality and morbidity in a large employed population, 1957–1983. *N Engl J Med* 312(16):1006–1011.

22. Rice, D. P., LaPlante, M. 1988. Chronic illness, disability, and increasing longevity. In *The Economics and Ethics of Long-term Care*, ed. S. Sullivan and M. E. Lewin. Washington, D.C.: American Enterprise Institute for Public Policy Research.

23. Rice, D. P. 1983. Sex differences in mortality and morbidity: Some aspects of the economic burden. In *Sex Differentials in Mortality: Trends, Determinants, and Consequences*, ed. A. D. Lopez and L. T. Ruzicka. Miscellaneous Series No. 4. Canberra: Department of Demography, Australian National University.

24. National Center for Health Statistics. 1983. Sex differences in health and use of medical care: United States, 1979. *Vital and Health Statistics*, Series 3, No. 24, DHHS Pub. No. (PHS) 83-1408. Washington, D.C.: Government Printing Office.

25. National Center for Health Statistics. 1981. Health characteristics of persons with chronic activity limitations: United States, 1979. *Vital and Health Statistics*, Series 10, No. 137, DHHS Pub. No. (PHS) 82-1565. Washington, D.C.: Government Printing Office.

26. National Center for Health Statistics. 1987. Use of nursing homes by the elderly: Preliminary data from the National Nursing Home Survey. *Advance Data from Vital and Health Statistics*, No. 135, DHHS Pub. No. (PHS) 87-1250. Hyattsville, Md.: National Center for Health Statistics.

27. McConnel, C. E. 1984. A note on the lifetime risk of nursing home residency. *Gerontologist* 24(2):193–198.

28. National Center for Health Statistics. 1978. *Health, United States, 1978*. DHHS Pub. No. (PHS) 78-1232 and 83-1232. Washington, D.C.: Government Printing Office.

29. President's Commission for the Study of Ethical Problems in Medicine and Biomedical and Behavioral Research. 1983. *Securing Access to Health Care*, Vol. 1. *Report*. Washington, D.C.: Government Printing Office.

30. Kleinman, J. C., Gold, M., Makuc, D. 1981. Use of ambulatory medical care by the poor: Another look at equity. *Med Care XIX* 10:1011–1029.

31. United States Health Care Financing Administration. 1984. Access to health care among aged Medicare beneficiaries. Series B, Descriptive Report No. 3, DHHS Pub. No. 84-20203. Washington, D.C.: Government Printing Office.

32. Berk, M. L., Bernstein, A. B. 1982. Regular source of care and the minority aged. *J Am Geriatr Soc* 30(4):251–254.

33. Davis, K. 1975. Equal treatment and unequal benefits: The Medicare program. *Milbank Memorial Fund Q* 53:466–468.

34. Ruther, M., Dobson, A. 1981. Equal treatment and unequal benefits: A re-

examination of the use of Medicare services by race, 1967–1976. *Health Care Financing Rev* 2(3):55–83.

35. Kane, R. L., Kane, R. A. 1980. Long-term care: Can our society meet the needs of its elderly? *Annu Rev Public Health* 1:227–253.
36. Harrington, C., Newcomer, R. J., Estes, C. L., and Associates (eds.). 1985. *Long Term Care of the Elderly: Public Policy Issues.* Beverly Hills, Calif.: Sage Publications.
37. Hodgson, T. A., Kopstein, A. N. 1984. Health expenditures for major diseases in 1980. *Health Care Financing Rev* 5(4):1–12.
38. Lubitz, J., Prihoda, R. 1984. The use and costs of Medicare services in the last 2 years of life. *Health Care Financing Rev* 5(3):117–131.
39. National Center for Health Statistics. 1983. Expenditures for the medical care of elderly people living in the community throughout 1980. *National Medical Care Utilization and Expenditures Survey,* Data Report No. 4, DHHS Pub. No. (PHS) 84-20000. Washington, D.C.: Government Printing Office.
40. Scitovsky, A. A. 1984. The high cost of dying: What do the data show? *Milbank Memorial Fund Q* 62(4):591–608.
41. Fries, J. F. 1980. Aging, natural death, and the compression of morbidity. *N Engl J Med* 303(3):130–135.
42. Kramer, M. 1980. The rising pandemic of mental disorders and associated chronic diseases and disorders. *Acta Psychiatr Scand* [Suppl. 285] 62:382–396.
43. Gruenberg, E. M. 1977. The failures of success. *Milbank Memorial Fund Q* 55(1):3–24.
44. Schneider, E. L., Brody, J. A. 1983. Aging, natural death, and the compression of morbidity: Another view. *N Engl J Med* 309(14):854–856.
45. Manton, K. C. 1982. Changing concepts of morbidity and mortality in the elderly population. *Milbank Memorial Fund Q* 60(2):183–244.
46. Rice, D. P., Feldman, J. J. 1983. Living longer in the United States: Demographic changes and health needs of the elderly. *Milbank Memorial Fund Q* 61(3):362–396.
47. United States Bureau of the Census. 1983. Provisional estimates of the population of states, by age and sex: 1980 to 2000. *Current Population Reports,* Series P-25, No. 937. Washington, D.C.: Government Printing Office.
48. Rice, D. P. 1985. The health care needs of the elderly. In *Long Term Care of the Elderly: Public Policy Issues,* ed. C. Harrington, R. J. Newcomer, C. L. Estes, and Associates, 41–66. Beverly Hills, Calif.: Sage Publications.
49. Rice, D. P., Estes, C. L. 1984. Health of the elderly: Policy issues and challenges. *Health Aff* 3(4):25–49.

Part Two

Paying for Services

Cost containment. No debate on national health policy is considered complete these days without the use of that resonant phrase. Interwoven into the concept are questions with far-reaching implications for an aging population. Must a measure of equity be traded for a soupçon of efficiency? Can a commitment to accessible care be squeezed into the straps of an austerity budget?

Consumers, providers, and policymakers agree—in theory, at least—that the elderly are entitled access to health care that will enable them to live out their years with dignity. Crouched beneath that pithy sentiment, however, are a multitude of pragmatic concerns. What will it cost to provide equitable care, and who will pay for it? How is responsibility best shared between the public and private sector? Among formal and informal caregivers? To ground the answers to those politically sensitive questions in hard facts, this section first reviews current systems of financing and evaluates their strengths and shortcomings, then it analyzes strategic reforms recently implemented or currently under debate.

Inevitably, we begin with a look at Medicare, generally acknowledged to be one of the most important pieces of social legislation enacted in the postwar period. Until Medicare's passage in 1965, the elderly were excluded from the prevailing system of employment-linked health insurance. Since that year their access to acute care has improved manyfold, but

27

weaknesses still riddle the system. Fears that Medicare faced imminent bankruptcy have faded in light of a robust national economy and changing hospital reimbursement policies, but some experts warn that the day of reckoning has merely been postponed.

The urgent need for long-term care (LTC), for which adequate financing mechanisms have yet to be developed, also receives considerable attention here. While the myth that families are abandoning their elderly relatives is debunked, increased longevity has heightened the demand for services required by a growing population with multiple and chronic health problems. Today, most public funding for LTC is institutionally biased; several contributing writers discuss the need to tear down bureaucratic impediments that restrict the reallocation of funds to community-based care.

Because successful policy experiments must be based on accurate information, Charlene A. Harrington's detailed description of the major public programs for the aged is a vital jumping-off point for our discussions on finances. Expanding on the demographic and socioeconomic characteristics spelled out in Part One, she talks about how and why health-care delivery is changing and notes that state and local governments—rather than the Feds—are currently sponsoring most new initiatives in the field.

Complementing Harrington's analysis of structured systems is Francis G. Caro's discussion of alternatives to institutionalization. Well-financed community-based LTC is the linchpin of independent living for the elderly, who may require personal and housekeeping services, housing subsidies, day programs, mental health services, life-care communities, and hospices, each of which is described here.

Given the flaws in financing current health-care delivery systems, a number of writers take up the battle cry of reform. The second part of this section starts with a description of the revolution that took place in 1983, when Medicare implemented a prospective payment system (PPS) to reimburse hospitals. George L. Maddox and Kenneth G. Manton unravel the workings of the PPS, and its companion, diagnosis-related groups, rooting the innovations in their sociocultural context. Every strategy for financing health care has its limitations, warn the authors, because the capacity to plan geriatric care rationally is constrained by social values and organizational limitations.

Linda H. Aiken then analyzes the Advisory Council on Social Security's 1984 recommendations to Congress. By taking a no-holds-barred look at hospital and physician reimbursement strategies, prepaid capitation arrangements, financing of medical education, and beneficiary cost-sharing schemes, the council touched off a still-raging national debate about Medicare's future.

Catastrophic coverage under Medicare has emerged as one of the major legislative health-care initiatives in the last decade. This legislation represents the most significant expansion in benefits for elderly people since Medicare was first introduced. Diane Rowland, Barbara Lyons, and Karen Davis assess the issues involved in enacting a catastrophic health plan, including the need for catastrophic coverage, and discuss the congressional debate that preceded passage of the Reagan Administration's legislation.

In their scramble to finance long-term care, health policy experts have turned to the private sector, a long-familiar player in the U.S. health-care delivery system. Judith Feder and William Scanlon describe the private sector's role in developing reverse annuity mortgages, expanding private LTC insurance, and establishing life-care communities and social health maintenance organizations. The only alternative to private financing, contend the authors, is a system of federal insurance.

The rocky terrain of national health insurance is probed by Philip R. Lee and Carroll L. Estes, who argue that public financing builds equal access to adequate care. Rather than eyeing policies for the elderly in a vacuum, they call for a more coherent and goal-oriented health-care system in which a role is allocated to the public and private sectors and to federal, state, and local governments.

Two

The Structured Approaches

Charlene A. Harrington

Our nation's health-care delivery system is extremely complex, and it is one of our largest industries, representing 10.9% of the gross national product in 1986[1] and having a labor force of more than 6 million people in 1985.[2] Between 1970 and 1980, employment in health care grew at a rate more than twice that of general employment.

The rapid increase in spending for health-care services has focused national attention on policies and activities to contain costs. As long as resources for health care were not constrained, the distribution of economic resources was not a major social concern.[3] As governmental resources have become more constrained in the 1980s, public policy changes have been directed toward reducing public expenditures by changing how health care is financed publicly. These changes have affected both health-care providers and consumers. They have also had profound effects on the health-care delivery system and on professional practice. Thus, economic issues have increasingly become a primary concern for health-care consumers, providers, employers, third-party payers, and public policy makers.

This chapter describes trends in health-care spending patterns in the United States for the total population and for the aged. The major public programs for the aged are examined. Recent policy changes in financing are also discussed, along with their effect on the delivery system. Finally, cost containment and new models for financing care are examined.

National Health-Care Expenditures

The nation spent $458 billion on health care in 1986, an amount that represents an 8.4% increase over the previous year.[4] Of the total expenditures, $404 billion were for personal health-care services, $24.5 billion were for program administration and insurance, $13.4 billion were for governmental public health activities, and $16.3 billion were for research and the construction of medical facilities.[5] The major concern in health care is the high growth rate in total expenditures beyond the rate of general inflation. Real per capita health-care spending increased by three times between 1950 and 1980.[6] The projections for health care in the future are that expenditures will continue to increase above the rate of inflation (although at somewhat less than the rate over the past decade) and that expenditures will continue to be an increasing proportion of the gross national product (estimated to be $1.529 billion and 15% of the gross national product in the year 2000).[7]

Reasons for Growth Rates

Analysis of the total cost increase nationally during 1985–86 showed that 11% of the increase was due to population increases, 32% to general inflation, 35% to other factors (such as the intensity of services and increased consumer consumption), and the remaining 22% to medical care price inflation.[8] Because medical price increases, excluding general inflation and other factors, were without substantial justification, provider prices have become a major target for cost reductions.[8]

One reason for the price inflation is the way that health care is financed. Since government and third-party insurers and payers pay directly for a large proportion of health care, the true cost of services is obscured; therefore, consumers have little incentive to be cost conscious.[8] Most third-party payments were paid on the basis of actual costs after services were delivered (cost-based retrospective reimbursement), although recent changes have been made that adopt prospective reimbursement (setting payment rates in advance). The retrospective or cost-based reimbursement approach encouraged providers to increase costs to increase revenues. Furthermore, health insurance premiums and out-of-pocket payments for health care are excluded from taxable income for the most part, which again does not encourage cost consciousness.[8]

Costs of Care for the Aged

The elderly account for a greater share of the total health-care dollar than do any other age group.[9] In 1977, individuals age 65 and older spent 3.5

times what the average person spent,[10] and the current ratio is considered higher than that in 1977.[11] This higher spending occurs because the aged have a greater number of disabilities and higher health-care utilization than do other groups. The aged also use more hospital services than do other groups, and hospital costs are higher than the costs for other health-care services. Moreover, the proportion of the aged is growing within the population as a whole, so they require more services. Spending on behalf of the aged nearly tripled during 1977–84, when the increase in spending averaged 13% per year.[12]

Sources of Payment

Sources of payment for the nation's personal health-care dollar in 1986 were as follows: Medicare paid for 19%, Medicaid for 11%, other governmental programs for 10%, private health insurance and other private funds for 31%, and the remaining 29% was direct out-of-pocket payments by consumers.[13] Medicare and Medicaid are the two major public programs that pay for health-care services.

Of the estimated expenditures on behalf of the average aged individual in 1984, two-thirds came from governmental and third-party payers.[14] The remaining one-third was paid by the aged themselves. Much of the aged's direct costs (25%) are for Medicare copayments, premiums, and deductibles paid directly out of pocket. Another 7% of the spending is for private health insurance (including Medigap policies).[15]

The direct per capita payments by the elderly have been estimated to more than triple between 1977 and 1989.[16] The elderly's health-care payments are rising faster than their incomes. Between 1984 and 1989, their out-of-pocket costs were estimated to grow at twice the rate of their incomes.[16] In 1965, before the adoption of Medicare and Medicaid, the elderly were using 15% of their income for health care. This amount decreased to 12% in 1977, then increased to 15% in 1984, and it is expected to reach 18.4% by 1989.[16] In contrast, in the nation over all, average expenditures were 11.6% of the household budget.[17]

Types of Expenditures

The nation as a whole has spent a large proportion of its health-care dollars on institutional services. In 1986, 39% of the total health bill was for hospital care and 8% was for nursing home services. The proportion of total dollars spent on institutional services increased from 37% of the total in 1950 to the present level of 47%.[18] The proportion spent on services for physicians (20%) remained fairly stable. Of greater concern is the fact that the proportion spent on other institutional services, including other professional services, drugs, medical supplies, eyeglasses, and appliances, dropped from 24% in 1950 to 14% in 1986.[18]

The greatest proportion of health expenditures for the aged is also for institutional services. An estimated 45% of the per capita spending for the aged is for hospital care. Another 21% is spent on nursing home care (a rate much higher than that for other groups).[19] Physician expenditures are estimated to be 21% of the total bill and other health-care expenditures are about 13%, including home health care, drugs, appliances, and other services.[19]

Financing Public Programs for the Aged

One major public concern is that the government has been paying a greater percentage of the total health-care bills. In 1965, public programs paid for 26% of the total costs, but in 1986, the government was paying for about 41%.[7] The growth in public payments occurred after the adoption of the legislation enacting the Medicare and Medicaid programs in 1965. In 1986, the federal share of health spending was 29.5%, compared to 12% from state and local funds, whereas in 1965 the funds were equally distributed between federal and state and local government.[7] The increases in total costs have threatened the solvency of public programs, and thus become a major public policy issue.

Medicare

Medicare, created by Title XVIII of the Social Security Act in 1965, is a federal insurance program to provide health-care benefits to the aged. In 1973, the program extended coverage to the permanently disabled and their dependents who are eligible for the Old Age, Survivors, and Disability Insurance program (OASDI) and to those individuals with end-stage renal disease. Medicare has two parts. Part A is supported by a portion of the Social Security withholding tax (FICA) collected from employers and employees. Part B, a voluntary program, is supported by monthly premiums paid by beneficiaries and from the federal general fund. Part A, the Hospital Insurance Trust Fund, pays for inpatient hospital services and posthospital skilled nursing services. Part B, Supplementary Medical Insurance, covers physician services, medical supplies and services, home health services, outpatient hospital services and therapy, and a few other services.[20]

The Medicare program requires premiums, copayments, and deductibles. Until the enactment of the Medicare Catastrophic Coverage Act of 1988, the hospital insurance portion required deductibles equal to the average cost of one day of hospital care ($520 in 1987) and the user paid co-insurance for each day of care beyond 60 days of hospital care ($130 in 1987) and beyond 20 days of nursing home care ($65 in 1987).[21] The copayments increased by 17% annually between 1977 and 1983, primarily due to increases in hospital care.[22] Beginning in 1989, catastrophic coverage eliminates the day limits and co-insurance on hospital care, and the deductible is limited to a single annual amount ($564 in 1989). Also, co-insurance charges are eliminated after the eighth day of care in a skilled nursing facility, and coverage is extended to 150 days of care per year. For Part B, the annual deductible is currently $75, and the co-insurance is 20% of most charges.[21] In addition, if a physician does not accept assignment (direct reimbursement by Medicare for the total charge), the beneficiary must pay the bill directly to the physician and cover the total amount over that paid by Medicare.[22] Beginning in 1990, the Catastrophic Coverage Act establishes a maximum limit on the enrollee's share of approved charges for physician services and supplies covered under Part B ($1,370 in 1990), after which Medicare will pay 100% of approved charges.

In 1986, nearly 31 million aged and disabled persons were enrolled in Medicare, which paid out $76 billion.[20] Although Medicare is a major program for the aged, it paid for less than half of the total bills of the aged because it excludes most long-term benefits and because it requires deductibles, premiums, and copayments.[23] Medicare spent 68% of its dollars on hospital care and another 25% on physician care.[24] Medicare funded a limited amount of nursing home care ($.6 billion in 1986), or less than 1% of the total Medicare budget. Medicare payments for skilled nursing facilities represented less than 2% of the total nursing home revenues in 1986.[20] The eligibility regulations for nursing home services are severely restricted to those who have short-term illnesses. Home health-care expenditures were $2 billion in 1986.[25,20] Home health-care expenditures in the Medicare program grew from $60 million in 1968, almost doubled between 1980 and 1982, and tripled by 1984. Eligibility under Medicare was made less restrictive in 1982, but it is still restricted to those who are homebound and need professional health-care services.[26] In spite of these changes, Medicare home-health expenditures are still only 3% of total home health expenditures.[20]

Medicaid

Medicaid, Title XIX of the Social Security Act, was enacted in 1965. It provides benefits through federal matching funds to states. In 1986, the state-administered Medicaid program provided health-care services for 22 million low-income persons and their families.[27] The program covers those individuals who are aged, blind, or disabled who receive benefits from the

Supplemental Security Income (SSI) program and those individuals and families who are eligible for income support from Aid to Families with Dependent Children (AFDC). States have broad options in covering various groups under the program, so wide variability in eligibility exists across states. In 1982, Medicaid was available nationally to only 64% of those individuals below the poverty level because of restrictive state eligibility policies.[27]

States are required to cover nine basic services: hospitals, skilled nursing, physicians, laboratory and X-ray costs, home health, early and periodic screening, diagnosis and treatment, rural clinics, family planning, and nurse-midwives where licensed. States may provide other services as optional benefits. The program's expenditures on various services vary by state, but the majority of funds (73%) are spent on institutional services.[24] States have also funded alternative programs, such as home health, adult day health care, personal care, and other health-related services.

Medicaid benefits are strongly oriented toward medical as opposed to social services. In 1986, only $1.5 billion (less than 3.5% of the total spending) went to home health care, while $16 billion was spent on nursing home care.[25] Although all states offer home health benefits, states can impose restrictions on their use. Eighty percent of all national Medicaid home health-care expenditures was spent by New York state.[26] Excluding those services provided through demonstration programs and/or waivers, 24 states offered personal care benefits in 1987.[28] Only six state Medicaid programs covered adult day health care on a statewide basis in 1987.[29,28] Most states did offer home- and community-based care on a demonstration basis as a substitute for nursing home care, but these programs limited the number of enrollees in most states.

In 1986, Medicaid spent $44 billion of federal and state funds.[5] Medicaid paid for 13% of total health-care spending for the aged and 42% of total nursing home expenditures. While the elderly represent only 15–17% of all Medicaid recipients, they account for 40% of total program expenditures.[30]

Social Services

Since the early 1960s, the government has assumed an extensive role in financing social services, through a variety of programs. The Social Service Block Grant (SSBG) provides federal money to states for state and local programs.[31] The programs are primarily targeted to those individuals who have low incomes, but the federal eligibility, service, and reporting requirements were eliminated in 1981. States provide services oriented toward encouraging economic and personal self-sufficiency, protection from abuse, prevention of inappropriate institutionalization, and arrangements for noninstitutional services.

The SSBG program, enacted as Title XX in 1974 and modified into a federal block grant to the states in 1981, gives states broad discretion in developing social services. However, it funds only those individuals who are eligible for AFDC or SSI programs. Federal contributions were limited to $3.0 billion in 1981, and then reduced by about 20%, to $2.4 billion, in 1982. Federal funds for the SSBG were $2.5 billion in 1983 and were raised to $2.7 billion for 1984, $2.6 billion for 1985, and $2.7 billion for 1986 and 1987.[32] Thus, the increase in the SSBG did not keep pace with inflation after the 1982 cutbacks. While accurate statistics are not available, it is estimated that in 1982, $575 million in federal SSBG funds (21%) were spent on services for the aged, primarily for homemaker services.[31] Because state data on the services provided, client characteristics, or utilization and expenditures are generally not available, the program may be vulnerable to future federal and state budget cuts.

Programs for the Aging

The Older Americans Act of 1965 (OAA) established a system of state and local social and recreational programs for the elderly. In 1972, further social and nutritional services were added to the program. This federal program was funded at about $1.2 billion for 1987 to provide such services as home health care and homemakers, home repairs, information and referral, and legal, nutritional, outreach, transportation, and other services.[32]

The OAA targeted funds to those elderly in need of supportive services who are not necessarily eligible for SSI, Medicaid, and other programs. State and area agencies on aging have discretion in providing meals, transportation, homemakers, day care, and other services. The program has always been limited and was reduced dramatically in 1981.[33] Title III-B of the OAA funds supportive services and senior centers. It received $270 million in 1987. Title III-C of the OAA provides congregate and home-delivered meals. In 1987, financial support for these services was $348 million and $74 million, respectively.[32]

Income-Maintenance Programs

The federal government has been supportive of basic income-maintenance programs. The federal SSI program, passed in 1972, provides a minimum income for the aged, blind, and disabled who are poor (with incomes below $1700 annually).[32] States may supplement the basic federal payment. The program covers those without Social Security or with minimal Social Security benefits. The importance of SSI is that it provides a minimum living allowance for many, and in most instances also allows an individual to qualify for eligibility in the Medicaid program. In 1985, 4.2 million people received federally administered SSI payments. In 1986, the maximal SSI monthly benefit was $336 for an individual and $504 for a couple.[34]

OASDI, which comes under the Social Security program, provides benefits to the aged and the disabled and their dependents. In 1985, the OASDI program provided a total of $186 billion in benefits, of which $167.4 billion went to 33.1 million beneficiaries of Old Age or Survivors Insurance (e.g., retired workers and their dependents or survivors) and $18.8 billion went to 3.9 million beneficiaries of Disability Insurance (i.e., disabled workers and their dependents). These programs are financed through the payroll tax for Social Security, which assesses a flat rate on earnings up to a ceiling. In 1985, the average monthly benefit for a retired person under the Old Age Insurance program was $479, the average monthly benefit for elderly widows and widowers under the Survivors Insurance program was $433, and the average monthly benefit for a disabled worker under the Disability Insurance program was $484.[34] Since about the mid-1970s these Social Security programs had been operating at a deficit; however, Congress corrected this problem in 1983 through the approval of higher premiums and reduced benefits.

In spite of these major income-maintenance programs, the percentage of the total population living in poverty has steadily increased, from 11.7% in 1979 to 14% in 1985.[35] The poverty rates vary considerably, with 37% of blacks impoverished, compared to 11.4% of whites. Female-headed households have a poverty rate of 33.5%, and 20% of families with children under 18 live in poverty.[35]

Private Financing of Health Care

Individuals who are not eligible for public funds must pay for their care directly or through some type of health plan (a third party). Private third parties are financial agents who handle health payments. They include Blue Cross and Blue Shield plans, commercial insurance companies, prepaid plans (health maintenance organizations), or self-insured plans. In 1986, private third parties, including private health insurers and others, paid for 30.4% of total health bills through the disbursement of $123 billion in benefits, while they earned an estimated $141 billion in premiums.[36] Most health insurance pays for only hospital and physician services, so other types of health care, such as drugs, must be paid for directly.

It is estimated that in 1984 nearly seven out of every ten older persons had supplemental medical insurance policies.[37] Among the Medicare beneficiaries with private insurance, 82% had one plan and 17% had two or more policies.[37] Of those with supplemental health coverage, 54% had Blue Cross/Blue Shield, 45% had commercial insurance, and 6% were enrolled in health maintenance organizations (HMOs) or other health plans.[37] Most policies covered the same services covered by Medicare, as well as those services not fully paid for by Medicare. Most policies did not cover nursing home or long-term care services. For example, only 41% had policies that covered drugs outside the hospital.[37] Congress is currently studying a number of proposals that would provide long-term care insurance under Medicare.

Out-of-Pocket Expenses

The aged and disabled with chronic illnesses rely heavily on informal support services. It is estimated that 70–80% of long-term care (LTC) is provided by informal sources.[38] Those who need formal services generally must pay for such services directly. As noted above, Medicare and private insurance cover little of nursing home and LTC services.

Few older people can afford the $70–100 per day for nursing home care or $70 per day for home health care that is charged in some areas of the country. Many who need care in a nursing home require care over an extended period of time. As a result, many older persons are forced to spend their entire savings, thereby impoverishing themselves. Between 25% and 67% of patients who enter a nursing home subsequently use up their resources and become eligible for Medicaid.[21]

The Effects of Health Financing on the Delivery System

The model for financing health and social services for the aged described above has been based upon separate programs at the federal and state levels. Each program has its own financing mechanisms, service-delivery system, and constituencies. Although the model has been successful in getting political support for public funds, it is not an efficient model for financing care. It has led to fragmentation in program funding and inequities among programs and target groups. System redesign to develop a more effective service model is greatly needed.

The current financing system separates the financing of LTC services from the acute-care system by having different payers pay for the services, that is, Medicare and Medicaid. Some policymakers even argue for separating the programs further by providing block grants to states for LTC services.[39] On the other hand, the creation of separate delivery systems for chronic and acute illnesses is not rational, cost-effective, or equitable.[40] Persons with chronic conditions need both LTC services and acute illness medical care. Delivery of a full range of services within one comprehensive system is essential for ensuring continuity of care and access. Fragmentation in financing and service delivery could worsen under a bifurcated approach wherein both systems are reluctant to incur the high cost of caring for chronic patients. Integrated service delivery allows funds to be shifted more easily to providers who offer a full range of services that are the most appropriate and least expensive. For example, if hospital and nursing home utilization is reduced, the cost savings could be directly applied by the provider to alternative LTC services in the community and home.

The primary LTC service financed by public programs is nursing home care. Nursing home expenditures are a growing concern to public policy makers because of increases in costs and problems with the quality of care and life. The supply of nursing home beds has not kept pace with the growth in the aged population, so access to nursing home services is limited in some areas. In 1986, an estimated 14,456 facilities had 1.5 million nursing home patients.[41] Nursing homes are the second largest employer of health personnel. Only about 5% of the total aged population is institutionalized at any point in time, but one in five persons living past the age of 65 will spend some time in a nursing home.[42] State Medicare programs, which are the primary payers of nursing home care, have begun to reduce Medicaid nursing home reimbursement rates.[43] Thus, some facilities discriminate against admitting Medicaid patients, require patients to sign agreements guaranteeing private payment for specified time periods, and even evict those patients who spend-down their resources and become Medicaid patients.

Home health care is a growing part of the health industry, but still is less than 3% of Medicare and Medicaid expenditures.[20] In 1984, there were an estimated 4703 Medicare-certified agencies nationwide. Since 1983, when Medicare reimbursement was changed to a prospective diagnosis-related rate, the number of agencies has grown rapidly. The Medicare policy change encouraged earlier discharge of patients from hospitals and greater use of home health care.[44]

The shortage of other community-based LTC alternatives to nursing home care, such as adult day health care, is an even more serious problem,[44] resulting directly from the current financing system. The fact that Medicare and Medicaid programs primarily finance institutional and physician services, and limit funds for alternatives, results in a lack of funding for these programs. The Social Services and Aging programs, which have funded alternatives to some extent, are severely restricted in their federal and state funding. Since private insurance provides almost no coverage for LTC, and Medicare coverage is extremely limited, initiatives to expand community-based alternatives have been left primarily to states.[40] Funding for alternatives has come from a combination of federal and state dollars.

At a time when public spending for LTC is problematic and alternatives have yet to demonstrate strong success in reducing costs, public policy makers are reluctant to expand alternatives. (For a more comprehensive discussion of community LTC options, see Caro, Chapter 3.)

Proprietary Ownership

An increasingly large percentage of the health-care industry is owned and operated by proprietary organizations, called the new medical-industrial complex.[45] Proprietary hospital chains comprise more than 15% of the total nongovernmental acute-care facilities and more than half the non-governmental psychiatric hospitals.[46] In addition, some nonprofit hospitals are managed on a contractual basis by profit-making corporations. Proprietary nursing homes represent about 75% of all nursing homes, and an increasing number are owned by large nursing home chains.[47] Home health-care agencies are also increasingly becoming owned by proprietary organizations, and about ten large companies control about one-sixth of the total market. Laboratory corporations have also grown to the point where about one-third are owned by profit-making companies, and about a dozen or more large corporations do a growing proportion of the total business.[45]

The growth of proprietary chains is fostered by the current financing system. While nonprofit corporations have tax advantages and access to tax-exempt bonds, proprietary corporations have been highly successful in raising capital through issuing stock, a means not available to nonprofit corporations. The investor-owned hospital corporations have been able to raise funds primarily because of the stability and predictability of their profits and their guaranteed revenues under cost-based reimbursement.[48] In addition, proprietary facilities receive favorable reimbursement from Medicare, and in some state Medicaid programs, the rate of return on equity to proprietary firms has reached as high as 22%.[48] As long as the financing of health care continues as it has in the past, these trends toward proprietary ownership and the expansion of large chains will probably continue.

Cost Considerations

Cost Containment

The major approach used by government to control its costs has been to cut program expenditures for each publicly financed program. Between 1981 and 1984, major cuts were made in Medicare, Medicaid, social services, and aging programs. Medicare's premiums, deductibles, and copayments have increased substantially since 1982.[49] These increases have had their most negative effect on the elderly who are poor and living on fixed incomes. Cost increases in the copayments and deductibles also result in rising rates for private Medigap coverage (insurance to cover costs not paid by Medicare).[50,51]

The most significant recent policy change in Medicare was made through the Social Security Amendments of 1983, which established prospective reimbursement for hospitals based upon the characteristics of patients. This method also changes payments from a per-day basis to a per-discharge basis, to give hospitals greater incentives to reduce utilization. (Prospective payment systems and diagnosis-related groups are examined in detail by Maddox and Manton, Chapter 4.) Medicaid and private third-party payers have all been shifting toward prospective payment for fee-for-service providers in an effort to control costs.

Rate Setting

The regulation of all-payer rates (regardless of the source of payment) has been used successfully in some states to control costs for hospitals but has not been seriously considered for LTC. Yet, it has potential benefit for both cost containment and improving access. An all-payer reimbursement system regulates charges for Medicare, Medicaid, private insurers, and private out-of-pocket payers. This approach has been used in four states and has been found to be effective in controlling hospital costs.[52] Congress is considering legislation that would mandate all-payer rates of hospitals in states that have been unable to control costs adequately.[53]

If LTC rates were set for all payers, nursing homes and other LTC providers would not have reason to select private patients over Medicaid patients, and access would improve. Minnesota is currently the only state that has legislation to prohibit nursing homes from charging higher rates for private patients than for patients supported publicly (Equalization Statute, implemented in 1978). This method has not been systematically evaluated, but anecdotal evidence suggests that it has improved acccess for public patients.[54] All-payer rate setting has yet another advantage. Private payers would not be forced to spend-down their incomes or to deplete their assets as quickly and would not become eligible for Medicaid as soon. Such a system might reduce overall costs, but in spite of its merits, regulatory approaches are strongly opposed by provider groups and have less political viability than competitive models.

New Models for Financing Health Care

Several interesting new models of financing and delivering health care and LTC have been funded by the Health Care Financing Administration (HCFA). Included are both brokered and consolidated models. Brokered models coordinate existing community-based services, primarily through the use of case managers or case-management teams, such as the National LTC Channeling Project.[55–57] A variation of this model uses prior authorization requirements for Medicaid nursing home placement and provides alternative services where possible (e.g., ACCESS in Monroe County, N.Y.). These projects have been successful in improving the coordination and delivery of services, but they have not demonstrated that they are cost-effective. The advantage of brokered models is that they build upon existing resources and do not necessitate the redesign of current provider organizations.

Consolidated service models provide direct services within the program. A single pool of public funds is usually established (for Medicare and Medicaid), and payment is made for a full range of services, including medical care, rehabilitative services, and social supports through a capitated fee instead of fee-for-service payments (e.g., On Lok, in San Francisco).[58] This approach provides greater incentives to control costs and allows for greater flexibility in the delivery of the most appropriate services without imposing constraints on reimbursement. Ideally, both models will continue to be tested, although new demonstration projects have been severely restricted because of federal cutbacks in research and demonstration funds for HCFA.

Health Maintenance Organizations

Most health-care services are paid for on a fee-for-service basis, although such financing provides incentives for higher utilization and costs. The prepaid health plans or health maintenance organizations (HMOs) are an alternative financing model that can achieve reductions in costs. HMOs establish rates in advance of service provision on a contractual basis for a specified range of services for each individual enrolled (i.e., capitation) rather than setting rates based on the units of service delivered. The enrollment is voluntary and the consumer pays a fixed monthly and annual payment, independent of the services.[59] Providers are placed at risk for the provision of services under this approach. In other words, providers must pay for additional costs incurred above the cost covered by the capitated rate.[59] This arrangement offers providers incentives to control costs and reduce utilization. On the other hand, incentives are also created for providers to be selective in the types of patients who enroll in the program and the types of benefits covered. In 1981, there were 260 HMOs in the country serving about 9.1 million individuals.[60] This number increased to 654 HMOs with 28 million members in 1987. Enrollment in HMOs is particularly prevalent in the Western and Eastern regions of the United States.

HMOs have traditionally excluded LTC benefits and have not sought aged or disabled enrollees, in part because Medicare would reimburse on only a fee-for-service basis. Another reason HMOs have avoided the aged and disabled is that they have been unwilling to assume the financial risks for these groups, which generally have higher utilization and expenses than other groups. These problems meant that in 1981 only 4% of those enrolled in HMOs were individuals on Medicare.[60] In 1982, changes in Medicare legislation allowed HMOs to be paid on a capitation basis, giving greater incentives to HMOs to enroll these groups. By 1986, 230 HMOs had 1.6 million Medicare enrollees.[61]

While Medicare enrollment in HMOs is expected to increase, additional incentives may be needed. Moreover, the aged and disabled need to be better informed about the benefits of enrollment in HMOs (e.g., better coverage, lower copayments and deductibles, fewer problems with billing, and less difficulty in finding a physician who is willing to take assignment of the Medicare patient).

Social Health Maintenance Organizations

Four new demonstration programs have been developed by HCFA and Brandeis University as prepaid LTC models (see Greenberg et al., Chapter 11). These social health maintenance organizations (SHMOs) are similar to HMOs except that they offer the LTC and social service benefits not usually included by HMOs.[62] SHMOs provide a complete range of social and health services, from acute care to home health and homemaker services. SHMOs are financed through capitation (i.e., with rates per enrollee fixed in advance), like HMOs. Clients enroll voluntarily and payments for enrollment may come from a variety of sources, including Medicare, Medicaid, and private sources. SHMOs are financially at risk because they must provide all benefits within the income from fixed, prepaid fees. If costs exceed revenues, the difference must be underwritten by the provider. Consequently, the system is designed to encourage cost-effective management of care.[63] Additional studies of SHMOs are needed to determine their effects on service delivery, access, quality, and costs.

LTC Insurance

LTC insurance has generated a great deal of interest in the past few years as a means of protecting individuals from impoverishment. In 1986, only 120,000 individuals were covered by LTC policies, issued by twelve companies.[64] These policies generally limit the amount of benefits, have deductibles, and are oriented toward nursing home care rather than home health care, thus reducing the policies' cost and marketability.[64] Meiners studied the market potential for LTC insurance and concluded that it is great.[65] Interest among consumers, insurers, providers, and government is new but gaining momentum, so this could be another approach to reducing the burdens of LTC for the elderly and their families.

The Politics of Health Financing

Public policy for financing health care in the United States is determined by the political process. Public policy makers make choices on overall revenue sources and spending limits that determine the resources available for governmental programs. Allocation choices are also made between health care, social services, income maintenance, Social Security, and other social programs, as well as nonservice programs, such as the military, agriculture, education, and other programs.

Decisions on resources allocated and on policies for the programs are heavily influenced by special interest groups. For example, the American Medical Association and the American Hospital Association are highly influential in the political process.[66] Another important organization in the political process is the American Health Care Association (representing nursing homes). Many other health-care trade associations are also involved in the political process. The history of decision making in health-care financing is closely intertwined with the actions and advocacy of these organizations, which contribute dollars, time, and influence to political campaigns, legislative actions, and regulatory efforts. These provider groups generally seek to maintain their current market share of the total resources and to continue the high growth in health-care expenditures. The current system is due to the success of the major provider associations in influencing policies, particularly those that favor fee-for-service funding of the major providers, high growth in expenditures, and the dominance of funding to hospitals, nursing homes, and physicians. To make substantial changes in the current financing and delivery of health care, business, labor, and consumer groups will need to be more politically effective than they have been in the past.

Advocacy and consumer groups for the aged are, of course, also involved in the political process. The aged, by virtue of their voting power and the legitimacy of their issues, have had a strong influence on the political process, although they are not organized as one block and do not make large amounts of political contributions.[67] Most advocacy and consumer groups for the aged have focused primarily on the maintenance of funding for the Older American Acts and protecting Medicare from funding cuts. Medicaid, the Social Services Block Grant, and Supplemental Security Income have received less active attention from advocates. Groups representing the elderly tend to have limited knowledge of financing issues and to be less involved in efforts aimed at shaping financing policies. New understanding of the fundamental nature of health and LTC financing may encourage greater activism by these groups.

Fiscal crises and cost containment have become dominant themes in LTC policy, as state and local governments seek ways to reduce costs. New program initiatives have been left primarily to the states, leading to gaps in services and inequities across regions. Public policies have primarily addressed short-range approaches rather than making fundamental reforms in the financing and delivery of services. New federal initiatives are needed to reform the current financing of health care and to protect the government and the aged from exorbitant cost increases. If reforms are not made to reduce the cost and to improve the delivery of LTC services, it is not likely that older Americans will have the type of health care they desire at an affordable price.

References

1. Division of National Cost Estimates, Office of the Actuary, United States Health Care Financing Administration. 1987. National health expenditures, 1986–2000. *Health Care Financing Rev* 8(4):1–36.
2. United States Bureau of the Census. 1987. *Statistical Abstract of the United States, 1987.* 109th ed. Washington, D.C.: Government Printing Office, 398.
3. Hicks, L. L., Boles, K. E. 1984. Why health economics? *Nurs Econ* 2:175.
4. See Ref. 1, p. 1.
5. See Ref. 1, p. 25.
6. Davis, C. K. 1983. The federal role in changing health care financing. Part I: National programs and health financing problems. *Nurs Econ* 12.
7. See Ref. 1, p. 24.
8. See Ref. 1, p. 17.
9. Waldo, D. R., Lazenby, H. C. 1984. Demographic characteristics and health care use and expenditures by the aged in the United States, 1977–1984. *Health Care Financing Rev* 6:25.

10. Fisher, C. R. 1980. Differences by age groups in health care spending. *Health Care Financing Rev* 1:65–90.
11. See Ref. 9, p. 1.
12. See Ref. 9, p. 10.
13. See Ref. 1, p. 29.
14. See Ref. 9, pp. 8–15.
15. See Ref. 9, p. 8.
16. United States Congress, House Select Committee on Aging. 1984. *Elderly Health Care Costs Projected to Rise Twice as Fast as Income.* (News release.) Washington, D.C.: Select Committee on Aging, 1–4.
17. See Ref. 1, p. 8.
18. Freeland, M. S., Schendler, C. E. 1984. Health spending in the 1980s: Integration of clinical practice patterns with management. *Health Care Financing Rev* Spring (5)168; and see Ref. 1, p. 25.
19. See Ref. 9, p. 11.
20. See Ref. 1, p. 13.
21. United States Senate. 1987. *Developments in Aging, 1986*, Vol. 1. Washington, D.C.: Government Printing Office, 185.
22. See Ref. 9, p. 23.
23. See Ref. 9, p. 15.
24. United States Department of Health and Human Services. 1987. *HHS News:* National health expenditures for 1986. July.
25. Waldo, D. R., Levit, K. R., Lazenby, H. 1986. National health expenditures, 1985. *Health Care Financing Rev* 8(1):1–21.
26. Reif, L. 1984. Making dollars and sense of home health policy. *Nurs Econ* 2:383–385.
27. Rymer, M. 1984. *Short-Term Evaluation of Medicaid: Selected Issues.* Cambridge, Mass.: Urban Systems Research and Engineering.
28. *Topical Law Reports. Medicare Medicaid Guide.* Volume 3-A. 1987 State Charts. Chicago, Ill.: Commerce Clearing House.
29. Vogel, R. J., Palmer, H. C. 1983. *Long-Term Care: Perspectives from Research and Demonstrations.* Washington, D.C.: Government Printing Office.
30. See Ref. 9, pp. 23–24.
31. Lindeman, D. A., Pardini, A. 1983. Social services: The impact of fiscal austerity. In *Fiscal Austerity and Aging,* ed. C. Estes and R. Newcomer. Beverly Hills, Calif.: Sage Publications, 133–155.
32. See Ref. 21, p. 361.
33. Newcomer, R. J., Benjamin, A. E., Estes, C. L. 1983. The Older Americans Act. In *Fiscal Austerity and Aging,* ed. C. Estes and R. Newcomer. Beverly Hills, Calif.: Sage Publications, 190.
34. United States Social Security Administration. 1987. *Social Security Bulletin: Annual Statistical Supplement. 1986.* SSA Pub. No. 0037-7910. Washington, D.C.: Government Printing Office, 11.
35. See Ref. 2, p. 443.
36. See Ref. 1, p. 34.
37. United States Senate. 1985. *Developments in Aging, 1984.* Vol. 1. Washington, D.C.: Government Printing Office, 178.

48   *Charlene A. Harrington*

38. United States Health Care Financing Administration. 1981. *Long-Term Care: Background and Future Directions.* DHHS Pub. No. (PHS) 81-20047. Washington, D.C.: Government Printing Office, 40.
39. Callahan, J. J., Wallack, S. S. 1981. *Reforming the Long-Term Care System.* Lexington, Mass.: Lexington Books.
40. Harrington, C., Newcomer, R. J., Estes, C. L., and Associates (eds.). 1985. *Long-Term Care of the Elderly: Public Policy Issues.* Beverly Hills, Calif.: Sage Publications.
41. Harrington, C., Swan, J. H., Grant, L. State Medicaid reimbursement for nursing homes, 1978–1986. *Health Care Financing Rev* 9(3):33–50.
42. Manton, K., Soldo, B. 1985. Dynamics of health changes in the oldest old: New perspectives and evidence. *Milbank Memorial Fund Q* 63(2).
43. Harrington, C., Swan, J. H. 1984. Medicaid nursing home reimbursement policies, rates, and expenditures. *Health Care Financing Rev* 6(1):39–49.
44. See Ref. 29, pp. 415–436.
45. Relman, A. S. 1980. The medical-industrial complex. *N Engl J Med* 303:963–970.
46. Institute of Medicine. 1983. *The New Health Care for Profit.* Washington, D. C.: National Academy Press.
47. Harrington, C. 1984. Public policy and the nursing home industry. *Int J Health Serv* 14(3):481–485.
48. Mark, B. A. 1984. Investor-owned and nonprofit hospitals: A comparison. *Nurs Econ* 2:240–245.
49. Harrington, C. 1983. Policy options for Medicare. *Nurs Econ* 1:187–192.
50. Carroll, M. S., Arnett, R. H. 1981. Private health insurance plans in 1978 and 1979: A review of coverage, enrollment, and financial experience. *Health Care Financing Rev* 3(September):55–87.
51. Feder, J., et al. 1981. Health. In *The Reagan Experiment*, ed. J. L. Palmer and I. V. Sawhill. Washington, D.C.: Urban Institute Press, 271–305.
52. United States General Accounting Office. 1980. Rising hospital costs can be restrained by regulating payments and improving management. *Report to the Congress by the Comptroller General.* Washington, D.C.: Government Printing Office.
53. See Ref. 21, p. 168.
54. Interagency Board for Quality Assurance. 1984. *Progress Report of Interagency Board for Quality Assurance.* Report presented to the Minnesota State Legislature. Saint Paul, Minn.: Interagency Board for Quality Assurance.
55. Zawadski, R. T. 1983. Community-based systems of long term care. *Home Health Care Serv Q* 4(3/4).
56. See Ref. 29, pp. 167–253.
57. United States General Accounting Office. 1982. The elderly should benefit from expanded home health care but increasing these services will not insure cost reduction. *Report to the Congress by the Comptroller General.* IPE-83-1. Washington, D.C.: Government Printing Office.
58. See Ref. 55, pp. 229–247.
59. Luft, H. S. 1981. *Health Maintenance Organizations: Dimensions of Performance.* New York: John Wiley and Sons.

60. Interstudy. 1987. *The Interstudy Edge, Summer 1987*. Excelsior, Minn.: Interstudy, 1–48.
61. Iverson, L. H., Polich, C. L. 1987. *1986 December Update of Medicare Enrollments in HMOs*. Excelsior, Minn.: Interstudy.
62. Greenberg, J. N., Leutz, W., Ervin, S., Greenlick, M., Kodner, D., Selstad, J. 1985. S/HMO: The social/health maintenance organization and long term care. *Generations* 9(Summer):51–55.
63. Harrington, C., Newcomer, R. J. 1984. Social health maintenance organizations: A new policy option for the aged and disabled. Working paper. San Francisco, Calif.: University of California Aging Health Policy Center.
64. See Ref. 21, p. 274.
65. Meiners, M. R. 1985. Long term care insurance. *Generations* 9:39–42.
66. Starr, P. 1983. *The Social Transformation of American Medicine*. New York: Basic Books.
67. Estes, C. L. 1979. *The Aging Enterprise*. San Francisco, Calif.: Jossey-Bass.

Three

Alternatives to Institutionalization: Community Long-Term Care

Francis G. Caro

The elderly are particularly susceptible to illnesses that require care for extended periods and that lead to permanent losses in functioning. Younger populations are usually expected to attain rapid and complete recovery from illness or injury, but among older people, recovery from acute illness is characteristically slower. More important, the elderly are vulnerable to a variety of chronic illnesses. Diabetes and arthritis are particularly good examples. Fortunately, professional health care may halt or diminish the progression of chronic diseases and may reduce the pain, discomfort, and disability they generate. However, elderly patients are likely to need particularly intensive rehabilitation if the restoration of their functioning is to be maximized. Particularly challenging are the diseases and injuries that leave the elderly with permanent impairments—leading, in turn, to loss in ability to function.[1] For example, despite intensive rehabilitation efforts, in a very old person a broken hip often leads to permanent limitations of mobility. In its most serious stages, Alzheimer's disease renders its victims totally and permanently incapable of caring for themselves.

Death, of course, is an important part of the health-care configuration for the elderly. It is generally expected that younger patients will recover from illness, but the elderly often do not. As aging progresses, the thrust of health care shifts from the promotion of recovery to the prolongation of life, or to the prevention of death.

This chapter looks at the implications of these health realities for service providers, focusing on the long-term care (LTC) needs of the infirm elderly and how they can be met outside institutional walls. Particularly among the very old, the presence of multiple chronic conditions must be taken into account in the treatment of acute health problems. When health problems are chronic, providers must shift their emphases from strategies that cure to those that help the patient live with the health problem. The limitations of natural recovery processes mean that more emphasis has to be placed on explicit rehabilitation strategies. Substantial long-term attention must be given to those who remain alive but with seriously diminished abilities to care for themselves. Finally, more emphasis must be placed on the management of circumstances surrounding death.

Special Needs of the Elderly

A particularly confusing concept is that much of the help needed by the elderly is not health care at all. The term *health care* usually refers to the diagnosis or treatment of health problems. Sometimes the term is reserved for the interventions commonly thought to require the specialized training and skills of health professionals. A loss of self-care capacity as a result of illness or injury creates a need for assistance with such activities as eating, dressing, bathing, toileting, mobility, and managing money. Those who live independently may need assistance with meal preparation, house cleaning, laundry, and shopping. These needs are real, labor-intensive, and costly when provided by paid personnel. These services are provided to the elderly because of health problems, yet they do not fit the conventional understanding of health care.

The LTC needs of the elderly are categorized in many different ways. Some define LTC as a distinct part of the health-care field. Others conceive of it as a set of services somewhat apart from health care. For some, the heart of LTC is the medical management of chronic disease, which involves medications, special diets, bandages, physical therapy, speech therapy, and so on.[2] Others see the core of LTC as assistance that responds to self-care deficits[3] and ensures that daily living needs are met.[4] Most providers of LTC are concerned with both the medical management of chronic illness and the response to functional deficits. How these concerns are balanced, however, can make an enormous difference.

If much of LTC is not health care, then what should it be called? Unfortunately, no fully satisfactory term is available to identify its non-medical aspects. Sometimes the terms *social care* or *social services* are used, but the phrases are so widely and loosely used that they lack specific meaning. The term *custodial care* is flawed by its passive connotations. The term *personal care* generates confusion because it may refer only to tasks that involve body contact, such as feeding, dressing, grooming, transfer, and toileting. When narrowly defined, *personal care* is distinguished from "noncontact" housekeeping tasks, such as meal preparation, cleaning, and shopping. Ratzka advocates *personal assistance* as more positive and less restrictive than other terms in current use.[5]

Another complication arises from the fact that functional abilities are situational. Elderly people survive in independent living situations for a variety of reasons: the division of labor within their household is manageable, their household is barrier-free and well equipped, or they live close to community resources. An elderly man may find himself in need of help when he loses his wife, who may have always handled all the cooking, shopping, and cleaning, or an elderly woman may be helpless financially after losing her husband, who may have taken care of all the couple's financial affairs. For the rural and suburban elderly, the ability to manage independently may be affected by the availability of transportation for shopping. For the urban elderly, the danger of street crime poses a significant barrier to free movement in the neighborhood, which is needed for complete independence.

In some cases, the ability to function independently is strongly linked to the availability of basic housing. Loss or lack of adequate housing can trigger a general disorientation and loss of functional skills. Resettling confused, homeless people into secure, comfortable residential environments can lead to the recovery of functional capacity.[6,7] Functional independence is premised on the availability of sufficient funds to meet basic living needs. Lack of sufficient funds to pay for housing, food, clothing, utilities, and transportation can severely undermine the older person's functional independence.

Unfortunately, the distinction between health care and social care is not simply a conceptual or academic matter. It greatly affects the allocation of resources and relationships among helping efforts. Simply put, health care enjoys much higher regard in this society than social care both because it is involved with life-threatening situations and because it brings in highly developed expertise to sustain life and to improve health. Social services have not been as successful in making a case for the importance of their mission. Although peripheral to the health-care sector's greatest sources of prestige, LTC enjoys greater societal respect when it is seen as part of the health-care system than when it is considered a social service. A practical result is the fact that third-party payments available for LTC are much greater when LTC is provided within a health framework.

The consequences of the attachment of LTC to the health-care sector are distinctly mixed. On the positive side, it encourages attention to the health and safety of its recipients, and it emphasizes the responsibility of providers for strategies that manage chronic disease, protect recipients

from health threats, and extend life. However, there are also several negative consequences. Supervision by health professionals and compliance
with health standards are expensive. For some recipients a strong health
emphasis is an unwelcome constraint, they are willing to take the health
risks associated with somewhat more independent lifestyles. Disproportionate amounts of scarce service resources may go for health care rather
than social care. The breadth of responsibility may overtax health-care
providers. Particularly in physician-dominated health care, the social care
needs of recipients may get insufficient attention. Finally, LTC may be
considered an enormously expensive drag on the health sector. The cost
issue is particularly serious for Medicaid. In 1983, 47.7% of Medicaid
expenditures were for LTC (with 96.3% of that amount for institutional
care).[8] From a traditional health perspective, such expenditures represent
public costs that should not be "charged" to the health sector, since they do
not serve major health purposes.

Care Settings

When LTC for the elderly emerged as a public issue, much of the focus was
on institutional care. In reality, institutions have always been of limited
importance as care settings for the functionally disabled elderly, but they
have received more than their share of attention because of their visibility
as well as their reliance on public financing.

Contemporary nursing homes are the result of several social and economic forces. In part, they reflect an effort to reserve hospital care for those
needing treatment for acute conditions. Those needing less-intensive institutional care had to be placed elsewhere. In part, residential care for the
elderly in this country also has its roots in county farms and poorhouses for
low-income, unattached adults. In time, separate facilities emerged for the
mentally ill, the mentally retarded, criminals, the chronically ill, and the
elderly. Other predecessors include private lodging houses, rooming
houses, and residential hotels that served low-income, unattached adults
in urban areas. As their clientele grew older and developed functional
disabilities, and as public funding opportunities developed, some residential facilities were converted into institutions. Those facilities that
qualified became nursing homes, to take advantage of the relatively high
rates of reimbursement. Eventually, the combination of large numbers of
functionally disabled elderly, substantial sources of third-party reimbursement for institutional care, and public fire and safety standards led to the
emergence of facilities specially constructed as nursing homes.[9] (Nursing
homes are examined in greater detail in Freeman and Vladeck, Chapter
12.)

Nationally, the number of nursing home beds has increased substantially in the past 20 years. The increases were particularly rapid in the 1960s and early 1970s, when the annual growth rate was 8.1% for nursing home beds. Continued growth of the nursing home population is expected. For the period 1985–1995, an increase in the nursing home population from 1.5 million to 1.9 million has been projected. (Estimates of future institutional expansion should be treated cautiously. Actual institutional expansion will be affected by the willingness of state regulatory agencies to authorize new beds, by third-party reimbursement rates, and by the availability of non-institutional services.) The use of institutions is strongly age related. Approximately 90% of those living in LTC institutions are elderly. Of those over 65 years of age, approximately 5% are institutionalized. Among those 65–74 years of age, only 2% are institutionalized. Among those 85 and over, 23% are institutionalized.[8]

Institutional LTC facilities have been widely criticized for deficient care, unsafe facilities, unfair profit taking by private operators, and high charges. Among the noninstitutionalized elderly, the prospect of nursing home placement tends to be viewed negatively.[10] Of course, institutional facilities vary greatly in the quality of service they provide, and everyone acknowledges the need for institutional care and the quality and integrity of some institutional operations. What is important for the purposes of this discussion is the dissatisfaction with institutional LTC that has sparked interest in noninstitutional LTC strategies.

Most LTC has always been provided by informal caregivers in private homes, particularly when our nation was a predominantly rural society in which multigeneration families often shared a residence. Traditionally, it was expected that families would address the LTC needs of those who survived to old age. Today, the caregiving capacity of families has been reduced by smaller family size, higher divorce rates, greater geographic distribution of families, and by the increased participation of women in employment outside the home. Nevertheless, families continue to have a major role in the provision of LTC. In fact, an estimated 80% of the LTC of the elderly in the United States is provided informally—mostly by relatives.[11] (See also Brody and Brody, Chapter 14, on this topic.)

In the past 15–20 years, interest in organized or formal noninstitutional LTC strategies has increased greatly. These services have arisen to meet the needs of the isolated elderly, and they are also designed to complement the help provided by informal caregivers.[12] (Sometimes the term *respite care* is used when a major aim of formal services is to provide relief to informal caregivers.)

The components of noninstitutional LTC are much more varied than those of institutional LTC. Characteristically, institutions are expected to provide total care of "patients" or "residents." Nursing homes, for example, manage chronic illness and provide personal care, housing, meal service, and activity programs. In contrast, some noninstitutional LTC services consist of a single component, such as home-delivered meals, housekeeping, or specialized transportation. In other cases, a package of services is provided, such as medical management, physical therapy, personal care, and housekeeping. In some instances all of the care is provided in the recipient's home, while in other cases the recipient is brought to a formal setting, such as a hospital, for some services. Usually, these are day programs in which transportation is part of the service package. In other instances, services are linked to housing, and the elderly recipients live in their own units in special housing configurations. Some services (e.g., housekeeping) are provided to them in their units. Other services may be available to them on the grounds, such as congregate meals and even intermittent nursing care.

Services may also be directed as much to concerned relatives as to the functionally disabled elderly. Home care is sometimes introduced to provide respite to an informal caregiver, or day hospital programs may be used to relieve a caregiving relative. Short stays in institutions are also sometimes arranged to enable an informal caregiver to take a vacation. Mutual support groups can help improve the skills and the morale of informal caregivers. Some relatives need counseling because of stress resulting from intensive caregiving or internal conflict resulting from the consideration of an institutional placement.

Providers of these noninstitutional service components are also highly diverse in their auspices and disciplinary perspectives. Among the important providers are home health agencies, with leadership provided by public health nurses. These agencies are often community based, but in other instances they are hospital based. In some cases, service components are sponsored by organizations with a primary interest in social services or housing, such as less formal home-care programs sponsored by churches. Sponsorship usually influences disciplinary leadership. Hospital-based programs are likely to be led by public health nurses or physicians. Home health agencies are directed by public health nurses. Social agency sponsorship usually means that social work is the dominant discipline. Church-sponsored programs are likely to be entirely nonprofessional.

Profit-making firms that are well established in the provision of nursing home care are increasingly important in the noninstitutional LTC domain. In a field once dominated by voluntary agencies, profit-making enterprises began with the self-pay market and eventually established themselves as eligible vendors for publicly funded services. Some voluntary agencies have found it advantageous to establish profit-making subsidiaries.

The interrelationship among home-care components may be extremely complex. Upon discharge from acute care in a hospital, an elderly patient may have home care arranged by a hospital-based home health agency. The hospital may contract with a community-based nursing agency for the actual in-home services, and the nursing agency, in turn, may subcontract with a third agency for home health aides who provide personal care and housekeeping services.

Due to the broad range of problems plaguing the elderly, and the diversity of disciplines potentially involved in providing services, leading to fragmentation among service providers, case management has emerged as an important strategy in noninstitutional LTC. (See Brody and Magel, Chapter 13, for a more detailed look at case management.) The limited ability of the functionally disabled elderly to negotiate a complex service system on their own, as well as difficulties in establishing eligibility for publicly funded services, contribute to the need for this specialty. Case management includes needs assessment, service planning, service negotiation, service monitoring, and periodic reassessment. When sufficient professional resources are available, assessment is sometimes done by multidisciplinary teams, which consist of a physician, a public health nurse, and a social worker. More often, assessment is done by a single professional, such as a nurse or a social worker, perhaps in consultation with other professionals. In some cases, service negotiation and service monitoring are performed by skilled nonprofessionals. Case management is usually part of the service of a formal organization; however, it is increasingly offered by professionals in private practice.

Limited aggregate data are available on the use of noninstitutional LTC. A 1982 national survey of Medicare recipients found that of those with functional disabilities, 5.5% relied exclusively on paid help and 20.6% used a combination of paid and nonpaid help.[13] A recent survey (conducted in the service-rich New York City environment) of low- and moderate-income noninstitutionalized elderly with functional disabilities found that 18% relied entirely on organized services and 23.2% used a combination of formal and informal care.[14]

Home care, like institutional care, is labor-intensive and relies extensively on women and nonprofessionals. Most workers are paid at or near the minimum wage. The availability of workers will affect future expansion of home care. In New York City, where home-care programs are highly developed, no difficulties have been experienced in attracting workers; recent immigrants from the Caribbean have been attracted extensively to the home-care field. In other labor markets with large numbers of women who are recent immigrants from developing countries, the experience is likely to be similar.

However, changes in immigration law in 1986 have reduced the availability of recent immigrants as long-term care workers. The legislation made it unlawful for employers to hire any alien who lacked work authorization. Further, the bill required that employers verify eligibility to work before hiring. In some areas, worker shortages have adversely affected delivery of home care. In Massachusetts, for example, where home care is well developed and a strong economy has created abundant employment opportunities for low-skilled workers, as much as 40% of the home care authorized in the state operated program has not been delivered in some regions because of worker shortages.

Federal efforts to control Medicare expenditures for hospital care are stimulating expansion of home care. Medicare reimbursement on the basis of a diagnosis-related group system provides hospitals with an incentive to discharge patients more rapidly. The availability of home-care programs with a strong health component provides a basis for accelerating hospital discharges. Advances in medical technology also contribute to the expansion of home care. Sophisticated equipment for the management of chronic illness previously available only in hospitals is increasingly available in forms suitable for use at home. Vastly improved electronic and mechanical aids for the physically disabled also make living at home feasible for people who previously required institutional care.

Several components of the continuum of services for the chronically ill and functionally disabled elderly warrant special attention.

Day programs for the chronically ill and functionally disabled elderly have both health and social service origins. As a health service, day-treatment programs are an extension of outpatient rehabilitation services. Patients are brought to a facility—either a hospital or a nursing home—on a regular basis, perhaps two or three days a week for much of the day. Patients receive not only therapeutic services but also a meal and an opportunity to participate in activity programs. Health-care providers play the lead role in approximately one-third of current programs. As a social service, day programs are an extension of the activities of senior centers. Some senior centers have built upon the midday meal and recreation programs they offer to the well elderly. To the elderly with significant self-care limitations, these senior centers offer supervised activities, a hot meal, and sometimes limited health monitoring on a regular basis for a portion of the day. An estimated two-thirds of current programs are closer to the social model in their origins.

From the consumer's perspective, day programs offer several benefits. Day health programs sometimes shorten hospital stays: patients receive rehabilitation on an outpatient basis that they otherwise would have received as a hospital inpatient or nursing home resident. Participants may also welcome the activities and social interaction associated with the program. For informal caregivers, day programs are welcome sources of respite. Caregiving relatives are assured that their spouses or parents are in good hands while they are free to engage in other activities. For health-care facilities, day programs can be useful as a way of extending the use of expensive rehabilitation facilities and in attracting future users of inpatient services.

The viability of day programs depends on several factors. Candidates for day programs usually also require care when they are at home. Day programs supplement in-home care provided by informal caregivers or organized services. The availability of adequate in-home care is the first condition for potential users of day programs. A second essential factor is the availability of transportation. When participants are ambulatory and transportation is provided by informal caregivers, this condition poses no problem. When participants have severe limitations on mobility and are geographically dispersed, complex and expensive specialized transportation services are needed. A third issue is third-party financing. When day services are provided in a health setting and include specialized transportation, they are expensive. Ironically, current public funding policies are more encouraging for day programs in more-expensive health settings than for those in less-expensive social settings. Although day programs are an attractive option in the spectrum of LTC services, they are less developed than either institutional or in-home services. The difficulties experienced by program administrators in meeting the conditions outlined here explain much of the relatively modest development of day programs.

The National Institute for Adult Day Care estimated that a minimum of 1200 centers are currently active, with an average daily census of 20. Nationally, an estimated 27,000 are served on any given day and 40,000 are served weekly.[15]

Continuing-care or *life-care communities* provide housing and a range of services, including LTC. These communities are designed to attract often fully independent and active elderly people, assuring them needed services as their self-care capacity diminishes. At the outset, residents have a living unit of their own that includes kitchen facilities. However, complete meal service is also provided. Housekeeping and personal assistance are available. A nursing facility is included for those with intensive LTC needs. When they move permanently into the nursing facility, residents give up their private living unit. Financial arrangements are integral to the concept of the life-care community. In exchange for an entrance fee and monthly payments, community members receive the use of a housing unit and specified services for life. Residents do not have any equity or ownership. Their agreement may include a provision for a partial refunding of the entry fee if they choose to leave within a specified period of time. In 1983, the National Consumers' League estimated that most entry fees ranged from $15,000 to $65,000. Most monthly fees were between $600 and $900.[16] The services covered by these fees vary. Characteristically, additional services are available at extra costs. In some cases the nursing facilities qualify for Medicare and Medicaid reimbursement. In other cases they do not. In 1983, the Senate Select Committee on Aging estimated that between 300 and 500 life-care communities were in operation, serving approximately 100,000 elderly. [17]

Life-care communities involve financial risks for both consumers and sponsors. Consumers make substantial initial payments for the assurance that extensive services will be provided if, when, and to the extent that they are needed. Consumers also take the risk that they will have the means to pay monthly fees, which may increase substantially. Sponsors must plan to have sufficient funds to meet their obligations. Predicting the scope of resident service needs and operating costs can be difficult. Some life-care communities have not been able to meet their financial obligations. Although many life-care communities are church affiliated, the churches may not assume financial responsibility if the community is unable to meet its obligations.

Because of the costs, life-care communities are an option for only the small proportion of the elderly who are affluent. Those without substantial equity in a home and without substantial pension income beyond Social Security are not likely to be able to afford continuing-care communities.

To a limited extent, programs that combine housing and LTC services are available for low-income elderly. New York State, for example, operates an Enriched Housing program for low-income elderly people with modest self-care limitations. Participants have their own living units, receive housekeeping services, and participate in daily congregate meals. Participants must be willing to sign over Supplemental Security Income (SSI) checks: they receive only a modest allowance for personal expenses. The state pays operators at the higher SSI rate received by adult homes. The program is not designed to serve those requiring extensive LTC services. Like the life-care communities, the Enriched Housing program provides some of the protection of an institutional program at the same time that residents retain an apartment of their own.

Hospice programs provide a special form of LTC for the terminally ill. Hospice care differs from traditional health care in two important respects: 1) the customary emphasis on cure is replaced by a primary concern with relief from pain, and 2) major attention is given to the psychosocial aspects of dying for both patient and relatives. The contemporary hospice movement has its origin in England, where the first formal hospice facility was opened in 1968. In this country, the number of hospice programs began growing rapidly after 1975. By 1982, there were over 800 programs serving some 50,000 patients annually, usually for periods of 35 to 60 days. [18]

Hospice services are provided in various settings: free-standing facilities, hospitals, and home-care programs. Some hospital hospice programs are housed in space of their own; others consist of teams of staff who work with patients wherever they are in the hospital. In this country, hospice care is most commonly provided through home-care programs. The vast majority of those served by hospice programs are cancer victims. The AIDS epidemic has resulted in a rapidly growing new population for whom hospice services are appropriate. Professional staffing of hospice programs is multidisciplinary, including physicians, nurses, social workers, psychiatrists, psychologists, and providers of personal assistance.

Because the hospice movement is as much a philosophy as an organized program, it has had an influence beyond formal programs. The approaches to pain management and psychosocial preparation for death promoted through the hospice movement have spread widely to other health and LTC settings. As a result, the terminally ill are likely to receive aspects of hospice care even when they are not participants in a formal hospice program.

The *mental health* component of services for the elderly is strikingly underdeveloped. In spite of widespread mental disorder among the elderly, mental health services are weaker for the elderly than for younger populations. Among the noninstitutionalized elderly, survey data reveal that 10–15% suffer from significant cognitive decline.[19] An equal number are estimated to have histories of affective disorders. Mental disorder is even more prevalent among the institutionalized elderly. The National Center for Health Statistics survey of nursing home residents in 1977 revealed that nearly 60% had a primary or secondary diagnosis of mental illness.[20] A more recent sample survey in upstate New York found that 64.2% of nursing home residents had significant behavioral problems.[21] The number of mentally ill elderly in nursing homes, in fact, now exceeds the number in mental hospitals.[22]

Mental disorders occur in several configurations. One group is made up of those with a chronic mental illness that emerged earlier in the life cycle and who have survived to old age. Those who experience the onset of a chronic mental disorder in later life constitute a second group. Those whose condition is situational (that is, a response to adverse conditions experienced in old age) are a third group. Specific cases, of course, are often difficult to classify; in some instances more than one category is applicable.

Although mental disorders are more prevalent among the elderly than among younger adults, the elderly are underrepresented among users of mental health services. Nationally, although the elderly make up more than 10% of the population, only 4% of the patients seen at outpatient mental health clinics are elderly, and only 2% of those treated at private psychiatric clinics are elderly.[23] In general, mental health professionals do not have a strong presence in nursing homes. Most direct care in nursing homes and other adult residences is provided by aides, who have little or no formal training. Medical care is provided by physicians, who rarely have formal training for work with the elderly. In spite of an extensive use of psychotropic medications, consultations with psychiatrists are rare. [23]

Contributing to the relative lack of professional attention to the mental health problems of the elderly has been a pessimism about the responsiveness of the mentally impaired elderly to treatment. Rather, loss of mental functioning has been seen as a normal and irreversible aspect of the aging process. Mental health professionals who work with the elderly challenge many of those assumptions. They report success in diagnosing and treating specific conditions. [24,25]

Part of the uncertainty about the role of mental health services in the care of the mentally impaired elderly stems from its similarity to the role of good social care. Mental health professionals working with the elderly often recommend interventions that encourage positive social interaction, participation in stimulating activities, and sensitivity to individual needs. These qualities are desirable also in the care of the dependent elderly, apart from their explicit importance for the treatment of mental disorder.

A major role for mental health services in the care of the elderly is the support of direct caregivers, formal and informal. Mental health professionals contribute through both consultation on individual cases and training. [26] A significant aspect of the mental health role is working with families. Mental health professionals serve families through advice on direct care strategies for a mentally impaired older person and through assistance to family caregivers in coping with the stress they experience as a result of their caregiving efforts. [27]

Financing Service

Third-party financing has been much better developed for the acute health-care needs of the elderly than for LTC needs. Because it is labor-intensive, LTC provided by formal services is very expensive. When provided in an institutional setting, LTC inevitably involves the cost of both the facility and its operation. Most elderly people cannot themselves afford to pay for institutional care or intensive home care indefinitely. Currently, neither public nor private income security programs for the elderly are designed to provide sufficient funds to pay for intensive health care or personal care. The elderly also tend to be reluctant to deplete their limited savings to finance LTC.

Public financing of institutional LTC is much more available than financing of noninstitutional LTC. Medicare finances only 1.9% of nursing home care. Medicaid, however, has come to be particularly important in financing nursing home care. In 1984, Medicaid provided financing for 43.4% of nursing home care. [28] Frequently, the elderly enter nursing homes as private-pay patients and convert to Medicaid financing after their own resources are depleted. For some low-income elderly with less severe functional disabilities, financing of institutional care is provided through the public income security stream (Supplemental Security Income) rather than through health-care funds.

Provisions for financing noninstitutional LTC are scattered and very incomplete. Medicare's home-care benefits cover patients with medical problems requiring the attention of a health professional. Eligibility is limited to those who are under the care of a physician, homebound, and in need of nursing or a therapeutic service. In 1983, Medicare home-health expenditures totaled $1.5 billion.[8] Medicare was the source of financing for 38.5% of the recipients surveyed in 1982 who received home care.[13] Since 1983, Medicare has also provided limited financing for hospice services. In 1985, Medicare hospice expenditures totaled $15 million.[28]

Medicare is not a source of financing for home care of the functionally disabled elderly with stable medical conditions. Several states provide relatively generous financing for the home care that Medicare does not cover. New York, Texas, and Oklahoma make use of Medicaid through an optional personal-care benefit to finance home care. In New York, the use of this option is extensive: in 1982, New York State accounted for 78% of the total Medicaid home-care expenditures.[14] Massachusetts and California are important examples of states that have drawn on federal Social Services Block Grant funds to finance home care. To a much lesser extent, some funds provided by the Older Americans Act have been used for financing home care. Some states provide financing for their own home-care programs for the elderly. The Massachusetts program, for example, is now entirely state financed.

The New York City Home Attendant and Housekeeper programs, the largest city-state home-care initiative, illustrate the potential scope of these programs. In 1984, the Home Attendant program served an average caseload of 28,940, at a public cost of $335.5 million. The Housekeeper program served another 9000 at a cost of $22.8 million.[29] Service authorizations for the Home Attendant program were remarkably extensive, averaging more than 50 hours per week. In exceptional cases, round-the-clock care is provided. Because the programs are financed by Medicaid, they are limited to the poor. Those with marginal incomes can qualify for partial financing through a spend-down provision. When their own monthly expenditures for approved forms of health care are equal to the difference between their income and the upper limit for Medicaid eligibility, Medicaid covers all additional approved health services, including home care. While this provision is helpful in extending third-party financing to some, it does not cover many with modest financial means.

The New York City Home Attendant program is particularly designed to serve the elderly who live alone and who can expect little help from informal caregivers. When home-care applicants live with relatives, home-care authorizations reflect expectations for significant participation of informal caregivers. When compared to other home-care programs, the New York City Home Attendant program is certainly atypical in the hours of care it provides. It is more common for state and local programs to provide only several hours of service per week.

Expenditures through other federal programs for the other LTC strategies discussed above are at much lower levels than are those for institutional care and home care. Current federal expenditures for adult day care are at least $33 million. Medicaid is the single most important source, accounting for more than half of the expenditures through public programs. The Social Service Block Grant and the Older Americans Act are also significant sources of funding for adult day care.[15]

The forms in which LTC financing is made available are significant. Usually, financing is linked to specific services, and health professionals are authorized to prescribe from a set of approved services. Providers are reimbursed on a fee-for-service basis. This approach, which places heavy responsibility on professional gatekeepers, implies limited consumer participation in decision making. The Veterans' Administration's Aid and Attendance program illustrates an alternative approach. The program provides cash payments to veterans with severe disabling conditions, and eligible veterans enjoy complete discretion in the use of the funds. When consumers control resources, they may develop LTC strategies very different from those prescribed by professionals. Consumers are more likely, for example, to employ helpers (including family members) directly and on a relatively informal basis. In so doing, consumers eliminate overhead costs (including fringe benefits) built into the fees of organized service providers. Of course, consumers forgo the protection provided by a formal service's training, supervision, record keeping, and insurance.

The result of current financing arrangements is a relationship between the level of affluence and the level of care received by the elderly. Predictably, the wealthy, who are not constrained either by Medicare's copayment requirements or by the limited scope of services covered by current LTC financing programs, can select programs in which they retain independent living but have ready access to a continuum of health and social care, both at home and in institutional settings. In states with more liberal Medicaid programs, the low-income elderly are also relatively well protected. Medicaid complements Medicare in these states as a source of financing for core health services and finances adequate institutional LTC. Furthermore, public funding is available for home care. However, elderly persons with modest means who cannot afford to pay for extensive LTC, who wish to continue living independently, and who do not qualify for extensive subsidized services are the clients most likely to find heavy complications in their pursuit of health care. (See Feder and Scanlon, Chapter 7, for an analysis of innovative ways to finance LTC.)

Discussion

We are in the midst of a period of great ferment in care of the elderly. The challenges of maintaining the functionally disabled elderly outside of institutions are particularly significant because of the large and growing number of functionally disabled elderly, the strong preference of the elderly to retain their independence, and the complex strategies required to sustain this population.

Over the past two decades, developments in the care of the functionally disabled elderly have been impressive. Much has been learned about the needs of the elderly and many service strategies have been developed. Third-party financing for services has expanded enormously.

At the same time, the field is challenged by many serious problems. High on the list is integrating diverse service components. A chronically ill older person may need several specialized forms of medical care, medications may be prescribed on a continuing basis to manage several distinct health problems, and therapy may be needed to maximize recovery from an illness or injury. Both personal care and housekeeping may be needed, and arrangements may be required to expedite hospital admission and to initiate home care upon discharge. An involved relative may need both respite and professional counseling because of the burdens associated with informal caregiving, and some household modifications may be necessary because of physical impairments. Usually, chronically ill, functionally disabled elderly people lack the ability to integrate such diverse services themselves; often, they may not have a relative or friend to do it for them. Among health professionals, only physicians have the authority to integrate all of the pertinent health strategies. Physicians, however, usually have neither the time nor the interest to attend in depth to social care problems. Case managers, whatever their disciplinary affiliation, rarely have an organizational base that gives them leverage over the full range of both institutional and noninstitutional services.

Another major question is how to balance public and private responsibility. To what extent should relatives be expected to provide LTC at home? To what extent should the elderly and their relatives be expected to finance formal LTC services? Under some circumstances, formal services substitute for informal services; paid workers do what was done previously by relatives or friends. Some policy advocates argue that publicly funded home care should not replace informal caregiving.[30] Others contend that extensive informal caregiving efforts can be unreasonably burdensome;

publicly funded services should be available to prevent an excessive burden on informal caregivers.[4] Since most informal caregivers are women, the issue is partially a women's issue, involving women's right to be relieved of traditional nurturing responsibilities so that they can work outside the home or pursue other activities of their own choosing.

Related is the question of self-payment for LTC. Many elderly people have some funds of their own that could provide partial payment for LTC. As coverage by private pension programs and Social Security improves, more elderly people can afford to live above a subsistence level. Some of the funds available for discretionary spending can be used for LTC. Many elderly people also have substantial equity in their homes. In principle, home equity conversion programs provide the elderly with a way of using the cash value of their homes without selling. A good deal of the reluctance of the elderly to deplete assets to pay for home care stems from the concern about what will happen to them after their assets are gone. Some of the willingness to use private money for institutional care is based on an expectation that when private resources are depleted, public funds will ensure continuing care. Life-care communities also attract the elderly because of their assurances about providing housing and some LTC services within financial parameters established in advance. An important limitation of nearly all publicly and privately financed home-care programs is that they make no commitment to providing fully adequate care for those who have exhausted their self-pay capacity.

Private LTC insurance is part of this picture. In principle, private insurance can cover some of the cost of both institutional and home care, through either individual or group policies. This coverage raises the question of the extent to which people should be expected to anticipate the risk of functional disability many years in advance and to protect themselves from some of the consequences.[31]

Another aspect of the private-financing question is the issue of family responsibility. For couples, the major question is the extent to which their common assets should be depleted to pay for LTC for one spouse. The functionally independent partner has reason to set aside some assets to protect herself or himself from indigence. Intergenerational financial responsibility is even more complicated. Adult children often are more affluent than their functionally disabled parent. Many voluntarily contribute to the costs of LTC. The question is whether they should be obligated to contribute and how much they should be expected to pay. In an earlier period, states regularly held relatives financially responsible for some of the costs of the institutional LTC of the indigent. These requirements gradually declined because of a mix of enforcement difficulties and a political climate favorable to publicly financed services. In the current, more conservative political climate, interest in making adult children take financial

LIBRARY ST. MARY'S COLLEGE

responsibility for the LTC of their parents is being revived. Even those who find the family-responsibility concept attractive must acknowledge that its enforcement is difficult. The problem is particularly great when LTC programs are state administered and responsible adult children live in other states. Of more immediate policy concern are elderly who seek to transfer assets to their relatives in anticipation of Medicaid financing of nursing home care. Recognizing the inevitability of destitution, the elderly characteristically prefer to keep assets in the family as much as possible. Public officials, of course, have reason to discourage the transfer of assets for the purpose of qualifying for public payment for nursing home care.

Another major question is how to allocate public funds for LTC to make a maximal contribution. Critics of current patterns of financing LTC contend that current systems reflect an institutional bias. They maintain that more would be accomplished through proportionately greater expenditures for home care. The argument is that home care is better for many elderly people, and on a per-case basis is often less expensive.

Other critics warn of the inefficiencies arising from an excessively medically oriented financing system. As indicated above, health care is more generously financed than social care, and efforts have been made to justify LTC as part of the health field to qualify it for the more adequate financing available there. However, with health financing comes the need for compliance with health standards. When the link to the health-care sector is artificial, compliance with health standards adds unnecessarily to costs.

The fragmentation of noninstitutional LTC funding also creates problems. Fragmented funding invites the development of small programs with narrow strategies. Therefore, consumers are faced with the need to learn about these discrete programs. Those with multiple needs, in particular, are likely to find it difficult to piece together a set of services that works for them. The use of services is also heavily influenced by service subsidies. More-efficient, unsubsidized services may be bypassed in favor of less-appropriate services for which third-party financing is available.

Funding fragmentation also contributes to a proliferation of job titles, which confuses consumers and frustrates workers. The problem is particularly serious for the in-home workers who are central to noninstitutional LTC. In New York City, for example, depending on the funding source, in-home workers are called home health aides, homemakers, housekeepers, or home attendants. Although the roles these workers play are very similar, the compensation and training requirements for various programs differ. Those who have qualified for more than one program sometimes work under one job title one day and another title the following day. Those who work within a single program framework often find it difficult to get assignments sufficient to give them a full work week. The development of a generic position for in-home workers that would benefit both consumers

LIBRARY ST. MARY'S COLLEGE

and employees is not likely as long as the field continues to depend on multiple funding sources with their own sets of regulations.

Funding is needed that permits a sensible allocation of resources across the range of health and social care strategies needed to sustain a chronically ill, functionally disabled older person. If better use is to be made of the public funds currently being spent, two major problems must be solved: 1) devising a system that both maximizes consumer choice and provides adequate public accountability, and 2) neutralizing the advocacy of those with a vested interest in current funding arrangements.

More adequate sources of financing will continue to be a major priority for home-care advocates. Several federal legislative proposals for major new programs to finance home care for the elderly have been introduced. Even in the 1970s, when federal domestic program initiatives were being considered, none of the home-care proposals attracted serious attention. Both the growth in the need for LTC and the growth of home-care programs have created further pressure for expanded third-party home-care financing. In 1987, for the first time, the late Representative Claude Pepper succeeded in bringing a bill calling for a substantial federal home-care program to the floor of the House of Representatives. Although the bill failed to pass, it signaled the emergence of a growing constituency for a major national publicly funded home-care program. However, in light of the current federal preoccupation with deficit reduction and avoidance of new taxes, substantial expansion of public financing for home care is not likely soon. Currently, private insurance offers greater promise for expanded long-term financing.

If a shift in the political environment makes expanded publicly funded home care a possibility in the future, a well-conceived rationale is advisable. In the 1970s, home-care advocates may have harmed their chances by justifying home care as a less-expensive alternative to institutions. Because good home care attracts clients who resist institutionalization, even "cost-effective" home-care programs add to aggregate public costs. Advocates should also be careful about proposing other rationales that may not stand up to evidence. In a series of federally funded demonstrations in the 1970s and early 1980s, home care did not consistently lead to reduced use of nursing homes or hospitals, improved physical or mental functioning, or reduced mortality.[32] An alternative is to justify publicly funded home care by the need to ensure decent solutions to the problems of daily living of the functionally disabled and to relieve relatives of unreasonable caregiving burdens. Home-care providers may find it difficult enough to meet these modest objectives. Advocates, however, may have to provide a great deal of public education to persuade policymakers that humane care by itself justifies substantial public expenditures.

In shaping proposals for more adequate publicly funded home care, policymakers will have to attend to the boundaries of the domain. LTC financing should not be expected to supplement inadequate public income-security programs or to cover basic housing costs. Eligibility criteria will have to be established that give attention to both the severity of the disability that triggers eligibility and the question of means testing.

The participation of informal caregivers will also need attention. A positive approach that assumes that the most physically proximate, close relatives want to participate in care may prove to be most productive. Publicly funded home care should then be seen as complementary to informal care. Explicit standards, well grounded in public opinion, regarding the caregiving effort expected of relatives will be helpful.

Another area requiring attention is quality standards for publicly funded services. An argument can be made for the universal application of the highest standards of service. However, for some conditions, the cost implications of applying the most sophisticated and expensive medical technology for all who might benefit are staggering. Quality standards for the social aspects of LTC have received less attention. The issues are less dramatic but are important both for the daily living experiences of the functionally disabled elderly and for the aggregate costs of services to the public. Except in the extreme, poor social care is not life threatening. Better social care should enrich life; it should not be expected to extend life. How much enrichment is the public obliged to provide to the functionally disabled elderly? Nursing homes that provide no more than the basics for survival have been harshly criticized. Better nursing homes invest great effort in enriching the lives of residents. Nursing home scandals have led to improved standards of care and more vigorous enforcement. However, the question remains whether the level of funding attached to Medicaid is sufficient to finance social care that meets a reasonable standard of decency.

As publicly funded home care expands and programs emerge with comprehensive care responsibilities, it is important that standards be developed for social aspects of home care. The public should not be expected to provide "ideal" care universally. At the same time, the care provided at public expense should be of better quality than "whatever is possible with the funds that happen to be available."

References

1. Koshel, J., Granger, C. 1978. Rehabilitation terminology: Who is severely disabled? *Rehabil Lit* 13:102–106.

2. Mundlinger, M. 1983. *Home Care Controversy: Too Little, Too Late, Too Costly.* Rockville, Md.: Aspen Systems Corp.

3. Eustis, N., Greenberg, J., Patten, S. 1984. *Long-Term Care for Older Persons: A Policy Perspective.* Monterey, Calif.: Brooks/Cole.

4. Caro, F. 1981. Objectives, standards, and evaluation in long-term care. *Home Health Serv Q* 2:5–26.

5. Ratzka, A. 1986. *Independent Living and Attendant Care in Sweden: A Consumer Perspective.* New York: World Rehabilitation Fund.

6. Baxter, E., Hopper, K. 1981. *Private Lives/Public Spaces: Homeless Adults on the Streets of New York City.* New York: Community Service Society.

7. Baxter, E., Hopper, K. 1984. Shelter and housing for the homeless mentally ill. In *The Homeless Mentally Ill,* ed. H. Lamb. Washington, D.C.: American Psychiatric Association.

8. Doty, P., Liu, K., Wiener, J. 1985. An overview of long-term care. *Health Care Financing Rev* 6(3):69–78.

9. Vladeck, B. 1980. *Unloving Care: The Nursing Home Tragedy.* New York: Basic Books.

10. Bell, W. 1973. Community care of the elderly: An alternative to institutional care. *Gerontologist* 13:345–354.

11. Brody, S., Poulshock, W., Masioccia, C. 1978. The family caring unit: A major consideration in the long-term support system. *Gerontologist* 18:556–561.

12. Frankfather, D., Smith, M., Caro, F. 1981. *Family Care of the Elderly.* Lexington, Mass.: D. C. Heath.

13. Liu, K., Manton, K., Liu, B. 1985. Home health expenditures for the disabled elderly. *Health Care Financing Rev* 7(2):51–58.

14. Caro, F., Blank, A. 1985. *Home Care in New York City: The System, the Providers, the Beneficiaries.* New York: Community Service Society.

15. National Council on Aging and the National Institute for Adult Day Care. 1986. *National Survey of Adult Day Care Centers: Preliminary Findings.* Washington, D.C.: National Council on Aging.

16. Spitz, L., Leader, S. 1983. *A Consumer's Guide to Life-Care Communities.* Washington, D.C.: National Consumers League.

17. United States Senate, Special Committee On Aging. 1983. *Life Care Communities: Promises and Problems.* Washington, D.C.: Government Printing Office.

18. Kutscher, A., Klagsbrun, S., Torpie, R., Debellis, R., Hale, M., Tallmer, M. (eds.) 1983. *Hospice U.S.A.* New York: Columbia University Press.

19. Reisberg, B., Ferris, S. 1982. Diagnosis and assessment of the older patient. *Hosp Community Psychiatry* 33(2):104–110.

20. Harper, M. 1986. Introduction. In *Mental Illness in Nursing Homes: Agenda for Research,* ed. M. Harper and B. Lebowitz. Rockville, Md.: National Institute of Mental Health.

21. Zimmer, J., Watson, N., Treat, A. 1984. Behavioral problems among patients in skilled nursing facilities. *Am J Public Health* 74(10):1118-1121.

22. Kramer, M. 1986. Trends of institutionalization and prevalence of mental disorder in nursing homes. In *Mental Illness in Nursing Homes: Agenda for Research,* ed. M. Harper and B. Lebowitz. Rockville, Md.: National Institute of Mental Health.

23. Cohen, G. 1980. Prospects for mental health and aging. In *Handbook of Mental Health and Aging,* ed. J. Birren and R. Sloan. Englewood Cliffs, N.J.: Prentice Hall.
24. Liptzin, B. 1986. Major mental disorders/problems in nursing homes: Implications for research. In *Mental Illness in Nursing Homes: Agenda for Research,* ed. M. Harper and B. Lebowitz. Rockville, Md.: National Institute of Mental Health.
25. Reifler, B. 1986. Alzheimer's disease in nursing homes: Current practice and implications for research. In *Mental Illness in Nursing Homes: Agenda for Research,* ed. M. Harper and B. Lebowitz. Rockville, Md.: National Institute of Mental Health.
26. Gurian, B. 1982. Mental health outreach and consultation services for the elderly. *Hosp Community Psychiatry* 33(2):142–147.
27. Brody, E. 1986. The role of the family in nursing homes: Implications for research and public policy. In *Mental Illness in Nursing Homes: Agenda for Research,* ed. M. Harper and B. Lebowitz. Rockville, Md.: National Institute of Mental Health.
28. Levit, K., Lazenby, H., Waldo, D., Davidoff, L. 1985. National health care expenditures, 1984. *Health Care Financing Rev* 7(1):1–36.
29. Community Council of Greater New York. 1986. A profile of long-term health care expenditures in New York City. *Res Notes* 62.
30. Greene, V. 1983. Substitution between formally and informally provided care for the impaired elderly in the community. *Med Care* 21:609–619.
31. Lane, L. 1985. The potential of private long-term care insurance. *Pride Inst J* 4:15–24.
32. United States General Accounting Office. 1982. The elderly should benefit from expanded home health care but increasing these services will not insure cost reduction. *Report to the Congress by the Comptroller General.* Washington, D.C.: Government Printing Office.

Four

Hospitals: The DRG System

George L. Maddox and Kenneth G. Manton

Attempts to reformulate the system of geriatric care delivery without appropriate reorganization of the general health-service system are doomed to failure. It is therefore important to consider the reorganization of geriatric care and the general health-care delivery system jointly. Recently, efforts to reshape the general health-care system have included the prospective payment system (PPS). The PPS strategy, promulgated as a general strategy for cost containment in Medicare, was described by Health and Human Services Secretary Heckler as "the most important change in Medicare history."[1]

The central question, however, may be not whether we can reshape the health-care system generally and the geriatric care system specifically, but whether we can achieve consensus about implementing a system of health care that ensures equitable access to care of acceptable quality, provided at a politically bearable cost to all citizens, including older adults. This chapter looks at the constraints on achieving the necessary consensus and at the information required for the implementation of effective policy and then describes the emergence of PPS and of diagnosis-related groups (DRGs).

The Sociocultural Context of Health Care

To understand the present and future of medicine and health care, "one has has to identify the ways in which people act, pursuing their interests and ideals under definite conditions, to bring the structure into existence."[2] Social structures (e.g., the health professions and the organization and delivery of health care) are products of processes in which social groups have chosen from a range of options. In his book on the social transformation of medicine, Starr documented medicine's evolution from a domestic activity into a vast industry successfully controlled by physicians who achieved "cultural authority" to exercise control.[2] He also documented the emergence of medical care as big business, a medical-industrial empire, in which health-care corporations are increasingly visible. Starr attached particular significance to 1) the failure of the United States, in contrast to countries of Western Europe, to develop national health insurance; 2) the dominance of the medical profession, which permitted physicians to control their own affairs, including producing an apparent surplus of physicians; and 3) public policy that stressed the primacy of private-sector responsibility for health care. These outcomes reflect social choices, but not necessarily choices based on reliable information regarding the implications for the provision of health care, especially in relation to access, quality, and cost.

A significant turning point in the restructuring of health care, according to Starr's argument, came in the 1970s as the public lost some of its confidence in the medical profession, faced a possible oversupply of physicians, and became greatly concerned about cost containment. The apparent failure of public regulation increased the probability that "instead of public regulation there [would] be corporate planning."[3] In a chapter titled "The Coming of the Corporation," Starr documented the move of an increasing number of physicians into salaried service, of hospitals into ambulatory care, and of insurance companies into arrangements with preferred providers with a variety of prepayment schemes, and a resurgent interest in for-profit health-care corporations.

The structure of medical practice and health care in the United States is not just *being* transformed, it *has been* transformed. As Ginzberg[4] argued, medical care has been "monetarized" to a significant degree and over a long period. Health care is now widely viewed as an economic product, not just a social good. Starr viewed the development of corporate medicine apprehensively in part because its outcome cannot be predicted confidently. He concluded with hope, "But a trend is not necessarily fate. Images of the future are usually only caricatures of the present. Perhaps this picture of the future of medical care will also prove to be a caricature. Whether it does or not depends on the choices Americans have still to make."[3]

Understanding the constraints placed on future options by past choices is important, and in this regard Anderson's comparative analysis of health care in the United States, Great Britain, and Sweden is particularly useful.[5] Democratic societies, Anderson argued, are concerned about distributing social resources equitably. Specifically, they are concerned about the equitable distribution of good-quality care at a politically bearable price. If, as experience suggests is likely to be the case, we cannot devise a system of care that promises unrestrained access to the highest quality care at a cost we are willing to bear, what trade-offs are we willing to consider?

Anderson argued that a successful health-care system must not only produce the desired outcomes but also operate in congruence with societal values, or, more specifically, the values of those with the power to make decisions. British, Swedish, and American methods of organizing and financing health care are distinctly different, for example, because of historical differences in social values regarding the role of government in the provision and control of health care, the responsibility and autonomy of providers and consumers of care, and the appropriateness of different incentives designed to affect the behavior of providers and consumers. These different values explain why the major conclusion from comparative study of health-care systems is that a variety of organizational and financial systems can work well. However, cross-national comparisons of health-care systems do not imply that the naive transfer of solutions from one society to another is a useful undertaking. A knowledge of the historical foundation of a society's health-care system helps us understand not only why it is as it is but also why a system that is successful in one society cannot be easily transferred to another society.

In a 1971 White Paper, the (then) United States Department of Health, Education and Welfare illustrated this point by outlining the basis for American preferences in organizing and financing health care that constrain current options:

> Given the choice between extending the activities of the Federal Government, and using the focus of the private sector to achieve an objective, the latter [is] preferred. Although "political," the choice can hardly be viewed as "partisan." Preference for action in the private sector is based on the fundamentals of our political economy—capitalistic, pluralistic and competitive—as well as on the desire to strengthen the capabilities of our private institutions to provide health services, to finance such services, and to produce the resources that will be needed in the years ahead.[6]

Thus, this view, stated in 1971 but clearly recognizable today, is that the provision of health care is primarily a private rather than a public responsibility. This view is the basis for accepting a fee-for-service system in which consumers or their intermediaries pay providers of care in a relatively free market. The White Paper's reference to competition is more difficult to interpret, but it suggests that the existing care system constitutes a relatively free market in which providers offer services that consumers choose to purchase. The paper suggested that the problems of the health-care system were organizational, and it recommended a trial of prepayment schemes (health maintenance organizations were used as an illustration) as an experiment in cost containment likely to achieve economical provision of adequate health care.

Anderson also argued that societal values affect not only the organization and financing of health care but also the planning process itself. Governments of societies with a "liberal democratic tradition" (Anderson's description of the United States, Sweden, and Great Britain) rarely make policy shifts in health and welfare programs and, in fact, are not ordinarily committed to integrated, comprehensive public policies. The preferred style of policy formation and implementation is accurately described as "disjointed incrementalism," which the British call "muddling through."[7] It emphasizes small corrections of policy based on feedback from current programs, rather than fundamental redirection of policy.

The checks and balances that are a fundamental part of federal– state– local negotiations constrain the formation, and even more the implementation, of public policy.[8] Furthermore, in the United States the responsibility for planning and the authority for allocating resources are separate. The federal government typically neither plans nor implements health care directly, but attempts to affect indirectly the availability, quality, and cost of the care offered and delivered through a regulatory strategy. In recent decades the government has emphasized fiscal control of reimbursement for services within existing fee-for-service arrangements, with the level of reimbursement established by prevailing local costs. This regulatory strategy, which appears to have had cost containment as its major concern, is judged by some observers[9] to have failed not only because it has not contained costs but also because it lacked the incentives that, on the basis of theory or experience, could have led to cost containment. Exceptions to this generalization are observed in recent federal encouragement of various health-care organizations offering relatively comprehensive care with capped budgets (e.g., prepayment schemes) and the recent emergence of DRGs.

The observed preference for incremental policy formation and planning makes the most recent attempt to promote a PPS as the dominant federal fiscal regulatory strategy particularly interesting. The general strategy of developing a PPS, represented by Medicare reimbursement through the DRG system, appears to violate the notion of disjointed incrementalism. That is, it represents a fundamental change in the mechanism for reimbursing acute medical care. Specifically, the particular institutions providing care are put at risk for the cost of care for each patient. The DRG system focuses directly on incentives to institutional managers and not on the physician providing care. Individual institutions must practice fiscal discipline without specific directives regulating costs for specific care situations. Thus the system is part of the general political consensus that prefers to regulate health-care costs without involving the government directly in the development of policies for specific care situations. Although this policy masterfully achieves political consensus in the short term, its eventual success will be determined by the technical ability to calibrate the reimbursement structure to the actual level of need for health care and by the provision of incentives to maintain appropriate access to quality care. The current DRG system anticipates real differences in individual need for health care and adjusts reimbursement to take into consideration case mix in the different DRG categories. For the DRG case-mix adjustment to function properly, several technical issues must be resolved. For health-care institutions to manage fiscal risk successfully, for example, the case-mix system must balance the pressure to increase the number of DRG categories (i.e., to increase their specificity) and the need to reduce the number of categories, to ensure more stable mean costs. A second technical problem involves developing procedures to assess the cost implications of accepting patients from populations in which the distribution of risks for being in one or another DRG category is unknown or poorly understood. This second problem is particularly relevant to geriatric care.

Typically, hospitals and similar health-care firms have not employed physicians and are not in a position to control prospectively the demand for services generated by physicians' orders on behalf of patients. By placing health-care firms at risk, a potential conflict of interest is produced between physicians and managers of health-care firms subject to DRG control. The proposed extension of the PPS to include physician reimbursement has implications for ameliorating or exacerbating conflict between physicians and health-care firms that remain to be explored. [10] Since hospitals, not physicians, currently are placed at economic risk, one might expect them to consider the employment of physicians as one way to merge the responsibility for planning and the authority for allocating resources. In this sense, a federal DRG strategy appears to accelerate the industrialization of health care as an economic product and to enhance the role of corporations in the provision of care.

Anderson's analysis of the problems of achieving equity in health care in liberal democratic societies stressed three concerns: cost, access, and quality. Federal interest in health-care policy in the United States, however, has increasingly focused on the first of these concerns, cost. The current DRG strategy has clearer implications for cost of health care as an economic product than for social concerns about access to and quality of care, particularly for older adults. A firm that knows for certain that a given DRG classification generates a predictable prospective payment and that also knows the imprecision of DRG classification has an incentive to select in advance, if it can, individuals likely to be in the least problematic DRG classifications. Since acute illness is more easily classified than chronic illness, and since the probability of chronic illness (in fact, multiple chronic illnesses) increases with age, it is difficult to imagine that health-care firms would prefer older patients.

The implications of the PPS for quality of care are more difficult to gauge. It can be assumed that the average health-care firm is committed to offering quality health care. In the absence of any consensus on standard "quality" geriatric health care, a DRG-type strategy will probably generate a variety of responses in the care offered. Only extensive research will sort out the actual long-term effects of this reimbursement policy on the quality of geriatric care. Certainly, using a case-mix strategy to determine reimbursement will require health-care firms to trade off among cost, access, and quality of care. Furthermore, without clear specification of the kinds of care particular professionals offer best in particular settings (inpatient, outpatient, community), firms have a new incentive to explore and experiment with how vertical integration of different components of care might control or reduce the cost of care.

Shifting responsibility to the private sector for ensuring that health-care firms consider the social as well as the economic good when they make trade-offs among cost, access, and quality may be beneficial. This shift is certainly consistent with our society's stated preference for placing responsibility for these decisions in the private sector. For health-care firms competing in an open market, however, the obligation to consider public welfare and training is ambiguous.

Anderson, in sum, was pessimistic about the ability of any society, particularly a society in the liberal democratic tradition, to plan and implement an optimal system of health care. At best, societies are in continual pursuit of a dream in which cost, access, and quality objectives can all be achieved. Pursuit of this dream is continual because the provision of health care involves as much art as science and because decisions about trade-offs among cost, access, and quality are often more political than scientific. The DRG strategy, we argue below, illustrates this point. The hope persists, however, that a rational, politically feasible solution for the problems of providing adequate health care can be found.

How DRGs Work

The current federal emphasis on DRGs as a strategy in national health-care policy is a particularly good illustration of limits of rationality in planning.

By focusing on fiscal control, this strategy does not directly attack the dominant fee-for-service procedure and does not tamper directly with freedom of choice in health care for providers or consumers. This strategy, examined in terms of the technical capacity to categorize patients, particularly geriatric patients, by their service needs illustrates well the limits of rationality in planning and implementing health care for older adults.

The Logic of Disease Classification

A basic requirement of the DRG strategy is the categorization of disease, that is, the generation of nosologic systems for diseases, including chronic degenerative diseases. Perhaps the most widely used disease classification system, and the system from which DRG classification is derived logically, is the World Health Organization's International Classification of Diseases (ICD), currently in its ninth revision. The ICD system employs a "linear" or unidimensional approach to the classification problem. That is, it tries to produce a unique classification for every disease. For acute disease processes, this classification often works reasonably well. However, for chronic degenerative diseases, especially among elderly persons, whose expression of disease is complex and who have a high prevalence of multiple chronic diseases, the linear approach to classification appears to work less well.

For example, ICD-9 involves approximately 10,000 different disease categories. Yet even with this number of categories, the ICD cannot adequately represent certain aspects of chronic disease, such as histologic type for neoplastic disease or the bacterial or viral agent in infectious diseases. Consequently, the ICD has developed a separate disease nomenclature for neoplastic disease (i.e., the ICD-0) and certain linked codes to represent the joint occurrence of disease. The proliferation of disease categories notwithstanding, many disease patterns still cannot be described simply. Furthermore, the available detail on disease progression, the ability to describe the joint occurrence of chronic diseases, and the ability to describe individual differences in disease expression are limited within the current ICD classification system.

The limitations of such a linear classification system should not be surprising given what we know about chronic disease processes. Indeed, the problems in developing such a system can be demonstrated empirically. Strauss et al.[11] studied the use of multivariate classification procedures to identify groups of chronically ill patients by discrete diagnostic categories. In their first assessment they took "textbook" descriptions of cases and submitted them to an analytic procedure that could relate cases to the variables on which they were grouped. For these synthetic data sets they found reasonable correspondence between empirical clusters of cases and the profile of symptoms associated with the diagnoses made for those clusters. When, however, they applied similar procedures to actual patient populations from two psychiatric clinics, the results were not as good; actual cases did not cluster well with respect to the symptoms defining specific diagnoses. Strauss et al. concluded that the logic of the diagnostic classification of symptoms poorly approximated the actual complexity of the profile of symptoms that real patients present. They called for development of analytic tools that can represent the actual heterogeneity of individuals within any given classification system.

The difficulties in applying discrete or "crisp" models of disease categories have been recognized in other scientific disciplines where complex phenomena must be evaluated and typed. These difficulties have led to the development of new concepts for the categorization of system attributes called *fuzzy set* theory.[12] The *fuzzy set* theory acknowledges that there are true differences between systems in which individuals can be located, so any given individual is never exactly within a given category. Instead, clusters have "fuzzy" boundaries that operate by measuring "how much" a given individual is in any particular category. The principles of *fuzzy set* theory are logically distinct from those in classical probability theory. For example, in probability theory one can determine the likelihood that a person is in a given group by using, say, discriminant analysis. In *fuzzy set* theory, one does not determine the probability that a patient is within a given group but determines the actual degree of membership of that case in one or more possible groups. The degree of membership is thus *not* a probability but an actual attribute of the individual. The primary distinction between *crisp* versus *fuzzy* clustering methods in describing cases is that, in crisp clustering methods, a person's not having all of the characteristics of a given group (or diagnosis) is attributed to the existence of random factors, whereas in fuzzy clustering the lack of correspondence is due to true individual differences. Thus the *crisp* versus *fuzzy* categorization of disease leads to very different views of the world. In a crisp, probabilistic world, rationality can ultimately appear to triumph because individual differences are assumed to be random. In a fuzzy world, rationality in classification must be limited because true individual differences exist and no simple procedure for categorization can fully capture them.

Dealing with Complex Classification

An alternate approach to dealing with the observed complexity of the world is to employ a hierarchy, rather than a linear logic, in developing disease classifications. Since linear logic fails in describing disease manifestation because categories must be endlessly generated to describe the complexity of disease expression, the Standardized Nomenclature of Pathology (SNOP) offers an alternate strategy. SNOP does not simply generate more categories on a single dimension, but uses a limited number of dimensions to generate a multidimensional description of disease. In particular, four dimensions (i.e., morphology, function, etiology, topography) are used to describe disease expression, with a disease (or disorder) actually being described in terms of a multidimensional "syntax." A similar type of multidimensional characterization is employed in the DSM-III system (American Psychiatric Association) for describing psychiatric disorders, where up to five dimensions can be employed to describe individual variation within a specific diagnosis. In a classification system, a hierarchy is generally more effective than a simple linear approach because it permits the description of a large number of diseases using a very small number of categories and a limited number of dimensions.

Practically, the ability of disease classifications to describe the actual manifestation of disease in procedures such as those employed in a DRG strategy is necessarily limited by the complexity of the real world. These problems are probably most serious for the geriatric and long-term care (LTC) populations. First, elderly populations have a high prevalence of multiple chronic diseases that may occur jointly with other diseases and interact in different ways. Thus the problem of categorizing older patients into "crisp" disease categories is greatly increased in complexity. Second, in a LTC population, diseases evolve in various nonacute stages in a very long-term process. Thus, an older person may not simply have a disease, but may illustrate a disease *process* that has developed to some identifiable degree. Third, the rate of explicit physiological change can be expected to accelerate at advanced ages. This accelerated aging can be expected to affect how a disease is expressed, including its rate of progression. Finally, several factors external to the disease process, such as an individual's economic and social resources and environment, will influence how the disease process affects individual functioning.[13]

Implications of Problems in Disease Classification for Describing Case Mix

The current system of health-care reimbursement based on diagnostic and service categories (i.e., DRGs) is affected by the limits to rationality in developing the nosologic systems just discussed.

The basic logic of the DRG system is that the type of diagnosed disease determines the reimbursable costs for care of a patient, with the reimbursable limits for a particular DRG category adjusted for regional wage differentials and for urban/rural differences. The performance of the DRG system is therefore linked to its ability to represent the real variation of costs among patients by the set of DRGs constructed.

Currently the 473 clinically meaningful DRG categories represent four dimensions of diagnosis, such as service type (e.g., renal transplant), age (e.g., above or below age 70), and the presence or absence of an auxiliary diagnosis. Since these dimensions are only partially represented in each of the 473 DRGs (e.g., not all diagnoses are divided on an age criterion), the logic of the DRG is actually linear, not hierarchical (i.e., the DRGs are not based on cross-classifications of the dimensions). The 473 DRGs were selected to be clinically meaningful and to explain as much of the variation in hospital costs as possible. The ability of the DRGs to explain the variation of patient costs was initially assessed empirically using the "autogroup" program, a modification of the Automatic Interaction Detection program developed by Sonquist and Morgan at the University of Michigan. The primary data used to construct the DRGs were the Medpar data, which are abstracts of administrative records on acute-care services reimbursed by Medicare.

Implementation of the DRG strategy has already raised several questions about its adequacy and the need for modification. First, will DRGs be able to reflect differences in costs due to the severity of disease? Second, should reimbursements be adjusted to reflect differences in the types of services delivered by different types of hospitals to patients with similar diagnoses? An attempt has been made to adjust for some of this difference by providing a cost adjustment for teaching hospitals. Third, will economic incentives in the DRG strategy encourage hospitals to adopt patterns of behavior that maximize fiscal return, to the detriment of the quality of care delivered? For example, hospitals may compete for patients with "profitable" diagnoses and avoid patients with less-profitable diagnoses. There may be fiscal pressure to discharge chronic patients prematurely. Fourth, will DRG reimbursement adversely affect health facilities other than hospitals? For example, the system may provide strong incentives for discharging terminal and chronic care patients to hospice programs and skilled nursing facilities in greater numbers than the current level of facilities and services can handle. Finally, if the logic of DRGs is extended to reimbursement under Medicaid, to physician reimbursement, to reimbursement by private insurers, and, possibly, to reimbursement of LTC facilities, the need to modify the strategy to cope with the questions just listed will become even more pressing.

The DRG strategy has implications that extend far beyond the problems of current reimbursement for health care to questions about clinical research, adoption of new medical technology, capital expenditures, and provision of various types of specialized care. Specifically, an activity like clinical research is often indirectly supported by the clinical base of a teaching hospital. The DRG strategy raises questions about the actual institutional costs of clinical research, the amount of clinical research that should be maintained, and how this research will be supported in the future. Similarly, the current DRG strategy also does not directly allow for the financing of new medical technology. Consequently, the DRG system will make increasingly explicit a range of decisions that must be made about the level of medical innovation that is desirable and how that innovation should be financed.

Increased Risk for Hospitals

Currently, the lack of carefully evaluated experience with DRGs prevents us from predicting confidently which of these or other problems will be manifest and to what degree. Only as the DRG system is fully implemented will the need for modification become clear. However, the basic logic of the strategy can be assessed in terms of concerns about the limits of rationality in the use of a linear, discrete disease classification system to describe accurately the health state of elderly chronically ill patients. The DRG system will be subject to two opposing pressures. The first is the necessity to increase the number of classifications to describe prospectively the costs of the individual patient. This problem is already manifest in proposals to adjust the DRG system to represent disease severity explicitly. The second is the nature of the DRG as a device for determining the level of risk in the reimbursement system. Since the DRG system determines the level of reimbursement prospectively, hospitals will be at risk for costs beyond that level. As the number of DRGs increases, the number of cases that can be expected within a DRG category decreases, so that the average cost per patient within a DRG becomes less stable. This clearly puts hospitals at increased risk. One possible response by the hospital is to transfer the risk to the individual patient, through a policy of selective admission and discharge. Other possibilities involve risk pooling, through "reserve" loading schemes, insurance, or the creation of large hospital corporations.

An additional element of risk within the DRG system is the dynamic operation of probability in the classical form of the "gambler's ruin" problem. Specifically, the longer one plays a game of chance, the larger the numbers of consecutive wins (or losses) that can be expected to emerge by chance. If a gambler plays long enough, then the probability of going broke approaches one. Similarly, assuming that the cost reimbursement for a DRG is exactly right (i.e., equal to the true average costs), in any group of hospitals one can expect some to emerge as winners and some to emerge as losers. The degree to which hospitals become winners or losers is a function of the variability of costs over patients. Table 4.1 presents a simplified, three-category DRG system, with the average cost, the standard deviations of cost, and the case-mix proportions for each category specified. If we imagine a group of 100 hospitals responding to patients in these three categories, then the maximum gains and losses associated with different numbers of randomly selected patients can be estimated (Table 4.2).

In Table 4.2 a simulation illustrates how the average earnings for the 100

Table 4.1.   A Hypothetical Three-DRG System[a]

DRG Categories	Mean Cost ($)	S.D. ($)	Case Mix (%)
DRG 257: Surgical—Total mastectomy for malignancy, age > 69 and/or DX2	3700	1500	50
DRG 172: Medical—Digestive malignancy, age > 69 and/or DX 2	3200	2600	33
DRG 7: Surgical—Peripheral and cranial nerve and other nervous system procedures, age > 69 and/or DX2	7500	3970	17

[a]Approximate mean cost, standard deviation, and case mix for group costs paralleling the 1981 Maryland hospital discharges for individuals age 65 and over.

Table 4.2.   Simulated Net "Winnings" of 100 Hospitals with Discharges from the Three DRGs Given in Table 4.1

Discharges (N)	Average "Winnings" ($)	S.D. ($)	Maximum Winnings ($)	Minimum Winnings ($)
25	540	12,411	23,385	−30,060
50	99	17,625	35,490	−49,695
75	1500	21,105	45,345	−51,675
100	1134	24,105	48,525	−88,965

hospitals varies moderately, ranging from a $540 gain with 25 discharges per hospital to a $1134 gain with 100 discharges per hospital (i.e., 50 discharges with DRG 257; 33 discharges with DRG 172; 17 discharges with DRG 7). The standard deviation of costs, however, increases from $12,411 to $24,105. The hospital with the maximum profit earns $23,385 with only 25 discharges and $48,525 with 100 discharges. The hospital with the maximum loss loses $30,060 with 25 discharges and $88,965 with 100 discharges. A comparable analysis of the implications of applying a DRG strategy to physicians' charges reaches a similar conclusion regarding the probability of winners and losers.[10]

The variability of costs shows that, even if the average DRG cost can be estimated accurately, there will be a risk of financial loss for some hospitals due to the probabilistic nature of the DRGs represented by the mix of patients in any given institution. Such loss is not necessarily a result of inefficient management; despite managerial efforts to rationalize actions, a DRG system includes a substantial risk of ruin by chance—a risk that can only be managed by transferring it to the individual patient or by pooling risk among institutions.

In addition to the questions about using diagnosis-based reimbursement, there are important substantive questions about the structure of the diagnostic categories that should be used in this system, especially in describing chronic morbidity for patients at advanced ages. First, an elderly patient frequently will be affected by multiple chronic conditions. The current DRG system can indicate only the simple presence or absence of auxiliary diagnoses. Second, age itself is an important indicator of the medical status of a patient. In the existing system, the dichotomous categorization of age above or below 70 years seems unlikely to represent adequately the variation revealed in longitudinal studies of aging. Finally, chronic diseases are processes. The current World Health Organization study of classification of impairments, disabilities, and handicaps recognizes the progression of the disease process itself and the correlated disability process.[14] A linear classification that inadequately represents the effects of progressive disease severity and related disability is unlikely to represent these other dimensions satisfactorily.

Prospective reimbursement could be a useful strategy for geriatric and long-term care if it employed a hierarchical, multidimensional logic in classifying disease, and a *fuzzy set* classification strategy to describe individual patients. Individuals would be described on multiple, continuous dimensions and would not be placed exclusively into single categories. With reimbursement for the individual patient based on a mixture of reimbursement factors for each dimension, a unique reimbursement level for each individual could be generated.

Future Changes in Health Care for the Elderly

While the historical and sociocultural analyses undertaken by Starr and Anderson would not necessarily predict specifically the PPS as the strategy of choice in the United States, the choice is certainly not surprising. The PPS, in the form of DRG, is consistent with the preference for fiscal control seen in federal health-care policy, particularly since 1980. The strong current emphasis on health care as an economic product is distinctive and warrants careful consideration. The emphasis is not new, since the PPS reinforces a long-term trend toward the "monetarization" of health care in the United States,[4] but lack of emphasis on health care as a social good is new in U.S. health-care policy.

The DRG strategy also illustrates and reinforces a long-standing preference for locating primary responsibility for organizing health care in the private sector. When the 1971 White Paper on health care was published, the major problems identified were organizational; the American health-care system was described as using relatively adequate available fiscal, personnel, and organizational resources inefficiently.[6] However, recommendations for reorganization were minimal, going little beyond favorable references to the idea of HMOs. A system of national health insurance was explicitly ruled out as politically unfeasible, a judgment confirmed by experience over the past four decades. During the 1970s, federal policy concentrated on constraining organizations through regulation while leaving the basic organization of health care and the economic incentives for providers unchanged. The DRG strategy is a major innovation that reshapes the economic incentives for providing health care and awaits the response of health-care organizations in the private sector.

One likely effect of this strategy is already evident—the reinforcement of the trend in the past decade toward corporate medicine. The capacity of large health-care corporations to integrate the fragments of a relatively uncoordinated system and to provide the fiscal security of pooled risks appears to be a safer, if not a safe, haven. Starr's characterization of the current situation is accurate: "Doctors are integrating 'backwards' into institutional service; hospitals are integrating 'forward' into ambulatory care; insurance companies are adopting new arrangements with 'preferred providers' to create hybrid prepayment plans."[15] Academic medical centers are exploring affiliation agreements, regional nonprofit multihospital systems are emerging, national for-profit hospital chains and diversified health-care conglomerates are thriving, and HMOs, independently and in chains, for profit and not for profit, are proliferating.

The eventual form that the health-care system will adopt under these conditions cannot be predicted. Current federal policy is designed to allow private-sector responses to run their course. In the current organizational scramble, it is also impossible to predict with certainty how older persons in particular will fare. There is, however, realistic concern based upon the technical difficulties in accurately calibrating a case-mix system for geriatric and long-term care. Specifically, the primary incentive to maintain quality of care in the current system is that the DRG categories, being based upon diagnoses, will ensure that reimbursement levels for each category of care will be budget-neutral, in the sense that, in an appropriately calibrated system, there should be no fiscal disincentives to meeting the medical needs of the population. Unfortunately, under the best of circumstances, calibrating DRGs for acute care is a difficult technical task. The calibration problem is even more complex for elderly persons because of the known age-related risk of multiple disease processes, the interaction of multiple chronic diseases, and the psychosocial processes that affect functional capacity in later life. In the face of this increased age-related complexity, it would appear that the risk to the provider in managing elderly patients would be increased. Indeed, the fact that geriatric medicine is in its early stages of development suggests that the current status of clinical science in geriatrics is not adequate to guide the calibration of DRGs to deal with the geriatric patient. It is difficult to imagine, therefore, that the older patient would be a preferred patient unless and until DRG-based reimbursement can be adapted to factor in age-related risks satisfactorily. In the meantime, the most likely source of adequate geriatric health care will probably be very large firms capable of pooling very large risk groups. Certainly in the short run, this is likely to mean that geriatric health care will be a function of the geographic availability of and access to large health-care organizations. Current federal policy appears to be willing to accept some level of risk that geriatric care might be unavailable to some older patients.

What can one say about the evolution of the U.S. health-care system—especially in terms of its ability to provide high-quality medical care to the elderly? First, any system that views health care primarily as an economic good has intrinsic difficulties. Under the previous fee-for-service system, the demand for service was frequently determined by the health-care suppliers and not always by the consumer, whose information and rationality about a complex good like medical care are limited. This problem is even more apparent for the higher per capita consumers of medical care, that is, the frail elderly, and it extends to proposals for national health insurance[16] and to the provision of comprehensive services in prepayment plans, such as HMOs. Given its emphasis on fiscal control, the DRG system modifies the emphasis on health care as an economic good by fixing the reimbursement level for specified units of care. Thus the efforts of the provider are focused upon improving efficiency in the delivery of units of care and in reducing adverse complications of care. Naturally, the premise of any system of reimbursement can be violated by providers who attempt to "game" the system by selectively choosing patients with "profitable" diagnoses and avoiding contact with the most seriously ill. Constant monitoring of the performance of providers under the DRG system is warranted to minimize such "gaming."

What is more difficult in the logic of the PPS as a strategy for ensuring adequate geriatric care is to develop an adequate reimbursement strategy for LTC. Units of care in LTC settings and related appropriate cost structures cannot be defined on the basis of current experience. Consequently, an experience-based system will probably have to give way to a normatively based system. That is, given the fact that we do not have an integrated and well-defined system for providing LTC services to the elderly, we do not currently have data with which to calibrate an adequate case-mix reimbursement system. Thus the development of a PPS for LTC services will require more and extensive research to assess the implications of federal health-care policy for very impaired elderly patients. It also appears that the provision of LTC services is more complex than acute care. The longer time over which LTC services are delivered, age-related functional incapacity, and the availability of informal and community support services (marital status, family structure, housing, personal resources) help determine the need for a subset of LTC services. Reimbursing LTC services obviously requires an alternate case-mix calibration strategy involving the cautious "blending" of reimbursement levels.

In sum, in the United States, health care in general and geriatric care in particular are being fundamentally changed by a federal policy that currently focuses primarily on care as an economic product. How geriatric and long-term care will fare remain to be determined, but past preferences and choices have shaped the current health-care system and severely constrain the available options for this decade.

References

1. Inglehart, J. K. 1983. Medicare begins prospective payment of hospitals. *N Engl J Med* 308(23):1428–1432.
2. Starr, P. 1982. *The Social Transformation of American Medicine.* New York: Basic Books.
3. See Ref. 2, p. 449.
4. Ginzberg, E. 1984. The monetarization of medical care. *N Engl J Med* 310(18):1162–1165.
5. Anderson, O. W. 1972. *Health Care: Can There Be Equity?* New York: John Wiley and Sons.
6. United States Department of Health, Education, and Welfare. 1971. *Towards a Comprehensive Health Care Policy for the 1970's: A White Paper.* Washington, D.C.: Government Printing Office.
7. Maddox, G. L. 1971. Muddling through: Planning health care in England. *Med Care* 9(4):439–448.
8. Pressman, J. L., Wildavsky, A. W. 1973. *Implementation.* Berkeley, Calif.: University of California Press.
9. Havighurst, C. C. 1982. *Deregulating the Health Care Industry.* Cambridge, Mass.: Ballinger.
10. Mitchell, J. B. 1985. Physician DRGs. *N Engl J Med* 313(11):670–675.
11. Strauss, J. S., Gabriel, K. R., Kokes, R. I., Ritzler, B. A., Van Ord, A., Tarana, E. 1979. Do psychiatric patients fit their diagnoses? Patterns of symptomatology as described with the biplot. *J Nerv Ment Dis* 167:105–112.
12. Clive, J., Woodbury, M. A., Siegler, I. C. 1983. Fuzzy and crisp set theoretical-based classifications of health and disease. *J Med Syst* 7:317–332. [See also Woodbury, M. A., Manton, K. G. 1982. A new procedure for analysis of medical classification. *Comput Biomed Res* 11:210–220.]
13. Luce, B. R., Liu, K., Manton, K. G. 1984. Estimating the long term care population and its use of services. *Long Term Care and Social Security.* ISSA Studies in Research, No. 21. Geneva: International Social Security Association. [For a general review of issues and evidence regarding the operation and

outcomes of the DRG strategy, see Worthman, L. G., Cretin, S. 1986. *Review of the Literature on Diagnosis Related Groups*. Santa Monica, Calif.: Rand Corporation.]

14. World Health Organization. 1980. *International Classification of Impairments, Disabilities, and Handicaps: A Manual of Classification Relating to the Consequences of Disease*. Geneva: World Health Organization.

15. See Ref. 2, p. 440.

16. Enthoven, A. C. 1980. *Health Plan*. Reading, Mass.: Addison Wesley.

Five

Keeping Medicare Financially Viable

Linda H. Aiken

Medicare faces bankruptcy by the late 1990s or just after the turn of the century unless program expenditures are reduced or revenues are increased.[1] The total Medicare reimbursement per enrollee increased at an annual rate of 13.6% from 1975 through 1985, more than twice the rate of economy-wide inflation.[2] Until 1982, when the Advisory Council on Social Security was charged to concentrate its review and recommendations on Medicare, little attention was paid to Medicare's looming problems. The council's report, sent to Congress in March 1984, formally began what promises to be a lengthy and heated national debate about the future of Medicare.[3]

Round 1 of the Medicare debate[4] provides a sense of what the important issues will be as Congress considers how to resolve Medicare's financial crisis. This chapter examines the recommendations of the Advisory Council on Social Security, which were influential in shaping the Medicare Catastrophic Coverage Act of 1988, and the diversity of views that emerged on each of the major options considered. This first formal round in the Medicare debate confirms that major groups in America are currently very far apart on the fundamental issues that must frame a strategy to preserve the beneficial features of Medicare.

The Problem

Part A and Part B of Medicare are financed through separate trust funds with distinct sources of revenue. Part A, the Hospital Insurance Trust Fund, is a pay-as-you-go system, financed by a payroll tax on 127 million workers and their employers for medical care for about 28 million people over 65 and 3 million disabled people under 65. In 1986, outlays for this part of Medicare were $44 billion. Under current law, general revenues cannot be used to make up any shortfall in the trust fund.

Since 1967, the per capita cost of Medicare hospital benefits has increased by 178%, but the wages of covered workers increased by only 12%.[5] Moreover, the ratio of taxpayers to beneficiaries dropped from 4:1 in 1965 to 3.3:1 in 1980, and it is expected to fall to 2.7:1 by 2015. Over the 1985 through 1995 period, Part A expenditures are projected to grow at an annual rate of 12.4% but revenues from currently scheduled payroll taxes are expected to increase by only 7.9%.[6]

Medicare outlays must be reduced by 13%, or revenues increased by 15%, or some combination of the two, to bring the Hospital Insurance Trust Fund into actuarial balance over the next 25 years.[1] To achieve this balance, the government has four available options: it can slow the rate of growth in reimbursement to hospitals and physicians, advance the age of eligibility, increase beneficiary cost sharing, or increase revenues.

Part B, the Supplementary Medical Insurance Trust Fund, is financed by monthly premiums and general revenues, with approximately 78% of costs financed through general revenues. Part B, at $27 billion, is the third largest federal domestic program, exceeded only by Social Security retirement and Medicare hospital insurance. Moreover, it is the fastest growing major domestic program, with outlays doubling every five to six years.[7] The major concern about Part B expenditures is the effect of the program on the record-high federal deficit.[8]

Moderating Increases in Provider Reimbursement

Hospitals

A central problem underlying Medicare's financial crisis is the rapid rise in hospital costs. Since 1967, hospital room rates have increased by more than 450%, nearly two and one-half times the rate of increase in the Consumer Price Index.

From its inception, Medicare reimbursed hospitals for the "reasonable costs" of caring for beneficiaries on a retrospective basis, but beginning in 1982, Congress enacted significant changes in hospital reimbursement policy to contain the rapid increases in Medicare's hospital costs. The Tax

Equity and Fiscal Responsibility Act of 1982 placed limits on the annual growth allowable in cost per hospital case. Then, the Social Security Amendments of 1983 adopted a more fundamental change in Medicare hospital payment policy by shifting from retrospective cost-based reimbursement to a system that sets prices in advance for each of 473 diagnosis-related groups (DRGs). (A detailed discussion of DRGs is presented in Maddox and Manton, Chapter 4.)

Now that the PPS (prospective payment system) is being implemented, a substantial portion of Medicare's financial problems could be solved by limiting the annual increase in payment per hospital admission to a rate that is more closely tied to the growth of inflation or the wages that determine the Program's income. Beneficiary groups strongly favor this approach. However, there are two very different points of view on the possible consequences of limiting hospital reimbursement. On the one hand are the proponents of more stringent payment limits, who argue that hospitals are inefficient and wasteful, and that improved productivity would result in ample resources to deliver high-quality care within current budgets. In support of this argument is evidence that many hospitals are faring well from a fiscal perspective, despite various cost-containment efforts. Hospitals experienced a growth in net revenue margins from 3.6% in 1981 to 6.2% in 1984.[9]

Others are not convinced that significant savings can be achieved without impairing beneficiaries' access to mainstream medicine or lowering the quality of care in American hospitals, now believed to be the best in the world. Concern about access derives from fears that once hospitals determine which diagnostic categories are less remunerative, they will discourage admissions of these types, making it difficult for the elderly to obtain needed care.

Prime targets for decreasing expenses are likely to be reductions in the number of employees or wage freezes, since the largest component of hospital costs is labor. Hospitals nationally employ 4.3 million people and are major employers in many communities. Efforts to reduce the work force or to freeze wages could be met with increased unionization, disruptive strikes, and increased unemployment in communities already hard hit by the economic recession. Cyclical shortages of hospital nurses have been linked to efforts to artificially restrain wage growth.[10]

Alternatively, if a large percentage of their limited resources is invested in labor, hospitals' buildings and equipment could deteriorate. Recent reductions in inpatient days have resulted in low occupancy rates for many hospitals and increased competition for a more limited number of patients. Many hospitals fear they will lose their competitive edge in the market unless they acquire the latest technology and maintain the physical plant. The 1983 prospective reimbursement legislation temporarily passed through capital costs, so this problem has not come to the fore yet. Eventually, however, it is anticipated that capital expenditures will be limited, and then hospitals will be forced to decide how to allocate limited resources between labor and capital acquisitions and renovations.

Experience in states with hospital rate control, although mixed on these issues thus far, suggests the consequences of limiting hospital reimbursement. Although rate-regulated states have succeeded in holding the annual rate of increase in hospital expenditures below the national average,[11] it is not yet clear how hospitals actually achieved those savings. Research undertaken in Maryland, which has one of the oldest hospital rate-regulation programs, suggests that nurses' salaries have not been adversely affected.[12] However, a study of all states with hospital rate regulation concluded that payment restrictions do tend to reduce wages, particularly at the bottom of the wage scale, and recent national data suggests that Medicare's PPS has had a dampening effect on nurses' wages.[13] New York's cost-containment program suggests the possibility that limited capital expenditures have resulted in deteriorating plants that now require major renovation to maintain the quality of care and to attract patients in a more competitive environment.

The extent to which hospital reimbursement can be limited without impairing quality and access or resulting in disruptive labor strikes will be a focus of continuing debate. Although the Advisory Council was troubled by the lack of information on the long-term effect of limiting reimbursement to hospitals, the absence of acceptable alternatives for financing Medicare led to a recommendation that the annual rate of increase in prices be limited to changes in the Hospital Input Price Index. This index is a measure of hospitals' costs of doing business, and includes six broad expense categories: payroll, employee benefits, professional services, depreciation, interest, and all others. In most years, the Hospital Input Price Index has increased more rapidly than the Consumer Price Index (CPI). In 1983, the Hospital Input Price Index increased by 6.9%, compared to the general inflation rate of 3.8%.

Under the prospective reimbursement legislation passed in 1983, the Secretary of Health and Human Services had the power to set the allowable annual increase in hospital payments per admission. The Trustees, in projecting future expenditures in 1983, assumed that the rate of increase would be set at the increase in the Hospital Input Price Index plus 1% to allow for the introduction of new technology and improvements in quality. Although the Advisory Council strongly supported the efficacious use of medical technology, they were concerned that technology and quality improvements should not always increase costs. The 1% allowance involved a considerable sum in actual dollars. If, as was recommended by the Advisory Council, beginning in 1988, hospital payment rates are limited to changes in the growth rate of costs faced by hospitals (Hospital Input Price Index), not allowing the extra percentage point, the savings through 1995 would be approximately $34.5 billion.

The Council also considered, but did not act on, a proposal to encourage states to set limits on all hospital rates. Strong views favoring and opposing state rate setting vary from preferences for free-market competitive approaches to strong regulatory solutions. Those in favor of hospital rate regulation fear that, under the current system, Medicare payments could diverge so much from hospital payments for privately insured patients that Medicare beneficiaries' access to mainstream hospital care would be impaired. Moreover, unabated increases in national hospital costs are likely to exert an upward pressure on the prices Medicare will have to pay.

However, in rate-regulated states, Medicare costs could be higher, depending upon the actual plan adopted, than the preferred rates the government can negotiate. For example, New Jersey's all-payer system, which served as the prototype for Medicare's DRGs, may lose its special Medicare waiver because the federal government believes Medicare costs are higher than they would be under the national prospective pricing system. The New Jersey plan includes, among other provisions, a special pool to finance hospital care for the uninsured poor to which Medicare and all other payers must contribute. While the federal role in hospital rate setting will continue to be debated, an increasing number of states, facing their own budget constraints and pressures from business coalitions, are moving toward some form of hospital rate control.

Medical Education

Considerable controversy emerged during Council deliberations on the appropriate role for Medicare in medical education. Currently, Medicare reimburses hospitals for a share of the costs of training residents and to a lesser extent nurses and other health-care personnel, and provides an adjusted payment for teaching hospitals to cover indirect education expenses. In 1983, medical education costs reimbursed by Medicare's hospital insurance program amounted to $1.8 billion.

In 1983, Congress exempted medical education costs from inclusion within DRG rates and doubled the allowance for indirect medical education costs. In essence, Congress accepted evidence that teaching hospitals differed from community hospitals in terms of the severity of illness of their patients, the intensity of care required, and their greater consumption of resources. The actual costs of caring for patients in teaching hospitals were thought to exceed the average cost for patients in the same diagnostic categories in community hospitals.[14] It was presumed that teaching hospitals would not be able to recover their true costs under an unadjusted national prospective payment system, and their long-term financial stability would be threatened. Because it was difficult to assess directly the differential costs of caring for patients in teaching hospitals, the number of residents per bed was used as an operational measure of the complexity of care in adjusting payments for teaching hospitals.

Two opposing views emerged on the appropriateness of using Medicare funds for medical education. The differences between them stem largely from confusion about what medical education support actually implies in the context of the Medicare program. Those opposing medical education expenditures contend that it is inappropriate to divert service dollars to education when Medicare is facing bankruptcy. They point to recent studies suggesting that the supply of physicians is now adequate in most communities, and possibly even too large in some, and they note that teaching hospitals, with the assistance of Medicare, train physicians in specialties that are already oversupplied but produce few who specialize in care of the elderly. Some argue that Medicare pays twice for specialty training—once for residency stipends and again for the higher charges billed to Medicare by these same specialists once they are in practice. Moreover, they argue, higher costs in teaching hospitals are due to inefficiency, excessive ancillary use, longer lengths of stay, and overstaffing.

The opposing view is that most of what is called medical education is actually service dollars that could not be withdrawn without impairing quality of care in teaching hospitals. The differences in costs between community hospitals and teaching hospitals, it is argued, cannot be attributed to poor management practices, low staff productivity, or even inadequate collection policies, but to the increased costs of managing vastly more complex medical-surgical cases, conducting research, maintaining underfunded ambulatory services for the poor, and admitting a higher number of uncompensated inpatients.[15]

Both sides in the medical education debate scored points in the first round. The rationale for an educational subsidy seemed on weak ground in view of the abundant supply of physicians and other health providers. Moreover, some questioned whether the federal government should be able to stipulate the specialty distribution of the physicians trained if Medicare continues to pay a share of residency stipends. Some would argue that Medicare funds for residency training should be used for specialties that are currently undersupplied. If refinements in the DRG pricing system could be made to reflect differences in severity of illness more accurately, teaching hospitals might not require indirect medical education subsidies at current levels. However, given the considerable complexity of calculating DRGs now, many are skeptical that further refinements are feasible.

Medicare's costs attributable to medical education are expected to increase substantially due to the doubling of the allowance for teaching hospitals included in the 1983 prospective payment legislation, a move that may increase the vulnerability of the allowance to reductions as pressures to reduce trust fund expenditures increase. In view of Medicare's precarious financial position, the Advisory Council recommended termination of Medicare's support of medical education by 1987. If this recommendation is implemented, it could result in savings of $40.8 billion by 1995. The Council's recommendation has not been implemented but the Consolidated Omnibus Budget Reconciliation Act of 1985 contained several provisions that begin to limit Medicare funding for medical education.[16] However, it is clear that the issue of medical education and the preservation of teaching hospitals will continue to be debated.

Physicians

Since 1967, Medicare's Supplemental Medical Insurance (Part B) expenditures, 75% of which goes to physicians, have increased more than eightfold. Physician services are the fastest growing component in Medicare, increasing at a rate of over 18% per year since the mid 1970s to $19 billion in 1986. Federal government contributions to Part B are expected to soon exceed the federal share of Medicaid.

Rapid increases in physician expenditures cannot be attributed to increasing numbers of physician visits per beneficiary or days of hospital care, since these have remained relatively stable since 1970. Physicians' fees have risen faster than the CPI, especially since 1980, and they account for a significant portion of the increase in Supplemental Medical Insurance expenditures. However, about 40% of the increase is not explained either by the growing number of beneficiaries or by increasing fees. This residual seems to reflect an increasing intensity of services per encounter, that is, more services and more expensive care, and changes in billing practices.[8]

Physicians have been able to decide on a case-by-case basis whether to accept direct reimbursement from Medicare, requiring the patient to pay only the annual deductible and 20% co-insurance, or to hold the patient liable for full charges, including that portion in excess of Medicare-approved charges. At the time that they receive care, patients rarely know the extent of their personal out-of-pocket liability. This lack of knowledge leads to excessive worry, inability to plan their finances, and the purchase of inappropriate supplementary insurance. Currently, physicians accept assignment on approximately 55% of Medicare claims. Assignment rates vary on a statewide basis from less than 20% to over 80%. Fewer than 20% of physicians accept assignment for all their Medicare patients. In 1983, 80% of bills for physicians' services exceeded the rates Medicare considered reasonable. Of the $5.6 billion in "overcharges," $2.5 billion were paid by the elderly. The remaining $3.1 billion was not paid but was submitted to

Medicare, so that future reimbursement levels would be based on these higher charges. [17]

The public believes that doctors' fees are too high. [18] A recent survey commissioned by the American Medical Association shows that two-thirds of Americans believe doctors in general are too interested in making money, and one in four Americans thinks his or her *own* doctor is too interested in money. [19] There is strong sentiment that Medicare should limit payments to doctors and not allow additional charges to beneficiaries. Within current arrangements, limiting federal contributions merely shifts costs to patients who are now liable, through premiums, co-insurance, deductibles, and fees in excess of Medicare-approved charges, for 56% of total physician charges. [17]

The consequences of limiting physician payment are unpredictable, and politically volatile, so there is considerable disagreement about how to proceed. Passage of the original Medicare legislation was achieved through an historic compromise with physicians that is best summarized by the following passage: "Nothing in this title shall be construed to authorize any federal official to exercise any supervision or control over the practice of medicine or the way medical services are provided, or over the compensation of any institutions." (Section 102(a) of the Social Security Amendments of 1965, PL 89–97). Few would recognize the terms of that compromise today. The greatest concern regarding changes in physician reimbursement is that many physicians would refuse to participate in the program and therefore could seriously hamper elderly patients' attempts to obtain medical care, particularly in small towns and rural areas.

Experience with the Medicaid program is often offered as an example of what could happen if Medicare physician reimbursement were limited and physicians were not allowed to bill patients for additional amounts. Medicaid has not been nearly as successful as Medicare in integrating eligible patients into private medical practice. For the most part, Medicaid patients receive care in hospital outpatient or public clinics. Private physicians have been reluctant to participate in the program, and a relatively small proportion of private physicians account for the majority of office visits: some 14% of physicians provide care for 60% of all Medicaid patients treated in private offices. [20] Physicians seeing a high volume of Medicaid patients differ from the average American physician in that they tend to be older and non-Board certified, and to be graduates of foreign medical schools.

However, the number of practicing physicians will increase by one-third over this decade. The average physician derives nearly one-sixth of his or her annual income from Medicare, and some specialists receive as much as 35% from it. [8] Therefore, some groups are willing to risk more stringent limits on physician reimbursement, together with a revised assignment plan, on the assumption that not many physicians can afford to turn away the elderly. Proposals include mandatory assignment for inpatient physician fees and incorporating physician and hospital payment into a single DRG rate.

The Advisory Council took an intermediate position on assignment by recommending the establishment of a Medicare physician participation agreement. Participating physicians, whose names would be published in an annual local directory, would agree to accept assignment on all services to Medicare patients. Claims for reimbursement for services furnished by nonparticipating physicians would remain unassigned, and payment would always be made to the patient, who would be responsible for the physician's entire bill, including any amount in excess of Medicare's reasonable charge. The Council also recommended that streamlined billing and payment procedures be available to participating physicians. These recommendations were partially adopted on an interim basis in 1984 when Congress froze Medicare's payment rates. Physicians who signed "participating" agreements to accept Medicare's rates as payment in full were later exempted from the freeze as an incentive to increase assignment rates.[2]

There was strong consensus on the Advisory Council that Medicare's mandated reasonable-charge method of physician reimbursement has not been neutral in its effects on physicians' fees and practice decisions. Following previously established fee patterns has perpetuated payment differentials among geographic areas and medical specialties. Moreover, current payment rates result in incentives for hospitalization and surgical procedures rather than for less-expensive settings or treatment choices, and thus have major implications for Medicare's hospital costs as well as Part B expenditures. The Council acknowledged that prepaid capitation arrangements have been successful in containing physician and hospital costs and recommended that Medicare encourage the enrollment of beneficiaries in HMOs and other arrangements operating on predetermined, fixed budgets.

If reimbursement continues on a fee-for-service basis, the Advisory Council recommended the development of fee schedules to replace the reasonable-charge system. The fee schedules would be uniform with respect to specialty and practice location, would discourage fragmentation of billing, and would emphasize controlling the costs of physicians' services for those treatments and procedures most common among Medicare patients, such as cataract extraction, pacemaker implant, and total hip replacements. The Council also supported the concept of incorporating physician and hospital payment into a single DRG rate if it could be proven feasible. In 1985, Congress authorized the creation of a Physician Payment Review Commission to make recommendations for long-term changes in Medicare's mechanisms for paying physicians.[21]

Advancing Eligibility Age

Increasing longevity has provided a rationale for proposals to advance the age of eligibility for Medicare. Proponents of advancing the age of eligibility note that although eligibility for full retirement benefits and Medicare have always been linked, there is no longer a strong association between the two. For the past two decades there has been a trend toward earlier retirement, and now more than half of those entitled to monthly Social Security benefits retire before age 65 and before they are eligible for Medicare. In addition, in 1983 Congress increased the age of eligibility for full Social Security retirement benefits from 65 to 67 on a gradual basis beginning in the year 2000, with full implementation by 2027. (Reduced benefits can still be taken at age 62.)

Opponents of advancing the age of Medicare eligibility argue that insufficient information is available on insurance coverage for those retiring before they are eligible for Medicare. Such a proposal risks swelling the ranks of Americans without health insurance. The cost of purchasing health insurance for the interim years between retirement and Medicare eligibility could be very high. In 1984, the actuarial value of Medicare was estimated to be $2210 a year, which was roughly 20% of the average per capita income of an elderly person. A conservative estimate of the cost of comparable insurance purchased in the private market was $3400 a year (unpublished data from the American Association of Retired Persons). Moreover, although two-thirds of those currently in the 65 to 67 age group are able-bodied enough to work, about 24% of men are too disabled to engage in any gainful employment, and another 13% are limited in the kind or amount of work they can perform. Women have an even higher prevalence of work disability.[22]

The major consequence of advancing the age of Medicare eligibility would be to shift the costs of insurance from the federal government to employers, an action that would be strongly opposed in the business community. Moreover, the elderly fear that the resulting increased insurance premiums would act as a disincentive for employing older workers.

The critical financial state of Medicare ultimately led the Council to recommend advancing the age of eligibility to 67 by three months per year, beginning in 1985, until 1989, when the age would be advanced six months per year, reaching full implementation by 1990. This plan would save $74.7 billion for the Hospital Insurance Trust Fund through 1995, and almost $5 billion for Part B through 1989. Although it is unpopular with many interest groups, this proposal will probably receive serious consideration in the future because of its potential to significantly reduce expenditures.

Beneficiary Cost Sharing

Heated debate has already begun on whether the elderly should pay a larger share of their health-care costs. Medicare covers less than half of the elderly's total health expenditures. Moreover, their out-of-pocket costs have dramatically increased in recent years. On the average, the elderly spend almost as great a proportion of their incomes on health care now as they did prior to Medicare. However, the elderly have fared better economically than the rest of the population in recent years since their retirement incomes have been more insulated from the effects of inflation than the incomes of workers. The present value of Medicare benefits far exceeds tax contributions; for example, the value of Medicare benefits to an elderly couple reaching 65 in 1982 was more than 26 times their contributions in taxes.[23]

An equitable approach to cost sharing poses a number of problems. Although on the average the after-tax incomes of the elderly are favorable when compared to the rest of the population, half of the elderly have incomes within 200% of the federal poverty line. White elderly women are twice as likely to be poor as their male counterparts, black men are four times as likely, and black women are five times as likely.[24] Moreover, one person in five over age 72 is poor. The old-old not only are more likely to be poor but also are likely to need more medical care. Although there are some elderly who can well afford to pay more for their medical care, there are many who would find it difficult.

So far, means-testing Medicare has been soundly rejected, for varying reasons. One reason is the fear that the public would not continue to support a mandatory payroll tax without universal eligibility.

Most cost-sharing proposals have advocated increasing coinsurance and deductibles. Proponents of this strategy argue that increased cost sharing will reduce discretionary use of health services, and thus the savings achieved would be even greater than the additional amounts paid by the beneficiaries. However, the vast majority of the elderly have supplemental insurance that covers copayments, reducing the likelihood that increased co-insurance will influence their use of health services.[25] Moreover, co-insurance and deductibles place the greatest burden on those who have the most illness and the old-old, whose resources are apt to be limited.

A premium-based approach to cost sharing offers the potential for equitably distributing the cost burden among all of the beneficiaries and limiting the amount any single individual would pay. For example, a premium of $4 a month, or $48 a year, paid by all beneficiaries would yield revenues in excess of $1.4 billion annually, for a cumulative total of $33 billion over the period 1984 through 1995.

The Advisory Council supported the premium-based approach to cost sharing, and designed a restructured benefit package to provide cata-strophic hospital coverage, impose an overall limit on out-of-pocket ex-penditures for Medicare-covered services, simplify the benefit structure, and distribute cost sharing equitably.

Until enactment of the Medicare Catastrophic Coverage Act of 1988, Medicare provided hospital care for up to 90 days in a benefit period, plus a one-time reserve of 60 covered days, and for 100 days at a skilled nursing facility. The patient was liable for an initial deductible based on the average cost of a day of hospitalization ($400 in 1985), co-insurance of one-fourth of the deductible for hospital days 61–90 in a benefit period, one-half of the deductible for each lifetime reserve day, and one-eighth of the deductible for days 21 through 100 in a skilled nursing facility. Benefits were not tied to a specific time period but to a "spell of illness," defined as the period beginning at hospital admission and ending when the patient has been out of a hospital or skilled nursing facility for 60 consecutive days.

This entire structure was poorly understood by beneficiaries. Moreover, it violated the major principle of insurance—protection from financial ruin. The risk of substantial financial loss, added to the overly complicated and poorly understood benefit structure, created a large demand for private supplemental insurance—which is equally complicated. Approximately 65% of Medicare beneficiaries purchase private Medigap policies, with annual premiums ranging from $300 to $800. More than 10% have more than one private policy, and 3% have more than two.[26] In 1984, the elderly spent an estimated $8 billion on supplemental insurance.[23] These policies generally cover co-insurance, and, in some cases, deductibles and un-limited days of inpatient care. Some of the more expensive policies also provide additional coverage, such as for prescription drugs. Few cover physician fees in excess of Medicare-approved charges.

Medigap insurance has been fraught with problems. Beneficiaries' lack of understanding of Medicare coverage and their fear of financial ruin due to catastrophic illness make them vulnerable to insurers who offer inade-quate or unnecessary supplemental coverage. Moreover, many insurers have overhead costs of up to 40% of the premium, compared to Medicare's administrative expenses of less than 5%. The same type of coverage, of-fered as part of Medicare, could therefore be provided for significantly lower premiums.

The Advisory Council recommended a restructuring of the basic Medi-care benefit, with the option of buying catastrophic coverage through increasing the Part B premium. Otis Bowen, the chairman of the 1982 Advisory Council on Social Security, became Health and Human Services Secretary in 1985 and focused White House attention on Medicare cover-age gaps. Bowen proposed unlimited hospital care and a $2000 annual limit on out-of-pocket costs in return for a $6 monthly premium paid by all beneficiaries. Congress enacted the Medicare Catastrophic Coverage Act of 1988, providing coverage for unlimited days of hospital care after a single annual deductible has been met, and limiting out-of-pocket spending for physician costs and supplies covered under Part B (to $1,370 per year in 1990). The improved coverage is financed by an increase in the monthly Part B premium for all enrollees, and a new supplemental premium based on federal income tax liability.

Even with the new catastrophic benefit, out-of-pocket expenditures still are perceived by the elderly to be high. There is no evidence to date that the expanded coverage has actually resulted in a decline in the purchase of private supplemental Medigap coverage, an outcome the Advisory Council hoped would be a result of its recommendation.

Increasing Revenues

Two related concerns underlie the debate over whether increased tax revenues should be used to finance a Medicare shortfall. The first concern is the inflationary effect of increasing revenues in the absence of reasonable cost controls within the program. Beneficiary groups have been outspoken in favor of more stringent cost controls on providers in lieu of increasing taxes. They realize that, ultimately, the cost of the program will influence its vulnerability in the political arena.

The second concern relates to differing perceptions of how much the nation can afford to invest in health services for the elderly. Public opinion polls consistently report widespread support for the Social Security program among Americans of all ages.[27] In fact, the majority of Americans polled believe that more resources should be invested in care of the elderly. In contrast, some economic analysts point with alarm to the increasing share of the federal budget devoted to the elderly, and the potential negative consequences of social welfare spending on the private sector, including reduced incentives for personal savings, which provide essential investment capital to stimulate economic growth.[5,23]

Although government spending has increased significantly in terms of total dollars since Medicare was initiated in 1966, the federal sector has grown only 0.9% in relation to the growth of the economy and has remained basically the same size over the past five years.[28] Moreover, in the past 20 years the United States has had one of the smallest and most slowly growing public sectors among industrial democracies.[29] Some believe that these trends do not provide a strong rationale for undertaking draconian cuts in the Medicare program for the purpose of saving the American economy.[30,31]

A number of revenue-generating tax options are under consideration for financing part of Medicare's budget deficit, including increasing payroll taxes, increasing federal excise taxes on tobacco and alcohol products, taxing employer-provided health insurance benefits, increasing general revenue subsidies, and reallocating the payroll tax rate between the Old Age, Survivors, and Disability Income Trust Funds and Medicare. A summary of the council's recommendations highlights some of the dilemmas associated with each option.

The council rejected further increases in payroll taxes, primarily because of their potential adverse effect on employment. Over the past decade, small employers have created a substantial portion of new jobs.[32] Increasing employers' contributions to the payroll tax act is a disincentive to the creation of new jobs, particularly marginal, lower-pay jobs. Moreover, the payroll tax places a proportionately higher tax burden on low-income persons, since there is a maximum wage ($43,800 in 1987) subject to taxes.

General revenues derived from graduated income taxes would be less onerous for low- and middle-income workers, and there is a precedent for their use in Medicare, since over 75% of Part B is currently financed from general revenues. Moreover, in contrast to Social Security retirement benefits, which are related to the amount contributed by the worker, there is no direct financial relationship between worker contributions and Medicare benefits, a fact that weakens the rationale for the payroll tax. However, in view of the historically high federal deficit, the council rejected increased Medicare reliance on general revenues at this time. The council chose not to debate the need for increasing income taxes to reduce the federal deficit, but this option obviously will receive continuing consideration.

As a compromise, the council recommended the establishment of user taxes on alcohol and tobacco products to finance part of hospital insurance benefits, on the basis of well-established relationships between use of these discretionary products and increased health-care costs.[33] Federal excise taxes on alcohol had not been increased in 30 years. As a result, the price of distilled spirits in constant dollars was only half what it was in 1960.[34] The federal excise tax on cigarettes, which has not been changed since 1951, was doubled for three years only in 1982. However, states object to increased federal excise taxes that might diminish their revenues, and, although state taxes on alcohol and tobacco have increased, they have not kept pace with inflation either. On the average, the total revenue raised by all states on alcoholic beverages in 1982 accounted for only 3.4% of total state revenues, and tobacco taxes accounted for 5%. Doubling the tax on alcohol and extending the current cigarette tax, with an added increase of 50%, would yield at least $100 billion in additional revenues for the Hospital Insurance Trust Fund by 1995.

The council also recommended taxing employer contributions to health insurance that exceed $70 per month for an individual and $175 per month for a family. The current tax exemption encourages first-dollar insurance coverage and removes any incentive for patients and their providers to use health services cost-effectively. An estimated $20 billion or more in additional federal income taxes would have been collected in 1983 if employer health plan contributions were treated as taxable income. Wages subject to Social Security payroll taxes would also increase, producing over $7 billion in additional tax receipts for the Hospital Insurance Trust Fund through 1995.

Income tax changes were not considered by the council because of the difficulty in allocating increased revenues from the general treasury to the Medicare trust fund. However, income tax changes are a vehicle for placing a greater share of Medicare's financing burden on the elderly, who could therefore pay more for their Medicare coverage without it being necessary to establish an unpopular means test. Eliminating the $1000 personal exemption for people age 65 and older would raise approximately $2.4 billion a year in additional revenues. [25]

The Social Security Reform Act of 1983 was an attempt to provide a stable financial base for the Old Age, Survivors, and Disability Income (OASDI) programs for 75 years. Several legislative changes were made that increased revenues to the OASDI Trust Funds, and very large surpluses are expected to accumulate, beginning in the 1990s and peaking in about 2005. The surpluses will eventually be required to finance the OASDI programs beyond the year 2020. However, many political realists wonder if Congress will be tempted to reallocate those funds, amounting to as much as $2.2 trillion, [35] to bail out Medicare, instead of making unpopular program modifications. The first step made by Congress in resolving the recent shortfall in the OASDI programs was to borrow from the Hospital Insurance Trust Fund. Hence, despite the crisis in Medicare's fiscal problems, it might be possible to "muddle through" for a while longer in the American political tradition of making small incremental changes.

Discussion

Since the completion of the work of the Advisory Council on Social Security, several actions have been taken consistent with council recommendations. Most notably, Congress enacted legislation to provide catastrophic hospital coverage financed through a premium, as proposed by the council (see Chapter 6 for a complete discussion). Ceilings were established for annual increases in hospital payments that are closer to the Hospital Input Price Index. A temporary freeze on physicians' fees was enacted, along with a variation of the council's all-or-nothing assignment concept that provides financial incentives to encourage physicians to accept direct Medicare payment. Although Congress increased federal excise taxes on liquor, it did not earmark the resulting revenues for Medicare, and it did not extend the cigarette tax increase passed in 1982. Part B premiums were increased to ensure that 25% of the costs were borne by the beneficiaries.

The outlook for the Medicare hospital trust fund is considerably improved over earlier forecasts. The estimated date of the depletion of the trust fund has been revised from 1989 to 2006. A combination of an improved national economy and lower inflation, more stringent hospital reimbursement policies, and changing patterns of hospital utilization account for the more favorable forecast. However, after taking into account these factors, outlays are still projected to grow faster than revenues beginning in the early 1990s, leading ultimately to a depletion of the trust fund. Moreover, lower-than-expected rates of growth in hospital expenditures are being offset by rapid increases in expenditures for physician services.

Thus, while some progress has been made, Medicare's financial crisis appears to have been postponed rather than solved. Medicare's problems are clear. The alternative solutions have been identified. Only the political alignments necessary to hammer out solutions are missing.

Despite the present polarization on solutions, a national consensus persists that the Medicare program is one of the nation's most successful policy innovations. Since Medicare was passed 24 years ago, its track record in improving the quality of life for elderly citizens has been one of this country's most stunning national successes. This is good news, particularly at a time when Americans have become increasingly skeptical about the country's abilities to solve many of the serious problems facing it. The challenge ahead will be to use resources effectively to preserve these gains and to push ahead farther to improve the lives of Americans of all ages.

References

1. Trustees of the Federal Hospital Insurance Trust Fund. 1987. *1987 Annual Report*. Washington, D.C.: Government Printing Office.
2. Congressional Budget Office. 1986. *Physician Reimbursement under Medicare: Options for Change*. Washington, D.C.: United States Congress.
3. Advisory Council on Social Security. 1984. *Medicare Benefits and Financing*. Washington, D.C.: Government Printing Office.
4. Aiken, L. H., Bays, K. D. 1984. The Medicare debate: Round one. *N Engl J Med* 311:1196–1200.
5. Petersen, P. S. 1983. A reply to critics. *NY Rev Books* 30(4):50.
6. United States House of Representatives, Committee on Ways and Means,

Subcommittee on Health. 1984. *Proceedings of the Conference on the Future of Medicare.* Pub. No. 29–323–0. Washington, D.C.: Government Printing Office.

7. Trustees of the Federal Supplementary Medical Insurance Trust Fund. 1987. *1987 Annual Report.* Washington, D.C.: Government Printing Office.

8. United States Senate, Special Committee on Aging. 1984. *Medicare: Paying the Physician—History, Issues, and Options.* Pub. No. 31–792–0. Washington, D.C.: Government Printing Office.

9. Freko, D. 1985. Admissions fall but margins are up in 1984. *Hospitals* 59(9):71.

10. Aiken, L. H., Mullinix, C. F. 1987. The nurse shortage: Myth or reality? *N Engl J Med* 317:641–646.

11. Sloan, F. A. 1983. Rate regulation for hospital cost control. *Milbank Memorial Fund Q* 61:195–217.

12. Atkinson, J. G., Schramm, C. J. 1982. Hospital cost containment and nursing. In *Nursing in the 1980s: Crises, Opportunities, Challenges,* ed. L. H. Aiken. Philadelphia, Pa.: J. B. Lippincott.

13. Admiche, K. W., Sloan, F. A. 1982. Unions and hospitals: Some unresolved issues. *J Health Econ* 1:31–108.

14. Horn, S. D. 1983. Measuring severity of illness: Comparisons across institutions. *Am J Public Health* 73:25–31.

15. Bergen, S. S., Roth, A. C. 1984. Prospective payment and the university hospital. *N Engl J Med* 310:316–318.

16. See Ref. 1, pp. 13–15.

17. United States House of Representatives, Select Committee on Aging. 1984. *Paying the Doctor: The High Cost of Physician Services for the Elderly.* Unpublished report.

18. Blendon, R. J., Altman, D. E. 1984. Public attitudes about health care costs: A lesson in national schizophrenia. *N Engl J Med* 311:613–616.

19. American Medical Association. 1983. *Physician and Public Opinion on Health Care Issues.* Chicago, Ill.: American Medical Association.

20. Mitchell, J. B., Cromwell, J. 1980. Medicaid mills: Fact or fiction. *Health Care Financing Rev* 2:37–49.

21. United States Congress, Office of Technology Assessment. 1986. *Payment for Physician Services: Strategies for Medicare.* Washington, D.C.: Government Printing Office.

22. Feldman, J. J. 1983. Work ability of the aged under conditions of improving mortality. *Milbank Memorial Fund Q* 61(3):430–444.

23. Keisling, P. 1983. Protection from catastrophe: The Medicare reform we really need. *Washington Monthly* 15(8):39–43.

24. United States Bureau of the Census. 1983. America in transition: An aging society. *Current Population Reports,* Series P-23, No. 128. Washington, D.C.: Government Printing Office.

25. Link, C. R., Long, S. H., Settle, R. F. 1980. Cost sharing, supplementary insurance, and health services utilization among the Medicare elderly. *Health Care Financing Rev* 2:25–31.

26. McCall, N. 1983. *Medigap: Study of comparative effectiveness of various state*

regulations. SRI International. Unpublished Final Report. Prepared for Health Care Financing Administration, Contract 500-81-0500.

27. Navarro, V. 1982. Where is the popular mandate? *N Engl J Med* 308:1516–1518.

28. Congressional Budget Office. 1982. *Balancing the Federal Budget and Limiting Federal Spending: Constitutional and Statutory Approaches*. Washington, D.C.: Government Printing Office.

29. Estes, C. L., Newcomer, R. J. 1983. *Fiscal Austerity and Aging*. Beverly Hills, Calif.: Sage Publications.

30. Munnell, A. H. 1983. A calmer look at Social Security. *NY Rev Books* 30(4):41–45.

31. Estes, C. L. 1983. Social Security: The social construction of a crisis. *Milbank Memorial Fund Q* 61:445–461.

32. Greene, R. 1982. Tracking job growth in private industry. *Monthly Labor Rev* 105:3–9.

33. Luce, B. R., Schweitzer, S. O. 1978. Smoking and alcohol abuse: A comparison of their economic consequences. *N Engl J Med* 298:569–571.

34. Cook, P. J. 1981. The effect of liquor taxes on drinking, cirrhosis, and auto accidents. In *Alcohol and Public Policy: Beyond the Shadow of Prohibition*, ed. M. H. Moore and D. R. Gerstein. Washington, D.C.: National Academy Press, 255–285.

35. United States Social Security Administration, Office of the Actuary. 1983. *Long-Range Projections of Social Security Trust Fund Operations in Dollars*. Actuarial Note No. 117. Washington, D.C.: Government Printing Office.

Six

Catastrophic Coverage under the Medicare Program

Diane Rowland, Barbara Lyons, and Karen Davis

The enactment of the Medicare program in 1965 extended basic health insurance protection for hospital and physician services to almost all elderly Americans. Medicare coverage played a major role in increasing access to care for the elderly population and contributed to improvements in their health and longevity.[1] Yet, over time, the scope of Medicare coverage and the extent to which elderly people are not covered in times of serious illness emerged as a major policy concern. These concerns ultimately resulted in the current legislation that expands Medicare to provide catastrophic protection.

The Medicare Catastrophic Coverage Act of 1988 (P.L. 100–360) became law on July 1, 1988. It is the most significant expansion in health insurance benefits for elderly people since the enactment of Medicare itself. It provides for full coverage of hospital care under Medicare, limits out-of-pocket spending for covered services, provides assistance through Medicaid to low-income beneficiaries, and adds new benefits to Medicare, most notably coverage of outpatient prescription drugs. The new law provides expanded protection to all 32 million elderly and disabled Medicare beneficiaries. It limits hospital costs for 2.2 million beneficiaries, protects over 2 million beneficiaries with physician costs exceeding $1370 each year, and assists the over 5 million beneficiaries with prescription drug expenses in excess of $600 per year.

Catastrophic medical costs are broadly defined as large and unpredictable health-care expenses associated with major illness or serious injury. The debate on catastrophic coverage highlighted problems in the level of protection for acute-care needs as well as brought increased awareness of Medicare's lack of coverage of long-term care services. The substantial co-insurance for services covered under Medicare coupled with the lack of coverage of prescription drugs, dental care, and other services can result in financial burdens of a catastrophic level for many elderly people.

To protect themselves from the financial burden for health care, many elderly persons turn to private insurance policies to fill in some of Medicare's gaps and help with cost sharing. For some of the poorest elderly people, the Medicaid program fills in Medicare's cost sharing, pays the Part B premium and provides additional benefits. However, coverage from supplementary programs most often only partially fills Medicare's gaps and proves inadequate in the face of true medical catastrophe. Moreover, 20% of Medicare beneficiaries have no supplementary coverage and rely solely on Medicare.[2] For these 5 million beneficiaries, Medicare protection is the sole source of financing when illness strikes.

This chapter examines the adequacy of Medicare coverage of hospital and physician care for the elderly population and the proposals to expand Medicare to include catastrophic coverage. The first section describes the benefits available under the Medicare program and identifies the gaps in coverage. The second section reviews the proposal for catastrophic coverage advanced by the Reagan Administration and the Congressional response. The third section outlines the new law providing catastrophic protection under Medicare, and the final section assesses the effects of expanded Medicare coverage and discusses the future policy implications.

The Need for Catastrophic Coverage

Medicare provides health insurance coverage to persons age 65 and over who are entitled to receive Social Security or Railroad Retirement benefits. About 97% of all aged persons are covered. Since July 1973, Medicare has also covered individuals who have been permanently and totally disabled for two years or more, and persons with end-stage renal disease. In 1988, 29 million elderly and 3 million disabled people were enrolled in Medicare.[3]

The Medicare program was modeled after private insurance plans for the under-65 population and designed to meet the acute-care health needs of the elderly population. The program consists of two parts: Hospital Insurance (Part A) and Supplementary Medical Insurance (Part B). Part A covers short-stay hospital care and provides limited coverage of posthospital care in skilled nursing facilities (SNFs) and home health services. Part B covers physician, outpatient hospital, home health and some ambulatory services. Medicare does not cover most preventive services, outpatient prescription drugs, dental care, routine eye examinations, eyeglasses, hearing aids, or long-term institutional services.

Part A coverage is automatic for Social Security and Railroad Retirement beneficiaries. It is financed primarily through Social Security payroll tax contributions. Those covered by Part A may voluntarily enroll in Part B by paying a monthly premium, set at $22.80 in 1988.[3] The premium covers about 25% of Part B costs and the remainder is financed by general revenues. Almost all people eligible for Part A also elect to be covered for physician services under Part B.

Medicare Benefits Prior to Catastrophic Coverage

Although Medicare offers protection against health-care spending to almost all elderly Americans, the protection it offers is not comprehensive. The Medicare benefit package is prescribed by law, with the scope of coverage and beneficiary cost-sharing levels carefully specified (Table 6.1). Limits on covered benefits and cost-sharing requirements can leave beneficiaries liable for large medical bills.

Hospital coverage is one of the most important benefits Medicare provides to elderly beneficiaries. Reflecting the acute-care orientation of Medicare, coverage of short hospital stays is fairly extensive. Part A covers inpatient hospital care for 90 days of any illness. A new illness is defined to begin when the beneficiary has not been in a hospital or nursing home for 60 continuous days. In addition to the 90-day coverage during a spell of illness, Medicare also provides a 60-day lifetime reserve.

The beneficiary pays a deductible upon admission to the hospital that is indexed to the cost of one day of hospital care. The amount of the deductible has increased rapidly since the introduction of the Medicare Hospital Prospective Payment System (PPS) in October 1983. The increase reflects both hospital inflation and the sharp decline in the average length of stay that occurred with the implementation of the new payment system. The shorter length of stay makes the cost of a day of care relatively more expensive than before. The deductible was $536 in 1988 and is projected to increase to $600 by 1990.[3,4]

Coverage of long hospital stays is less adequate. The limit of 90 days' coverage of any illness plus a 60-day lifetime reserve can be exceeded in severe cases. In addition, the cost-sharing levels on extended hospital days are steep. The beneficiary pays one-fourth of the deductible for the 61st–90th day of hospital care ($134 per day in 1988), and one-half of the deductible for each of the lifetime reserve days ($268 per day in 1988). Although the number of beneficiaries with hospital stays exceeding 60 days is small, the costs associated with a long stay can be very high.

Table 6.1.   Medicare Benefits before Catastrophic and Cost-Sharing Requirements, 1988

Coverage	Beneficiary Payments

Part A

Coverage	Beneficiary Payments
Inpatient Hospital Services	
Per spell of illness:	
First 60 days	$536 deductible
61st-90th day	$134 daily co-insurance
60 lifetime reserve days	$268 daily co-insurance
Posthospital SNF Services	
First 20 days	None
21st–100th day	$67 daily co-insurance
Home Health Services	None
Hospice Services	Subject to durational limits and copayments for outpatient drugs and respite care

Part B

Coverage	Beneficiary Payments
Physicians' services and other medical services	Premium—$274 per year
	$75 deductible
	20% co-insurance
	Amounts in excess of reasonable charges on unassigned claims (balance billing)

Source: Ref. 3.

For physician services, the beneficiary is responsible for the first $75 of services, as well as 20% of all Medicare allowable charges, and any physicians' charges in excess of those allowable by Medicare. Physician services under Medicare are provided on an "assigned" or "unassigned" basis. When a physician accepts assignment, he or she agrees to accept the Medicare allowable charge as payment in full for the services rendered. Thus, if assignment is accepted, the Medicare beneficiary's out-of-pocket costs are limited to the deductible and 20% co-insurance. If the physician does not accept assignment, the beneficiary must also pay charges in excess of what Medicare allows.

To encourage physicians to accept assignment of claims, a Medicare participating physician program was established in 1984. Under this program, physicians agreed to accept assignment on all services in return for more rapid claims processing and higher allowable charge levels under Medicare. Participating physicians are listed in a directory. Nonparticipating physicians are permitted to continue to accept or refuse assignment on a claim-by-claim basis. As of January 1987, 30.6% of the physicians providing care to Medicare beneficiaries had signed agreements to be participating physicians.[5]

Nursing home coverage under Medicare is geared to recuperation from hospital care and is limited to short-term stays in SNFs following hospitalization. Medicare coverage is a postacute, rather than long-term care, benefit. There is no deductible for SNF care, but the beneficiary is required to pay a co-insurance charge that is set at one-eighth of the hospital deductible for the 21st–100th days of SNF care ($67 per day in 1988). Because the SNF co-insurance amount is based on the inpatient hospital deductible, which has increased sharply, the beneficiary's share of SNF costs has increased much faster than actual SNF costs and exceeds the cost of a day of SNF care in some areas of the country.

Home health care is also a Medicare benefit, but it is covered only when a beneficiary can be shown to need intermittent skilled nursing care or physical or speech therapy. Guidelines permit daily skilled nursing visits up to eight hours per day for up to 21 days. There is no co-insurance, limitation on the number of home health visits covered, or prior hospitalization requirement. However, many chronically dependent Medicare beneficiaries do not qualify for home health benefits because their care needs are custodial rather than skilled in nature. The skilled care requirement essentially limits the use of home health care to those recovering from an acute illness episode.

Lack of coverage of any outpatient prescription drugs is a notable gap in Medicare's acute-care coverage. Inpatient prescription drugs are generally covered by Medicare, but coverage of outpatient drugs is limited to those injected by a physician or nurse. The trend toward earlier hospital discharge of Medicare patients resulting from implementation of prospective payment for hospital care means that the cost of drugs that previously would have been covered during a hospital stay has now been shifted to the beneficiary.

Gaps in Medicare Coverage

Despite coverage by Medicare, many elderly and disabled beneficiaries face serious financial burdens in meeting their health-care expenses. Medicare meets less than half of all health expenditures for elderly people, but is clearly important in financing hospital and physician care (Table 6.2). It pays for 75% of the elderly population's hospital bills and nearly 60% of physician care. Medicaid, the health financing program for the poor, provides assistance to supplement Medicare for some of the low-income elderly population. It funds about 13% of the aged's personal health-care expenditures overall and almost 50% of their nursing home expenditures.

Elderly people themselves are responsible for the remaining third of health-care expenses. Twenty-five percent is paid by direct out-of-pocket payments associated with obtaining and receiving services and 7% is cov-

Table 6.2.   Percent Distribution of Personal Health-Care Expenditures per Capita for People 65 Years of Age or Over, by Source of Funds and Type of Service, 1984

Source of funds	Type of Service				
	Total care	Hospital	Physician	Nursing home	Other care
Total per Capita	100.0	100.0	100.0	100.0	100.0
Private	32.8	11.4	39.7	51.9	65.3
Consumer	32.4	11.0	39.6	51.2	64.8
Out-of-pocket	25.2	3.1	26.1	50.1	59.9
Insurance	7.2	7.9	13.5	1.1	4.9
Other private	0.4	0.4	0.0	0.7	0.5
Government	67.2	88.6	60.3	48.1	34.7
Medicare	48.8	74.8	57.8	2.1	19.9
Medicaid	12.8	4.8	1.9	41.5	11.4
Other government	5.6	9.1	0.7	4.4	3.4

Source: Data from Ref. 8.

ered by private health insurance plans for which elderly persons enroll and pay premiums. Seventy-two percent of Medicare beneficiaries have private insurance to supplement Medicare, but the average premium cost for such coverage in 1987 was $500 to $600 per year.[6] In addition, all beneficiaries who are enrolled in Part B are required to pay a monthly premium ($22.80 in 1988).

In 1987, out-of-pocket spending for liabilities in connection with Medicare-covered services alone were estimated to average $561 per elderly Medicare beneficiary.[7] This spending includes $456 for Medicare cost sharing and $105 for extra billing for physicians' services not provided on an assignment basis. This does not include out-of-pocket spending for services not covered by Medicare or premiums for Part B coverage or Medigap insurance. Premiums for Part B added another $214 in expenses in 1987, resulting in an average of $775 for Medicare cost sharing and Part B coverage per beneficiary.

Most of the out-of-pocket liability for Medicare-covered services stems from physician care, because these services have 20% co-insurance and physicians can bill beneficiaries for the difference between their charges and Medicare's payment level. More than 50% of copayment costs incurred by Medicare beneficiaries are for physician services and related care. When extra billing for unassigned claims is included, more than 60% of out-of-pocket spending associated with Medicare-covered services is attributable to physician care.[7]

The highest out-of-pocket costs are, however, incurred by Medicare beneficiaries who have a hospital stay. The 22% of the Medicare population with an inpatient hospital stay during the year incur 70% of the out-of-pocket costs.[7] In 1987, a beneficiary with one hospital stay incurred, on

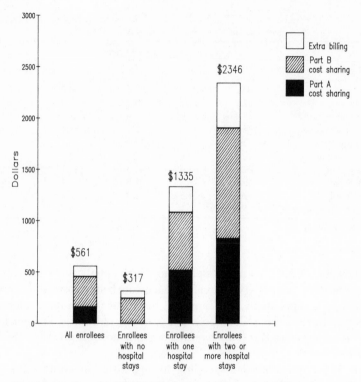

Figure 6.1. Out-of-pocket liabilities per enrollee under Medicare by use of services, 1987 (in dollars). *Source:* Data from Ref. 7.

average, $1335 in out-of-pocket liabilities, compared to $317 for a benefi-ciary without a hospital stay (Figure 6.1).

The greatest financial burden is faced by those with multiple hospital stays in a year. Almost one-third of hospitalized Medicare beneficiaries are rehospitalized during the year. A second hospital stay during the year added another $1000 to out-of-pocket costs, reflecting the payment of a second hospital deductible plus additional physician co-insurance.

The benefits not covered by Medicare also contribute heavily to the financial burdens faced by elderly people. In 1984, per capita spending per elderly person was $4202.[8] Of this amount, $1059, or one-fourth, was paid by the elderly themselves. Almost three-fourths of out-of-pocket spending by elderly beneficiaries was for services that Medicare does not cover or offers only as a limited benefit (Figure 6.2).

Medicare offers minimal protection against the costs of nursing home care and almost no protection for the costs of custodial care services re-quired by chronically ill persons over an extended time period. Less than 5% of hospital discharges result in a Medicare-covered SNF stay. Nursing

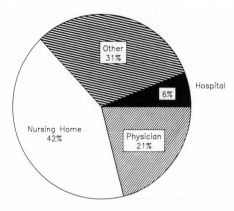

$1,059 per aged person

Figure 6.2. Distribution of annual average out-of-pocket spending by the elderly. *Source:* Data from Ref. 8.

home care costs an estimated $22,000 per person per year and half of all nursing home expenses for the elderly population are paid out of pocket.[8] For those who do not require nursing home care, out-of-pocket spending for prescription drugs, personal care at home, eyeglasses, hearing aids, and dentures can also be burdensome.

These out-of-pocket costs are not inconsequential and average about 15% of income.[9] However, out-of-pocket expenses are not spread evenly over all aged persons. The heaviest financial burdens are concentrated on the sickest and frailest elderly people, many of whom have low incomes. Elderly persons with incomes below $5000 spend, on average, 18% of their income on out-of-pocket medical care expenses, compared to 4% for those with incomes of $20,000 or more (Table 6.3). Although many elderly people elect to purchase private insurance to help cover out-of-pocket expenses, the cost of a supplemental policy can be too high for those with lower incomes.

Table 6.3. Annual Out-of-Pocket Spending by Elderly for Medical Care as a Percent of Income, 1986

Income Level	Percentage of Income Spent on Medical Care
Under $5000	18
$5000–$9999	12
$10,000–$14,999	9
$15,000–$19,999	7
$20,000 and above	4

Source: Ref. 3.

Assistance from Other Programs

The combination of cost-sharing charges for covered Medicare services coupled with the potential for high out-of-pocket payments for uncovered services has led the majority of Medicare beneficiaries to purchase private insurance coverage to supplement the program's benefit package. This protection, frequently referred to as "Medigap" coverage, is purchased by an estimated 72% of Medicare enrollees, at an average premium cost of $500–$600 in 1987.[6]

The principal protection offered by most of these policies is coverage of Medicare's deductibles and co-insurance charges. Some Medigap policies cover a limited number of additional services not covered by Medicare, such as prescription drugs. Few policies protect against extra billing above Medicare-allowable charges by physicians or the costs of long-term institutional care.

Medicaid serves as a supplementary program for the low-income elderly population. Medicaid was enacted in 1965 as a companion piece of legislation to Medicare to provide federal assistance to the states in financing medical care for poor people, both elderly and nonelderly. For elderly poor people who are Medicare beneficiaries, Medicaid pays the Medicare cost-sharing requirements and Part B premium and provides additional benefits.

Medicaid is essentially Medicare's safety net. Once covered by Medicaid, an elderly person faces little risk of high out-of-pocket expenses. In addition, physicians who treat Medicaid patients may not bill these patients for any charges not paid by Medicare or Medicaid. This means that all services to Medicaid beneficiaries are expected to be accepted on an assigned basis. Many states also cover a range of additional services through Medicaid, such as prescription drugs and dental care.

The problem is that Medicaid does not supplement Medicare for all poor elderly people. Eligibility limitations coupled with variations in scope of coverage among states leave over two-thirds of poor elderly people, 2.2 million people, without Medicaid to fill in gaps in Medicare and provide additional assistance with out-of-pocket costs.[10]

About 5 million (20%) of elderly Americans have no protection other than Medicare against health-care costs. This group must pay out-of-pocket for all Medicare cost-sharing and for medical services not covered by Medicare. As a result, the aged with only Medicare coverage are the group most at risk for catastrophic out-of-pocket liabilities.

Low-income elderly persons are the most likely to rely solely on Medicare for health insurance protection. Almost half of those with no coverage to supplement Medicare have incomes below 150% of the federal poverty level; over 22% of the Medicare-only population are poor and another 22% are near-poor. This means that those who are least able to afford out-of-pocket spending for medical care are the most likely to be without assistance to fill in Medicare's gaps.

The adequacy of health insurance coverage is obviously closely related to health status. Elderly people in fair or poor health are not only more likely to require medical care, but also are more likely to be without private insurance to help with Medicare cost sharing than are elderly people in better health. The most serious financial burden for medical care falls on those elderly people who have low incomes, poor health, and inadequate insurance. Among poor elderly people in fair or poor health, 28% have only Medicare coverage. [10]

Scope of insurance coverage also appears to influence use of services. Health-care expenditures for poor and near-poor elderly people differ substantially by insurance status. Aged persons with Medicare only consume the lowest level of medical care services while those who are covered by Medicaid and Medicare consume the highest level. [10] Those elderly persons with private insurance to supplement Medicare use less care than the Medicaid-covered population, but almost twice as much care as the poor aged who rely solely on Medicare coverage.

Providing Catastrophic Protection

The inadequate protection against catastrophic acute health-care expenditures led to pressure to expand Medicare coverage. The push for catastrophic coverage was initiated by the Reagan Administration's study of the burden of catastrophic expenses from illness, and a legislative proposal in February 1987 to provide catastrophic coverage under Medicare. Congressional interest in improving care for elderly and disabled Medicare beneficiaries resulted in swift action in both the House and Senate. Proposals to improve Medicare coverage received bipartisan support, despite concern over the federal deficit and the need to limit budget spending.

The new legislation providing for expanded coverage of catastrophic care under Medicare is a sweeping reform that restructures the scope and improves the adequacy of Medicare benefits. It fills many of the gaps in current benefits that have resulted in large out-of-pocket costs for beneficiaries with serious illness. It accomplishes the goals of the original administration proposal, but it goes beyond the scope of that proposal to offer new benefits and expanded protection.

Administration Proposal

The momentum for expanding Medicare to include catastrophic care began, in part, with the 1982 Advisory Council on Social Security. Chaired by a physician, former Indiana Governor Otis Bowen, the council exam-

ined the financing and adequacy of the Medicare program. Its recommendations, released in December 1983, included a proposal to provide catastrophic coverage under Medicare by covering all hospital care and limiting
out-of-pocket costs for Part B.[11]

In the fall of 1985, President Reagan tapped Dr. Bowen to be Secretary
of the Department of Health and Human Services, the federal agency with
responsibility for Medicare. Dr. Bowen brought his concern for the need for
catastrophic coverage under Medicare with him to the department and
made Medicare reform a priority of the Reagan Administration.[12]

In his State of the Union message in February 1986, President Reagan
directed Secretary Bowen and the Department of Health and Human
Services to undertake an examination of the burden of catastrophic illness
for all age groups and to report recommendations to him. Secretary
Bowen's report, delivered in the fall of 1986, identified three major components of catastrophic coverage: acute catastrophic protection for the elderly, long-term care protection, and catastrophic protection for the general population.[13] It resulted in an administration-sponsored legislative
proposal to expand Medicare coverage.

The president submitted the administration's proposal (H. R. 1245/S.
592)[14] to the Congress on February 24, 1987. The proposal incorporated
the Medicare catastrophic coverage recommendations contained in the
Bowen report, but did not address coverage for the nonelderly population
or long-term care. However, given the restrictive budgetary environment
and the administration's commitment to reduce domestic spending, the
proposal for expanding coverage for elderly people was a major departure
from administration policy and a breakthrough for advocates of program
improvement.

The administration's proposal restructured Medicare benefits and set a
limit on annual out-of-pocket spending for Medicare-covered services under Part A and Part B. Part A co-insurance for inpatient hospital days and
covered SNF days was eliminated, and the maximum number of hospital
deductibles was set at two per year. To limit liability for beneficiaries, the
proposal provided a $2000 annual limit on co-insurance and deductibles for
Medicare-covered services. However, beneficiaries would continue to be
liable for all expenses for services not covered by Medicare and excess
billing by physicians who do not accept assignment.

The catastrophic plan was to be financed by an additional premium paid
by program beneficiaries, initially set at $59 per year and indexed annually.
The full cost of the expansion was to be financed by this increase in the
Medicare Part B premium. The proposal did not vary the amount of the
premium by income. The principle was that the entire cost of the expanded
coverage was to be borne by the elderly and disabled Medicare beneficiaries
who would benefit from the new coverage. The administration estimated

that 1.4 million beneficiaries would incur expenses related to Medicare-covered services in excess of $2000 in 1987 and would therefore directly benefit from the proposed legislation.

Congressional Action

Congressional action on catastrophic care followed quickly. Hearings on gaps in Medicare coverage and the need for catastrophic coverage were held by the major legislating committees in Congress during 1986 and 1987. Legislative proposals were developed and considered in both the House of Representatives and the Senate during 1987. The House catastrophic bill (H. R. 2470)[15] was passed on July 22, 1987. The Senate approved a similar, but less expansive, catastrophic bill (S. 1127)[16] on October 27, 1987.

Both the House and Senate bills endorsed the need for improvements in the Medicare basic benefit package, but went beyond the administration's Medicare proposal in scope and comprehensiveness of benefits, limits on cost sharing, and provision of additional benefits. The Congressional bills also moved to relate financing burdens to income by using a supplemental income-related premium in combination with the flat Part B premium.

The bills differed in specifics rather than overall approach to benefit reform. The House bill included a more generous expansion of existing benefits, a broader drug benefit, and a lower cap on out-of-pocket spending for Part B services than did the Senate bill. The House bill also added new benefits, such as respite care, and provided direct assistance to the low-income population through mandated Medicaid improvements. Both bills employed an income-related supplemental premium to finance some of the expanded and new benefits, but the method for setting the premium liability as well as the distributional effects were notably different in the two bills.[17]

The joint House-Senate conference committee to resolve differences between the two versions of the legislation began in March of 1988 and completed its work in June. The final conference agreement reconciling the differences between the House and Senate bills incorporates key elements from both approaches.

The Medicare Catastrophic Coverage Act of 1988

The Medicare Catastrophic Coverage Act of 1988 offers improved Medicare coverage against the cost of serious illness to Medicare's 32 million aged and disabled beneficiaries. It expands coverage for existing Medicare benefits, adds new coverage for prescription drugs and routine mammography examinations, and relates the premium contribution to income after

Table 6.4. Key Medicare Provisions of the Catastrophic Coverage Act of 1988

Item	Legislative Provision
Inpatient Hospital Care	
Deductible ($564 in 1989)	One per year
Days covered	365 days per year
Copayments	None
Physician and Other Outpatient Services	
Deductible	$75.00
Copayments	20% of charges within limits allowed by Medicare
Cap	$1370 per year on charges within limits allowed by Medicare
Charges exceeding Medicare limits	Patient pays all
Skilled Nursing Facility Care	
Days covered	150 days per year
Copayments	$20.50/day (1989) for first 8 days
Requirement for prior hospitalization	Prior hospitalization not required
Prescription Drug Coverage	When fully implemented in 1993, Medicare pays 80% of costs above $710; in 1991, Medicare pays 50% of costs above $600
Respite Care	80 hours per year of home health services to relieve unpaid care providers, for certain beneficiaries
Home Health Care	Up to 38 days of care per illness, 7 days per week
Hospice Care	Extension beyond 210 days when patient recertified as terminally ill
Mammogram Coverage	Covers mammogram every other year
Financing	
Part B Premium	Additional premium of $4 per month in 1989, increasing to $10.20 in 1993
Income-Related Premium	New supplemental premium, administered through tax system, paid only by those with income tax liability of at least $150 (about 40% of all enrollees)

Source: Ref. 4.

payment of a flat premium. The scope of Medicare coverage as a result of the new provisions is summarized in Table 6.4.

Expanded Benefits

The 1988 legislation improves coverage for current Medicare hospital benefits by eliminating the current limits on covered hospital days and repealing the co-insurance requirements on extended hospital stays. Beneficiaries are still required to pay a hospital deductible, but the deductible is limited to a single payment per year (estimated at $564 in 1989). Thus, Medicare will now cover an unlimited number of days of inpatient hospital care after payment of a single annual hospital deductible. This provision limits hospital costs for the 2.2 million beneficiaries who pay more than a single hospital deductible each year. [18]

The legislation also improves extended care assistance under Medicare by restructuring the SNF benefit and co-insurance. Co-insurance for SNF care is no longer related to the hospital deductible. Instead, co-insurance is set at 20% of the national average per diem Medicare reasonable cost for SNF care, estimated to be about $20.50 per day in 1989. The new co-insurance is imposed on the first eight days of covered SNF care each year. After the first eight days, co-insurance is eliminated. In addition, the three-day prior hospitalization requirement for SNF benefits is eliminated and coverage is expanded from 100 to 150 days of care per year.

The legislation also expands the Medicare home health benefit and the hospice benefit. Home health care is expanded to permit care on a daily basis for up to 38 consecutive days and can be continued if deemed necessary by the physician. The current limitation requiring that care be "intermittent care" and not exceed five days per week for 21 days is overridden. The new law also provides that hospice care can be extended beyond the current 210-day limit if the beneficiary is certified as continuing to be terminally ill.

Ceiling on Out-of-Pocket Costs

A major feature of the catastrophic legislation is the maximum ceiling on out-of-pocket expenses for covered services under Part B. The legislation provides that after a beneficiary has incurred out-of-pocket expenses of over $1370 (in 1990) for Part B services, Medicare would pay 100% of the reasonable cost of any additional Part B services. In future years, the cap would be indexed, to maintain the percentage of Medicare enrollees exceeding the cap at 7% per year. Currently there is no limit on out-of-pocket spending for physician cost sharing. Approximately 2.2 million elderly and disabled beneficiaries have medical expenses in excess of the $1370 cap. [18]

Out-of-pocket expenses under Part B subject to the new cap include the Part B $75 deductible and the co-insurance of 20% required on Part B services. The $1370 limit applies only to Medicare-approved charges. Beneficiaries are still responsible for out-of-pocket costs associated with extra billing by physicians and for uncovered services, as well as for the prescription drug deductibles and co-insurance amounts.

New Benefits

The catastrophic legislation provides coverage of outpatient prescription drugs for the first time under Medicare. With the new benefit, Medicare will pay 50% of the cost of outpatient prescription drugs in excess of $600 per year in 1991. In 1992, Medicare's share of the costs increases to 60%, and in 1993, to 80%. Thus, when the benefit is fully phased in in 1993, the beneficiary will pay 20% co-insurance for drug expenditures in excess of the deductible. The deductible will be increased in future years to keep the percentage of beneficiaries helped by the provision at a constant 16.8%. This provision will assist 5.4 million beneficiaries.[4]

The new legislation also adds a respite care benefit for dependent beneficiaries. Under this provision, up to 80 hours per year of assistance from an outside aide is available to provide respite for families caring for beneficiaries at home. This benefit is available only to beneficiaries whose physician or drug expenditures exceed one of the catastrophic spending caps. It is notable that this is the first nonskilled long-term care benefit added to Medicare.

Mammography examinations as a preventive health measure are also added to Medicare by the new legislation. For women age 65 and over, mammography screening examinations will be covered every other year. For disabled Medicare beneficiaries, an annual screening is provided for women from ages 50 to 64. Younger disabled women are covered for baseline examinations with rescreenings every other year, or more frequently, if indicated. Again, coverage of a preventive service is new for Medicare.

Low-Income Provisions

The legislation is especially noteworthy in terms of the new protections it offers for the low-income elderly population. Medicaid supplemental coverage for the elderly and disabled is expanded by covering all poor elderly and disabled beneficiaries under the Medicare buy-in provision. States are required to pay Medicare premiums and cost sharing for elderly and disabled Medicare beneficiaries with incomes up to the federal poverty levels ($5770 per year for a single individual in 1988). Cost sharing covered by Medicaid includes both amounts for current benefits and new requirements from the catastrophic legislation. States can either fill in the Medicare deductible and co-insurance for prescription drugs or offer drug coverage through Medicaid.

Coverage up to the poverty level is phased in as a percentage of poverty between 1990 and 1993, and will provide assistance to 2 million low-income beneficiaries.[18] In addition, the legislation also requires states to extend coverage to pregnant women and infants up to 100% of the federal poverty level by 1990.

The legislation also liberalizes Medicaid rules for retention of income and assets by a spouse, living at home, of a Medicaid-eligible nursing home patient. The spouse of someone who must be in a nursing home and who needs Medicaid assistance may keep at least $786 of monthly income (122% of poverty for a two-person family) and at least $12,000 in liquid assets before income and assets are counted as available to help pay for nursing home care. By 1992, the monthly income set-aside increases to $970, approximately 150% of the federal poverty level. This provision will help to prevent spousal impoverishment.

Financing and Costs

The financing approach is one of the most creative and controversial aspects of the legislation emerging from Congress. In both the House and Senate bills, as well as in the original Reagan Administration proposal, the expanded and new Medicare benefits were financed by the Medicare beneficiaries themselves. The new legislation retains this approach, relying on the Medicare population to finance the benefit improvements. They are financed by a combination of an increase in the current Part B premium paid by all enrollees and a new supplemental premium that is related to income and collected through the income tax system.

The increase in the flat rate premium covers about 37% of the cost of new benefits. The flat premium will increase by $4 per month in 1989 to pay for expanded coverage. This premium increase will be added to the regular Part B premium of $24.50 that is paid by all beneficiaries. By 1993, the additional flat premium will be an estimated $10.20 per month.[4]

The new income-related supplemental premium covers the remaining 63% of benefit expansion costs. Beneficiaries will pay $22.50 for every $150 of federal income tax liability, up to a maximum income-related premium of $800 in 1989. The 60% of beneficiaries who pay less than $150 in income taxes per year will not be required to pay any supplemental premium. By 1993, the supplemental premium will rise to $42 per $150 of tax liability and the maximum payment will rise to $1050.[4]

The financing of catastrophic coverage is an important precedent in two respects. First, the reliance on premium financing rather than payroll tax or general revenue financing requires the elderly beneficiaries to pay for the new Medicare benefits, rather than having those costs borne by the non-elderly. This is a departure from the social insurance nature of Medicare Part A, which calls for employees and their employers to set aside a fixed percentage of earnings during their working years to pay for health benefits after retirement. In addition, for the first time in Medicare's history, higher-income elderly and disabled beneficiaries will be asked to pay a higher premium for coverage.

The new legislation is estimated to result in the increased spending of almost $30 billion under Medicare between 1989 and 1993. Virtually all of these costs will be financed by the new premiums paid by the elderly and disabled population. The low-income protections under Medicaid, however, will be financed by general revenues and state tax dollars for Medicaid. The increased Medicaid costs for states will be offset by savings resulting from broadened Medicare coverage.

Assessment of Catastrophic Coverage under Medicare

The final bill enacted by the Congress and signed into law by the president is a sweeping expansion in benefits for elderly and disabled people. The new legislation remedies the gaps in coverage for those with severe illness, adds prescription drug coverage, provides limited assistance for long-term care, and introduces progressive financing. It sets a controversial precedent for future financing reforms and opens the door for examination of other benefit improvements, most notably long-term care.

The major effect of the legislation is the improved protection it affords to Medicare's 32 million beneficiaries. Currently, people with long hospital stays, large doctor bills, and high drug expenses can incur thousands of dollars in health expenses that are not covered by Medicare. The catastrophic coverage legislation markedly reduces their burdens. It directly assists the 2.2 million beneficiaries who experience long or multiple hospital stays each year, over 2 million beneficiaries with high out-of-pocket costs for physician care, and the over 5 million beneficiaries with large drug expenses.[19]

The new law recognizes the need to provide special assistance with premiums and cost sharing for the low-income population. It mandates that, by 1993, state Medicaid programs cover these Medicare costs for all elderly and disabled beneficiaries with incomes below the poverty level. Currently, Medicaid covers less than one-third of poor elderly people.[10] This provision alone provides aid to another 2 million poor elderly people and ensures that all poor Medicare beneficiaries will be relieved of the current cost sharing and Part B premium obligations, as well as being protected against additional premium costs from the expanded catastrophic coverage.

The catastrophic plan provides important protection for the 6 million low- and modest-income elderly people who currently have neither Medicaid nor private Medigap insurance to supplement Medicare. They rely solely on Medicare to pay their health-care expenses and are most at risk of impoverishment from illness. The new $1370 limit on out-of-pocket spending for covered Medicare services provides catastrophic coverage for this group. Without this ceiling, an elderly person with an income of $10,000 who has only a moderate illness with one hospital episode could easily be required to pay $2500, one-fourth of his or her total income, for out-of-pocket medical expenses.

The 20 million Medicare beneficiaries who currently purchase private insurance coverage to supplement Medicare also stand to gain from the new measure. More extensive Medicare coverage should reduce premiums for private Medigap insurance or enable beneficiaries to purchase more comprehensive coverage at existing rates. Private policies will have to be rewritten in light of the new law. It is estimated that the new benefits in the bill could result in a reduction of about $35 per month in private insurance premium costs.[18] Thus, much of the increased cost for Medicare premiums should be offset by reduced payments for private coverage.

The net effects of the new benefits provided by the catastrophic legislation are protection for all elderly people with catastrophic expenses and reduction of the serious financial burdens on low-income elderly people. On the financing side, the cost of these new benefits is borne by Medicare beneficiaries as a group, with the greatest burden falling on higher-income elderly and disabled beneficiaries. As a result, the catastrophic provision redistributes total health-care expenses of beneficiaries away from the poor and sick to the relatively well-to-do.

The Medicare catastrophic protection reduces the risk of impoverishment from serious illness or injury for the nation's 32 million Medicare beneficiaries and provides an important and significant expansion of coverage for elderly and disabled Americans. Yet, as essential as this improved protection is for the beneficiaries with substantial medical burdens, the substantial catastrophic costs associated with long-term nursing home care remain unaddressed by this legislation.

Nursing home and community-based care for the frail elderly population continue to be priorities for legislative action. By bringing new attention to the high out-of-pocket payments many Medicare beneficiaries face for long-term care services, passage of the catastrophic coverage act could serve as a catalyst for long-term care reform in the future.

References

1. Davis, K., Rowland, D. 1986. *Medicare Policy: New Directions for Health and Long-Term Care.* Baltimore, Md.: Johns Hopkins University Press.
2. Congressional Budget Office. 1986. Testimony by Nancy Gordon before the

Subcommittee on Health and the Environment, U.S. House of Representatives, Hearing on Health Care for the Elderly, March 26. Serial No. 99–139. Washington, D.C.: Government Printing Office.

3. United States House of Representatives, Ways and Means Committee. 1988. *Background Materials and Data on Programs within the Jurisdiction of the Committee on Ways and Means.* WMC Pub. No. 100–29. Washington, D.C.: Government Printing Office.

4. Democratic Study Group of the United States Congress. 1988. Medicare Conference Report: Catastrophic Illness Protection. Fact Sheet No. 100–39. Washington, D.C.: Democratic Study Group of the United States Congress.

5. Burney, I., Paradise, J. 1987. Medicare physician participation. *Health Aff* 6(2):107–120.

6. Congressional Budget Office. 1987. *A Comparison of Selected Catastrophic Bills* (Study Paper). July 30. Washington, D.C.: Congressional Budget Office.

7. United States House of Representatives, Ways and Means Committee. 1987. *Background Materials and Data on Programs within the Jurisdiction of the Committee on Ways and Means.* WMC Pub. No. 100–4. Washington, D.C.: Government Printing Office.

8. Waldo, D., Lazenby, H. 1984. Demographic characteristics and health care use and expenditures by the aged in the United States, 1977–1984. *Health Care Financing Rev* 6(1):1–29.

9. United States Senate, Special Committee on Aging. 1984. *Medicare and the Health Costs of Older Americans: The Extent and Effects of Cost-Sharing.* Washington, D.C.: Government Printing Office.

10. Commonwealth Fund, Commission on Elderly People Living Alone. 1987. *Medicare's Poor.* Baltimore, Md.: Commission on Elderly People Living Alone.

11. Advisory Council on Social Security. 1983. *Medicare Benefits and Financing.* 1982 Report. Washington, D.C.: Government Printing Office.

12. Bowen, O., Burke, T. 1985. Cost neutral catastrophic care proposed for Medicare recipients. *Fed Am Hosp Rev,* 42–45.

13. United States Department of Health and Human Services. 1986. *Department of Health and Human Services Report to the President: Catastrophic Illness Expenses.* Washington, D.C.: United States Department of Health and Human Services.

14. United States Congress. 1987. H. R. 1245/S. 592 Medicare Catastrophic Illness Coverage Act. Administration bill. Washington, D.C.: United States Congress.

15. United States House of Representatives. 1987. H. R. 2470. Medicare Catastrophic Protection Act of 1987. July 22.

16. United States Senate. 1987. S. 1127. Medicare Catastrophic Loss Prevention Act of 1987. October 27.

17. Davis, K. 1987. Medicare financing and beneficiary income. *Inquiry* 24(Winter):309–323.

18. Congressional Budget Office. 1988. Final Cost Estimates on Conference Agreement on H. R. 2470.

19. Foley, T., Michel, R., Rostenkowski, D., et al. 1988. *Dear Colleague on Medicare Catastrophic Act of 1988.* June 1. Washington, D.C.: United States House of Representatives.

Seven

Paying for Long-Term Care

Judith Feder and William J. Scanlon

Except for the very rich, paying the bill for extensive long-term care (LTC) means financial catastrophe. While public or private insurance is available to protect against other catastrophes, such as extended stays in the hospital, neither private nor public insurance protects against the financial crisis of LTC. Current financing for LTC draws on individuals' own resources, backed up by Medicaid.

This pattern of financing reflects private insurers' aversion to the risks involved in addressing the LTC problem and government's limited willingness or ability to compensate for the lack of private insurance protection. The federal government has largely ignored the LTC issue, shifting responsibility to the states. As a result, both resources for and commitment to financing LTC vary considerably from place to place.

The problems of financing LTC are well known, but fiscal concerns have inhibited governmental intervention to solve them. Instead, attention has turned to the private sector as a prime source of LTC financing. This chapter describes what we can expect from the private sector in the financing of LTC. Private resources can be better utilized to finance LTC, but the

Another version of this chapter was presented at the forum "Strategies, Services, Structures," sponsored by the Office of Aging and Long-Term Care of the Hospital Research and Educational Trust, American Hospital Association, February 13, 1984. Preparation of the paper was funded by the Ford Foundation.

factors that have limited privately financed protection in the past will limit
that protection in the future. Given those limits, government remains
responsible for ensuring adequate financing for LTC. Although political
and fiscal barriers may inhibit the enactment of broad social insurance,
protection can be improved in the immediate future through incremental
changes in existing public programs. (A detailed overview of the nature of
long-term care services is found in Brody and Magel, Chapter 13).

Private Financing for Long-Term Care

The success of private financing for LTC depends largely on the resources of
actual and potential service users—the elderly or near elderly. Improvements in Social Security and private pensions have clearly strengthened
elderly citizens' financial positions, and further improvement can be expected over the coming decades. Despite these improvements, however,
about one-fourth of the elderly had incomes below $5000 in 1984 and
could hardly be expected to finance their LTC. Even in the year 2000, at
least 20% of the elderly will have no private pensions, and many pensioners
will have limited benefits. Women, in particular, will remain disadvantaged, since pensions may not extend to survivors.[1]

Although many elderly have limited incomes, some analysts believe it
will be possible to enhance the elderly's contributions to LTC financing.
Advocates of enhanced private financing promote two types of action:
mobilizing the elderly's assets—independent of income—to facilitate purchase of LTC services or insurance, and broadening the marketing of
affordable LTC insurance, which could spread the burden of financing LTC
beyond the individuals who actually need service. Efforts to make insurance affordable include initiatives to promote more efficient delivery of
LTC services. The various proposals have potential limits as well as merits
that should be kept in mind.

Mobilizing Individuals' Resources to Purchase Long-Term Care

Recognition of income limitations among the elderly has spurred interest
in unconventional means to mobilize the elderly's resources. Prominent
among these innovations are reverse annuity mortgages, which enable the
elderly to convert their home equity into income while continuing to live
in their homes.[2] Under such arrangements, an older person's home is
promised as repayment for a loan that is used to purchase an annuity that is
paid out in monthly installments, ideally over the remainder of the borrower's life. Repayment, or transfer of the home's ownership, occurs when
the borrower dies. An alternative arrangement with similar effects is the

sale lease-back, whereby the elderly actually sell their homes but use the proceeds to pay rent while they continue to live there.

These arrangements are attractive because most of the elderly, even the low-income elderly, own their own homes, many of which have appreciated substantially over the years. Eighty percent of all elderly people and 65% of the elderly poor are homeowners. Their average equity is estimated at over $50,000, a level reached even by about one-fifth of the poor elderly.[2] Analyses indicate that reverse annuity mortgages could improve the liquid financial resources of the elderly considerably. Jacobs and Weissert estimate that about one-third of all the elderly could receive over $2000 per year by converting their homes to annuities. Home equity is therefore worthy of consideration as a potential source of LTC financing.

Currently, lending institutions do not allow the elderly to make use of the equity in their homes. Lenders typically require that borrowers not only offer their homes as collateral but also have a steady and reliable source of income for the life of the loan. An elderly person who has already retired and who may die before the term of the loan is unlikely to satisfy these conditions.

Despite the advantages to the elderly of changing these practices, lenders may not be willing to offer reverse annuity mortgages. These new types of mortgages involve a marriage of the insurance and mortgage industries. For each, reverse annuity mortgages represent a departure from traditional practice. Mortgage lenders are not used to contracts with indefinite terms based on life expectancy. Neither mortgage lenders nor insurers are used to accepting real property as repayment. Reluctance to undertake new ventures is compounded by potential individual lenders' relatively small volume of loans. A single lender with a limited number of elderly borrowers could suffer severe losses from a few individuals' unexpectedly long lives.

If lenders are willing to offer reverse annuity mortgages despite these risks, they can be expected to take measures to protect themselves. For example, lenders may limit annuities to a fixed term, taking over the borrower's home at a specified time, whether or not the borrower is still alive. A less traumatic but still problematic protection would be the lender's undervaluing of the home. Lower valuations could reduce the utility of reverse annuity mortgages for LTC financing and would reduce the attractiveness of such mortgages to the elderly.

Advocates of reverse annuity mortgages have suggested addressing these problems through public mortgage insurance, which would reduce the risks lenders face and, therefore, the likelihood of undesirable lending practices. By providing mortgage insurance, the public sector might encourage development of reverse annuity mortgages and enable many elderly people to make use of their home equity. Such loans might be limited to persons needing LTC services who are likely to use the funds for that purpose. Enabling these persons to buy in-home services might forestall their use of a nursing home at government expense.

However, reverse annuity mortgages are unlikely to provide very many elderly with sufficient resources to finance the cost of nursing home care. Furthermore, relying on individuals to finance such costly and unpredictable needs runs counter to the typical approach to protection against catastrophe. It concentrates the financial burden of severe impairment, an unpredictable event, on the unlucky few who experience it, rather than spreading the financial burden among the many who *could* become impaired. When LTC need represents a catastrophe, insurance is the appropriate method of financing.

Expansion of Private Long-Term Care Insurance

Insurance works by collecting premium income from a large group of people and using that income to pay for the care received by a small proportion of the group. Unless insurers can be certain that the insured population is much larger than the population likely to get benefits, the policy becomes either too risky to market or too expensive for consumers to buy. Insurers have been reluctant to offer LTC insurance largely because they fear that only persons likely to use services will buy it.

In addition to fearing "adverse selection," insurers fear "moral hazard": the likelihood that, once insured, people will increase their use of service. Although all health insurance raises this possibility, its occurrence is more likely in LTC. Even the unimpaired might find the nonprofessional services making up LTC attractive, and limiting services to persons truly in "need" is very difficult. Higher use than anticipated, like adverse selection, raises the prospect of serious losses, and inhibits the development of private insurance policies for LTC.

Advocates of private insurance for LTC believe the fears of potential insurers are exaggerated. They argue that many elderly, not just the about-to-be-impaired, would purchase LTC insurance if it were available at a reasonable price. They also argue that policies can be designed to minimize moral hazard and keep prices reasonable by limiting coverage to nursing homes, excluding home care, and providing coverage only after an initial 90-day nursing home stay.[3]

Despite these arguments, insurers themselves remain wary of the LTC market.[4] In 1987, only about 400,000 LTC insurance policies were in force—double the number for 1986 but still representing a tiny store of potential elderly users.[5] Furthermore, even existing policies appear to be marketed in ways that limit insurers' risk of adverse selection and, accordingly, limit the population that can obtain protection. Insurers avoid poor risks by denying coverage for reasons of age or poor health status, and they seek good risks by focusing marketing efforts on relatively wealthy, healthy, and young elderly people.[6] These people are attractive to insurers because they are unlikely to need LTC for some time and they provide a steady stream of premium income.

For the population able to purchase insurance, insurers' efforts to protect themselves against moral hazard may also limit the policies' value. Reputable insurers are reluctant to offer policies that require careful monitoring and utilization control because of the expense and because of negative repercussions from not paying benefits that policyholders, however mistakenly, have come to expect. Hence they protect themselves against financial risk in other ways, including "capping" the total dollar value of benefits, limiting the number of days or visits covered, including large deductibles, specifying benefits in dollar amounts (indemnity benefits), rather than services covered, and raising premiums with age and over time.[7] Specifying indemnity benefits and raising premiums over time also protect the insurer against inflation, another major concern. These limits mean that even people who can get private LTC insurance face a financial risk if their expenses exceed covered levels.

Finally, if LTC policies follow the acute-care insurance model, purchase of an insurance policy would not guarantee the availability of benefits when need arises. In standard health insurance policies, failure to pay premiums for a given year brings an end to insurance coverage, regardless of how many previous years premiums had been paid. Thus, even healthy, relatively wealthy elderly may exhaust their ability to maintain their protection if they live a very long time. An alternative to this arrangement would be to model LTC insurance on various types of nonterm life insurance. Premiums on nonterm life insurance entitle policyholders to some benefits even if premium payments stop.

How attractive LTC insurance policies are to those elderly whom insurers are willing to insure also remains an open question. When the elderly buy standard health insurance, they are protecting themselves against an event, use of medical care, that has a reasonably high probability of occurring in any given year. When benefits are limited, for example to extended nursing home stays, a 65-year-old is very unlikely to need such care, not only in any single year for which premiums apply, but over a lifetime. A person who buys LTC insurance at age 65 might pay 10 years of premiums before drawing benefits, or might die without ever having received any benefits at all. If consumers view drawing benefits as an unlikely occurrence, policies will be marketable only if premiums are very modest.

Combining Insurance and Service Delivery

Innovation linking new forms of insurance and service delivery may alleviate some of the problems with traditional insurance. Providers of LTC can themselves become insurers by agreeing to provide an enrolled population *all* needed services in return for fixed fees, paid in advance. Since the provider *is* the insurer, this arrangement provides an incentive to keep service delivery in line with available resources, and controls on service use reduce some of the insurer's financial risks. But there are risks even with these arrangements, and protection is likely to remain limited in the population and benefits covered.

Two prominent examples of the insurance/provider arrangement are the social health maintenance organization (SHMO) and the life-care community. The SHMO, like the HMO, charges a fixed annual rate and provides all covered services as needed over the year. Unlike the HMO, however, the SHMO includes LTC as well as acute-care services and focuses its efforts on efficient overall care to the elderly. The hope behind the SHMO is that savings from more efficient acute-care delivery will support LTC at affordable rates.[8] (SHMOs are discussed in detail in Greenberg et al., Chapter 11.)

Life-care communities offer a different arrangement and different types of efficiencies.[9] In return for an entry fee (averaging about $35,000 in 1980) and a monthly fee (averaging about $560 in 1980), life-care communities agree to provide residents the full range of LTC services, as needed. By gathering large numbers of elderly in one place, life-care communities may be able to provide in-home services less expensively and, in many cases, forestall or prevent the need for more intensive care.

By delivering care more efficiently, SHMOs and life-care communities aim to mitigate the financial risks of insuring LTC. Neither's potential has been fully tested, but both appear to have some limitations. To keep capitation rates attractive and avoid financial risk, pioneer SHMOs have had to limit their nursing home benefits, exposing enrollees to continued risk.[10] Similarly, life-care communities restrict entry to the healthy and, with increasing frequency, are charging additional fees for intensive service.[11] Therefore, even their residents may face catastrophic costs when they need a lot of care.

Expectations for the Private Sector

Over all, then, what can the private sector contribute to LTC financing? Increased and more liquid resources may enable more elderly to purchase care as they need it and to purchase insurance in advance of that need. Simultaneously, innovations in service delivery may reduce the prices paid for services or insurance, thereby expanding the scope and duration of protection. However, private financing will also have limitations. Some people will have inadequate resources to purchase service and will have a combination of resource and health limitations that make them uninsurable in the private market, some will find insurance an unattractive investment, and some of the insured will face expenses that insurance will not cover. Clearly, public financing will need to cover the people and the essential services that the private sector leaves out.

Government's Role in Financing Long-Term Care

To those who believe that all persons, regardless of income, should have equal protection against the financial risks of severe impairment, the only adequate solution to LTC problems is a public insurance system, incorporated in or added to the Medicare program. Insurance spreads the cost of a catastrophic event beyond its victims, and only public insurance can be expected to finance both current victims and the poor, providing all individuals protection against catastrophic expenses. Moreover, only public insurance can be expected to risk the cost of covering the full range of LTC services, including in-home services that can maximize personal independence. Finally, only *federal* insurance can provide all impaired persons equal protection, regardless of their place of residence.

The argument for a public LTC program modeled on Medicare is buttressed by Medicare's successes, but burdened by its failures. Medicare has been highly successful in protecting the elderly against catastrophic acute-care expenses, thereby reducing financial barriers to using care, but has had great difficulty controlling the costs that accompanied its access gains.

Recognizing this fact, advocates of universal LTC insurance based on the Medicare model include in their designs arrangements to contain costs. Some have claimed that these arrangements could make service delivery so efficient that all persons in need of LTC could be served without an increase in total health-care spending.[12]

Even with improved efficiency, it is hard to believe that truly adequate LTC could be provided at no extra cost. Because so many people are currently unserved, new service will almost certainly produce extra costs. Experience indicates that offering new services does not reduce total cost, even if the new services are intended as cheaper substitutes for existing services, such as nursing homes for hospitals and home care for nursing home care. Expanding service not only allows some efficient substitution but also expands the population receiving care.[13]

Expansion of service and increased costs are particularly likely with LTC. Existing public programs barely provide for home care,[14] which advocates of public LTC insurance strongly support, and in many places nursing home care is not sufficiently available for those who need it. Research indicates that in the 10 states with the fewest beds per elderly person, 50% of those most in need of nursing home care (unmarried persons age 75 or older needing help in all aspects of personal functioning) were still in the community, compared to only 10% in the states with the greatest number of beds per elderly person.[15] Given the gaps a new program would have to fill, promising that a major new program will involve no costs at all seems unreasonable.

The likelihood of increased costs should not inhibit efforts to promote universal social insurance for LTC. As long as economic and political pressure impedes major increases in government spending, however, advocates of improved LTC financing should also pursue improvements in last-resort protection for those least able to cope in the current system: the poor and near poor. Although a means-tested program may not give these persons protection or service equal to that obtained by those better off, in the short term it may offer the most feasible way to improve the lot of people who need care they cannot afford.

Improvements should take two forms: 1) enhancement of Medicaid, the current program of last resort, to provide more equitable and adequate protection against the expenses of LTC; and 2) enhancement of Medicare to protect individuals against the catastrophic expense of even a short-term need for LTC services.

Medicaid's current problems derive from its limited eligibility and limited funds. Its tie to poverty is probably its most widely recognized problem. To become eligible for Medicaid, a nursing home resident must contribute all resources (except $25 per month) toward the cost of care. This contribution may not be unreasonable for a single individual becoming a permanent resident in the nursing home, but it is clearly a problem to a person whose spouse depends on shared income and savings and remains at home. Giving up shared income or assets may force that spouse to live near the poverty level or reduce the resources available to finance his or her present or future care needs.

Although they are serious, eligibility restrictions are by no means Medicaid's only limitations. Rising costs and constrained state budgets have made Medicaid cost containment a major issue in most states. In turn, efforts to contain costs have prevented Medicaid programs from covering a full range of LTC services and have inhibited access even to those services it theoretically covers.

Although the federal government offers to match state spending for in-home as well as nursing home services, states have been reluctant to take advantage of this option for fear of increased costs.[14] Economic concerns have also limited the availability of covered services to persons eligible for care.[16] In attempting to control nursing home costs, which absorb more than one-third of their Medicaid budgets, states have limited the supply of nursing home beds, either by paying low rates for Medicaid patients or by invoking certificate-of-need regulations to prevent expansion. Most states have not simultaneously tightened their eligibility rules to reduce the number of Medicaid-eligible persons seeking care. As a result, more Medicaid-eligible patients seek nursing home beds than there are beds available.

By limiting the total bed supply, states create a "seller's market," and nursing homes can favor more-profitable patients over less-profitable patients. Nursing homes prefer private-pay patients over Medicaid patients, who pay less than private rates, and they also choose among Medicaid patients. Because most Medicaid programs do not vary rates sufficiently to reflect differences in patients' care needs and care costs, nursing homes prefer patients who need less care. The Medicaid patient in need of the most intensive nursing home care, the patient most appropriately placed in a nursing home, has the hardest time finding a bed.

This population and the burden of caring for it are likely to increase because access barriers to Medicaid-eligible heavy-care patients are likely to worsen. Constraints on the bed supply will prevent it from keeping pace with the growth of the elderly population. Furthermore, competition for beds will grow as earlier hospital discharges, generated in response to Medicare's prospective payment system, create more short-term nursing home patients. Many of these patients will be attractive to nursing homes because they are private-pay, or because hospitals find it advantageous to reward nursing homes that take certain numbers of their discharges. This new demand for beds by short-stay patients will further limit access for long-term, heavy-care Medicaid patients.

Changes in federal Medicaid policy could alleviate the fiscal pressure that leads to inadequate protection and could actively promote broader Medicaid coverage. Excessive pressure to contain costs derives in part from an inequitable distribution of federal resources under Medicaid's current financing arrangements. Although federal matching funds compensate to some degree for variations in states' ability to pay, the federal government's share of Medicaid costs varies only with a state's per capita income. It does not vary with the different needs for care determined by the size and characteristics of different states' elderly populations. Were these factors incorporated in the Medicaid matching formula, states with a greater need for service would get more money, enhancing their ability to provide reasonable levels of care.

However, simply providing more money does not guarantee that it will be well spent. Federal incentives or standards potentially could influence eligibility, the scope of services covered, the methods of paying providers, and the mechanism for controlling use. The Medicare Catastrophic Cover-

age Act of 1988 assures equity across states by requiring federally determined minimum resource standards that better protect the income and
assets of spouses remaining at home. (The Medicare Catastrophic Coverage Act of 1988 is discussed in detail in Rowland, et al., Chapter 6.)
Promotion of access and efficiency may necessitate federal requirements
that rates paid to providers ensure minimum levels of access, that rates vary
with patients' care needs and reward investment in patient care, and that
pre-admission screening be used to ensure appropriate use of institutional
and noninstitutional care. Several states have already adopted payment
and review mechanisms to promote access to care and efficient service
delivery. More federal money and federal requirements or incentives would
help bring other states along.

These measures could substantially improve Medicaid's protection
against the costs of truly long-term care, but they would do little to protect
the individuals whose short-term need for LTC services following an acute
illness could also be catastrophic. Theoretically, Medicare provides that
protection, since it covers short-term skilled nursing or rehabilitation services after an acute stay, but in practice Medicare's protection is limited.
Currently, unless patients are receiving one or more clearly defined skilled
service, Medicare covers their care only as long as they are in need of skilled
service due to their "unstable" medical condition (either improving or
declining). Focusing on instability and the need for skilled care protects
Medicare against financing long-term maintenance care for an impaired
person who is neither dying nor getting better, but it also precludes coverage for recuperating patients in need of supportive personal care, not
skilled care. Therefore, although Medicare offers up to 150 days of care in a
skilled nursing facility, average coverage is less than 30 days. Similarly,
Medicare's home health benefit potentially covered 200 visits per person
before 1981 and today allows potentially unlimited coverage, but in actu-
ality provides an average of 23 visits per beneficiary.[17]

The termination of Medicare benefits does not necessarily mean an end
to patients' service needs. What ends is the narrowly defined need for
skilled care on which Medicare coverage depends. Need for service may go
well beyond that point. The average Medicare patient stays in the nursing
home 30 days beyond termination of Medicare coverage.[18] Need for home
care may also continue beyond termination of coverage, although there is
no information to confirm this.

Given Medicare's "skilled care" criterion and its effective enforcement
through claims review, even individuals whose need for assistance in personal care and support is short term are exposed to considerable financial
risk, particularly if they need care in a nursing home. Without committing
Medicare to LTC insurance, Medicare's short-term nursing home benefit
could be refined and expanded to truly protect the elderly from the finan-

cial catastrophe of recuperation from acute illness. Medicare could en-hance its protection by covering personal care services during recupera-tion, even when patients are not technically unstable and require no skilled services. The result would be a substantial but not uncontrollable expansion of Medicare coverage. At a minimum, benefits would probably increase from the 28-day average Medicare-covered stay to the 58-day average actual stay for patients receiving some Medicare coverage.

These marginal but significant adjustments to LTC financing are not, for the most part, in conflict with the development of innovations in private insurance and delivery. Better-off elderly people will take advantage of relatively expensive private insurance mechanisms, protecting their assets for posterity and reducing the pressure on public programs. Public and private insurance programs alike can take advantage of innovative delivery mechanisms (like the SHMO) that attempt to promote efficient service use. At the same time, public programs will provide more secure and equitable assurance that care will be available and affordable when people need it.

The overall system, however, will continue to be fragmented and to be characterized by heavy reliance on individual resources, a limited role for private insurance, and an extensive role for means-tested financing. The alternative to this fragmentation and inequity is a potentially costly social insurance program that many may favor in theory but has yet to gain support in practice.

References

1. Zedlewski, S. 1984. Microsimulation of the private pension system: Four pro-jections to the year 2000. In *Brookings Conference on Retirement and Aging, Fall 1982*. Washington, D.C.: Brookings Institution.
2. Jacobs, B., Weissert, W. 1984. Home equity financing of long-term care for the elderly. In *Long-Term Care Financing and Delivery Systems: Exploring Some Alter-natives*. Conference Proceedings, January 24. Washington, D.C.: Government Printing Office.
3. Meiners, M. R. 1983. The case for long-term care insurance. *Health Aff* 2(2):55–79.
4. Lifson, A. 1984. Long-term care: An insurer's perspective. In *Long-Term Care Financing and Delivery Systems: Exploring Some Alternatives*. Conference Proceed-ings, January 24. Washington, D.C.: Government Printing Office.
5. United States Department of Health and Human Services. September 21, 1987. *Report to Congress and the Secretary by the Task Force on Long-Term Health Care Politics*. Washington, D.C.: Government Printing Office.

6. Phillips, R. F. 1984. The Fireman Fund's experience. In *Long-Term Care Financing and Delivery Systems: Exploring Some Alternatives.* Conference Proceedings, January 24. Washington, D.C.: Government Printing Office.
7. See Ref. 5 and United States General Accounting Office. May 1987. Long-term care coverage varies widely in a developing market. Report to Chairman of Subcommittee on Health and Long-Term Care Select Committee on Aging, House of Representatives. HRD 87–80.
8. Diamond, L. M., Berman, D. E. 1981. The social/health maintenance organization. In *Reforming the Long-Term Care System.* ed. J. J. Callahan, Jr. and S. S. Wallack. Lexington, Mass.: Lexington Books.
9. Winklevoss, M. E., Powell, A. V. 1984. *Continuing Care Retirement Communities.* Homewood, Ill.: Richard D. Irwin.
10. Greenberg, J. N., Leutz, W. N. 1984. The social/health maintenance organization and its role in reforming the long-term care system. In *Long-Term Care Financing and Delivery Systems: Exploring Some Alternatives.* Conference Proceedings, January 24. Washington, D.C.: Government Printing Office.
11. Pies, H. E. 1984. Life care committees for the aged—an overview. In *Long-Term Care Financing and Delivery Systems: Exploring Some Alternatives.* Conference Proceedings, January 24. Washington, D.C.: Government Printing Office.
12. Somers, A. R. 1984. Long-term care for the elderly and disabled: A new priority. *N Engl J Med* 37(4):221–226.
13. United States General Accounting Office. 1982. The Elderly Should Benefit from Expanding Health Care but Increasing These Services Will Not Insure Cost Reduction. *Report to the Congress by the Comptroller General.* IPE-83-1. Washington, D.C.: Government Printing Office.
14. Cohen, J. 1983. *Public Programs Financing Long-Term Care.* Washington, D.C.: National Governors Association.
15. Weissert, W., Scanlon, W. 1983. Determinants of institutionalization of the aged. In *Project to Analyze Existing Long-Term Care Data, Final Report.* Vol. 3. Washington, D.C.: Department of Health and Human Services, Office of Assistant Secretary for Planning and Evaluation.
16. Feder, J., Scanlon, W. 1980. Regulating the bed supply in nursing homes. *Milbank Memorial Fund Q* 58(1):54–88.
17. Sulvetta, M. B. 1983. Causes of increased Medicare spending for home health. Working paper 1466–26. Washington, D.C.: Urban Institute.
18. National Center for Health Statistics. 1977. Unpublished statistics from *National Nursing Home Survey.*

Eight

Toward National Health Insurance

Philip R. Lee and Carroll L. Estes

Health care for the elderly should not be viewed in isolation from health care for the population at large. As the other chapters in this section make clear, public policy issues facing the American health-care system today are financing and costs. Reforms that focus exclusively on the elderly will not resolve current problems in either area.

There are few who doubt the need for reform in the organization and financing of health care. Disagreements arise, however, the moment a specific reform is proposed. Several basic approaches to health-care reform have been adopted in recent years: 1) the pluralist, procompetitive, or market approach; 2) the bureaucratic, or planning approach; and 3) the institutional or structural approach, which has had fewer advocates.[1] Proponents of each of these approaches argue that their proposed reforms will lead to cost containment, improved quality, or assured access. However, it is not easy to propose reforms that, while just and equitable, also provide patients with both reasonable access and adequate services at an affordable cost. A key issue related to the elderly is whether these objectives can be achieved through a continued age-segregated approach, as exemplified in the Medicare program, or whether an age-integrated approach will be required.

Goals of a National Health-Care Policy

The first step in designing a comprehensive but affordable system of health care is to agree upon goals or purposes. It is also essential to clarify the roles of the public and private sectors and the respective roles of the federal, state, and local governments.[2] Medicare's purposes were clear in the beginning: access to mainstream medical care for the elderly, protection for the elderly and their families against the high costs of health care, and support for the prevailing, fee-for-service model of health care. Today, health-care cost containment, particularly Medicare cost containment, appears to be the primary goal of federal health policy. Reducing the role of the federal government and decentralizing or transferring program authority and responsibility from the federal government to the state and local governments and to the private sector also were priorities of the Reagan Administration. This is exemplified by policies affecting Medicaid and by a range of domestic programs that were transferred to state responsibility, reduced in scope, or eliminated under the banner of "new federalism." In these policy shifts some of the broader goals of a national health-care policy have been obscured.

In its 1983 report, the President's Commission for the Study of Ethical Problems in Medicine and Biomedical and Behavioral Research provided an ethical perspective on, and a clear statement of, society's obligation related to health care:

> The Commission concludes that society has an ethical obligation to ensure equitable access to health care for all. This obligation rests on the special importance of health care: its role in relieving suffering, preventing premature death, restoring functioning, increasing opportunity, providing information about an individual's condition and giving evidence of mutual empathy and compassion. Furthermore, although life style and the environment can affect health status, differences in the need for health care are for the most part undeserved and not within an individual's control.

The President's Commission also observed:

> When equity occurs through the operation of private forces, there is no need for government involvement, but the ultimate responsibility for ensuring [that] society's obligation is met, through a combination of public and private sector arrangements, rests with the Federal government.[3]

In the present climate of rising health-care costs and cost containment, and with the growing emphasis on competition and the role of the marketplace in solving cost, access, and quality issues, doubt is growing about the nation's willingness to design and pay for an equitable system of health care.

The Rising Costs of Health Care

Translating the goal of equitable access to adequate health care for all into specific policies, programs, and services requires an understanding of the factors that affect the rising costs of health care. The structural conditions that have produced the rising costs represent the most formidable barrier to the adoption of a national policy for health-care financing consistent with the goals of the President's Commission for the Study of Ethical Problems in Medicine and Biomedical and Behavioral Research.

Several factors have led to increased spending for health care. These include the oversupply of physicians, the growth of complex technologies, the growth in the third-party payment system (public and private, including the incentives for the purchase of private health insurance), the financial incentives for physicians and hospitals to provide more and more services, and the lack of incentives for consumers or third parties to constrain costs.[4]

Physician Supply: A Major Factor in Future Cost Increases

Physician supply and the continued expansion of hospital resources (e.g., new technologies) remain unresolved problems related to controlling costs. Physician supply has been affected dramatically by federal and state policies since the early 1960s; as a result, the problem has been changed from physician shortage to oversupply and specialty maldistribution.[5]

Physician supply in the United States reached 444,000 in 1980, exceeding congressional goals and federal estimates of need. The Graduate Medical Education National Advisory Committee has predicted an oversupply of 70,000 physicians by 1990, representing a growth rate of 40% between 1978 and 1990.[6] Although anticipated population growth will moderate the increase to 30% on a per capita basis,[7] this rate of increase will exceed the rate of growth of the past two decades and will come at a time of slower economic growth and dramatic changes in health-care financing and organization. The result will be a significant reduction of the resources available to each physician.[8] These constraints are already being felt in areas of the country where physicians are in oversupply (e.g., San Francisco).

Over the past four decades there has been a trend toward fragmentation of medicine into more specialties and subspecialties, due to advances in biomedical research and technology. The decade ahead is likely to see a continuation of that trend. Significantly, health-care financing is a key factor in the growth and support of technology-based specialties and subspecialties, since present Medicare, Medicaid, and private health insurance physician reimbursement policies reward procedure-based specialties instead of primary care specialties. Furthermore, the new Medicare hospi-

tal reimbursement policy of "passing through" the costs of medical education is likely to aggravate the problem. The policy leaves decisions about
physician supply and the mix of specialties in the hands of medical schools,
teaching hospitals, and the chiefs of the very specialty services (e.g.,
surgical subspecialties) already in oversupply.

Currently, there is a vacuum in federal policies with respect to physician
supply, while Medicare and Medicaid policies take different and conflicting
courses with respect to physician payment. It is difficult to predict how the
conflicting trends in health policy—health-care cost containment through
state regulation of providers, increased emphasis on competition and market strategies at the federal level, and a continued increase in physician
supply due to a policy vacuum at both the federal and state level—will play
out in the next decade. Clearly, a coherent set of manpower policies are
needed that are integrated with policies related to payment for services and
the organization of care.

Health-Care Financing: The Role of the Individual and Third Parties (Public and Private)

If health-care costs are to be contained in the future, constraints must be
placed not only on physician supply and specialty distribution, but also on
other real resource inputs into health care.[9] In addition to the general
trend in the economy (e.g., inflation or the lack of inflation), a critical
factor in the growth of health-care resources and costs has been third-party
payments and the reimbursement policies of third-party payers.

Between 1950 and 1965, private health insurance coverage expanded
rapidly, increasing enrollment through employer-based plans and more
than doubling its share of health-care expenditures from 9.1% to 24% of
total health-care expenditures in the United States. Since 1965, the private health insurance companies' and other private third parties' share of
total health-care spending has stabilized at about 30 to 31% of personal
health-care expenditures. Private health insurance is limited primarily to
hospital and physician services and covers about 35% of hospital costs and
35% of physician costs.[10]

Direct out-of-pocket payments by individuals are also important. According to recent estimates from the Health Care Financing Administration, in 1987 direct payments by individuals accounted for approximately
25% of total health-care expenditures in the United States, while public
programs (e.g., Medicare, Medicaid, local government) accounted for
41%.[11] In contrast, consumers have paid only about 6% of total costs in the
United Kingdom, 8.5% in Sweden, and 12.5% in West Germany. In
Canada, France, and Australia, consumers have paid approximately
20%.[12]

The share of expenditures borne directly out of pocket varies by type of service. In 1987, consumers paid directly out of pocket approximately 9% of hospital costs, 49% of nursing home costs, 26% of physician services, 61% of dental services, and 75% of the cost of drugs and drug sundries. [11]

The changing nature of the economy, particularly the growth of jobs in the service sector and the 1981–82 recession, and the lack of national commitment to health care for unemployed, the working poor, and undocumented aliens have produced a growing population of uninsured and underinsured. According to data from the National Medical Care Expenditure Survey, 24 to 37% of the U.S. population under the age of 65 had inadequate health insurance coverage in 1977. Of these, 9% were uninsured throughout the year and an additional 9% were uninsured part of the year. Between 5% and 15% were considered underinsured. [13] Over the past decade, the situation has deteriorated. Although it might be expected that the number of insured would increase, data from the 1984 Census Bureau survey showed that approximately 17% of the population under age 65 years (or about 35 million people) lacked any health insurance, and the number had increased more than 20% between 1979 and 1984. [14]

A significant factor contributing to the increase in the number of uninsured was the policy change in 1981 (Omnibus Budget Reconciliation Act of 1981) that permitted states to reduce Medicaid eligibility. This change, coupled with Medicaid cutbacks in the late 1970s, has had serious consequences for the poor, particularly the working poor. Between 1975 and 1983 the proportion of low-income Americans insured by Medicaid fell from 63% to 46%. This drop occurred while the number of Americans, particularly women younger than 65 and children, living at or below 125% of the federal poverty level, was increasing. [15]

Another important development affecting health-care financing and access to care has been the emergence of the employer as the primary source of private health insurance premium payments. In 1980, employers paid 84% of private health insurance premiums, while employees paid only 16%. Because tax laws exclude employer contributions to health insurance (or health care) from employees' taxable income as well as from the pay on which employer and employee Social Security contributions are based, employer contributions for the purchase of private health insurance or for the direct payment of health services represent a tax subsidy to workers covered through their employers. [16] This subsidy, which is growing rapidly, became a target of the Reagan Administration's advocates of competition. However, all attempts to convince Congress to reduce or eliminate this subsidy have come to naught.

Health-Care Cost Containment: Competition or Regulation

The advocates of greater competition and greater reliance on the forces of the marketplace have proposed three approaches to contain health-care costs: managed competition, greater consumer cost sharing, and greater access of consumers to information on costs, availability of services, and scope of services.

One proposed solution is a consumer-choice health plan that promotes competition among health-care providers.[4] This approach and the proposals by those who advocate greater cost sharing by patients constitute the primary strategies for increasing competition in the health-services market.

A variety of regulatory strategies have been tried to control rising costs: hospital utilization review, health planning to control hospital bed supply, hospital and nursing home reimbursement controls through all-payer regulation or other controls at the state level, fee schedules for physicians, Medicaid eligibility reduction, and wage and price controls. By far, the hospital sector's best performance in terms of hospital spending occurred during periods of mandatory limits on hospital payments or the threats of those limits (e.g., the Economic Stabilization Program; the Medicare Prospective Payment System, based on diagnosis-related groups; and the Carter Administration's Hospital Cost Containment Proposal). States that have regulated hospital payments have slower growth in hospital expenditures than states that have stressed competition and deregulation.

Federal Policies

After a hospital cost-control measure was defeated in Congress in the late 1970s, attempts to stem rising costs began to focus on market reform models. This development found expression initially in the health-planning legislation enacted in 1979, which reflected two divergent Congressional attitudes: an antiregulatory, procompetitive sentiment; and a prodecentralization sentiment, which advocated the decentralization of existing planning and regulatory programs, with increased responsibility for state and local governments. Since Congress was not anxious to spend more money on health care, the procompetitive, market-reform approach was promoted as an effective means of cost containment. The procompetitive, antiregulatory, and prodecentralization ("new federalism") forces also exerted the dominant influence in the early 1980s when Congress passed the Omnibus Budget Reconciliation Act of 1981, the Economic Recovery Tax Act, the Tax Equity and Fiscal Responsibility Act of 1982, and the Social Security Amendments of 1983.[17,18]

The most important health policy change was the prospective payment of hospitals mandated in the Tax Equity and Fiscal Responsibility Act of 1982 and detailed in the Social Security Amendments of 1983. As Maddox and Manton discuss in Chapter 4, this policy shift moved Medicare from a cost-based system of hospital payment, based on insurance company audits of hospital financial reports, to a prospectively determined payment system based on price per case.[18]

While the federal government has advocated market-reform strategies, it has actually increased the regulation of hospitals (as the result of the Tax Equity and Fiscal Responsibility Act and the Social Security Amendments of 1983). Also, the greater flexibility given states to modify Medicaid policies as a result of the Omnibus Budget Reconciliation Act of 1981 has resulted in increased regulation to reduce Medicaid expenditures. In addition to advocating market reforms and the development of competing capitated health-care plans (e.g., health maintenance organizations), the Reagan Administration stressed vouchers and increased patient cost sharing in Medicare.[19]

State Policies

While procompetitive policies have been advocated at the federal level and in some of the western states, at least eight states have adopted mandatory hospital rate-setting policies based on per diem rate limits or global budgets.[20-23] Although it is not easy to classify or to describe the mandatory programs because some have just been adopted and others have been undergoing significant change, it is possible to describe the two different approaches to controlling the reimbursement of hospitals. The first approach, used for more than a decade in New York, is the formula method, which compares the cost of a unit of service (e.g., per diem expenditures) with the costs in a comparable group of hospitals. The second approach, the budget review method, used in Maryland, involves the establishment of a budget by the hospital followed by direct negotiations with the state rate-setting commission. The rate review can either be a line-by-line review of each hospital's proposed budget, or it can be based on a global budget with a percentage increase formula.

In some states hospital rates are fixed in advance for Medicaid patients only, while in other states all payers are included. Massachusetts has adopted a prospectively determined cap for all hospital revenues, calculated individually for each hospital. Each third-party payer is responsible for a portion of the hospital's total revenue (cap), depending on the proportion of hospital services used by its subscribers.[24] New Jersey regulates hospital payments for all payers on the basis of a per-case rate, using the diagnosis-related groups (DRG) approach. In contrast, Maryland and Connecticut attempt to control the entire hospital budget. Maryland and

Georgia use the DRG approach to classify hospitals into reimbursement groups.

Studies of state discretionary policy and long-term care by the Institute for Health and Aging at the University of California, San Francisco, have revealed markedly different policies among the states with respect to Medicaid eligibility, scope of benefits, and cost-containment strategies. Using prospectively determined reimbursement rates, as distinct from cost-based reimbursement, has proven to be one means of controlling nursing home expenditures. Several community-based alternatives to institutional care are being explored, but their cost-control outcomes are yet to be determined.[19]

In 1982, California acted dramatically to take advantage of the provisions of the Omnibus Budget Reconciliation Act of 1981 that provided states greater flexibility in the Medicaid program.[25,26] California has emphasized a competitive model for both Medicaid and the private sector. Faced with the relative failure of earlier Medi-Cal reform measures enacted in 1981, the legislature authorized the state to enter into contracts with hospitals on a bid or negotiated basis. It also abolished the Medically Indigent Adult Program and transferred that responsibility to the counties, with 70% funding in 1983. By 1987, state funding for the MIA program had dropped below 60% as county costs rose rapidly. Private health insurers were authorized to enter into contracts for alternative rates of payment with institutional providers and health-care professionals. This legislation has had a significant effect on medical practice and medical care in California, increasing dramatically the number of preferred provider organizations and other organizational and financing arrangements designed to curtail costs by restricting access to a limited number of providers.

Studies at the Institute for Health Policy Studies at UCSF reveal that the health-care system is in a state of extraordinary flux, particularly in urban areas, such as the San Francisco Bay Area.[27] It is difficult to imagine any stable pattern emerging in the near future. The changes in California, including a rapidly growing patient load within county (public) health systems, an increase in health maintenance organizations (44% of the non-Medicare, non-Medicaid population in the San Francisco Bay Area are enrolled), and a shrinking fee-for-service sector, fit the "three-tiered" system described by Thurow.[28]

Interstate Comparisons

A state-by-state analysis of personal health-care expenditures suggests that some states and some regions of the country have been able to provide personal health care at a far lower cost than have others.[29] The two areas of the nation that have the lowest per capita costs are the Southeast and the

Rocky Mountain region. The states with the highest per capita costs are California, New York, and Massachusetts, where very different cost-containment policies have been initiated. Although solutions to the problem of rapidly rising health-care costs are not readily apparent in preliminary cross-state comparative studies, these studies can contribute to an understanding of workable solutions to the access/cost dilemma and to the development of future policies.

International Comparisons

In addition to examining the different cost-containment approaches adopted by different states, much can be learned from international comparative studies of health-care systems, financing, and cost-control strategies.[12,30–33] For example, policymakers and the public in Canada, France, West Germany, and the United Kingdom, which have publicly funded health insurance systems, believe that the allocation of health-care resources cannot be left to market forces. Although the systems differ in these countries, the bulk of the funds to pay for health care comes from general revenues or social security taxes.[12]

In the United Kingdom, roughly 96% of the funds for health care come from public sources, primarily general revenue funds. The National Health Service (NHS) has defects as well as virtues, and it stirs frequent ideological debate about waiting lists and health-care rationing. Nevertheless, the British experience represents an unequivocal success in its ability to control costs through the allocation of hospital budgets. Although many believe that the NHS is underfunded, there can be no doubt that the British have been able to control health-care costs during the past 35 years. (A detailed look at the United Kingdom is contained in Williamson, Chapter 16.)

In Canada, France, and West Germany, from 75% to 80% of health-care expenditures are publicly financed. While Canada uses general revenues, primarily income taxes, to finance its provincial health insurance programs, West Germany and France finance their health insurance programs mainly through compulsory social security payroll taxes. France also has a deliberate policy of consumer cost sharing for physician office visits, prescription drugs, and short-term hospital stays. These direct out-of-pocket payments by consumers account for roughly 20% of total health-care expenditures.[12]

Cost containment has presented a problem for France, Germany, and Canada, but since the early 1970s Canada has been more effective than any other Western industrialized country except the United Kingdom in controlling health-care costs. Since the Canadian provincial governments shifted to global budgeting of hospitals, they have been able to limit annual expenditure increases to a predetermined amount.[34,35] Prior to 1971, when Canada's publicly funded medical and hospital insurance program was fully implemented, health-care expenditures had been rising more rapidly in Canada than in the United States.[36,37] Since 1971, however, health-care expenditures have been contained to a remarkable degree. In 1971, 7.5% of Canada's GNP was attributed to health-care expenditures; in 1981, this figure was 7.9%, rising to 8.5% by the mid-1980s. In the United States, health-care expenditures as a percent of GNP rose from 7.8% to 10.5% during the same period.

The key to Canada's success has been control of the real inputs (employees, beds, and technology) in the hospital sector.[34] A recent analysis of hospital cost containment in the province of Ontario[35] confirms this. Global budgeting has resulted in a reduced number of employees, as hospital workers' wages have continued to rise. The number of beds (ratio of beds to population) and the introduction of new technologies have been controlled through separation of the operating and capital budgets. Capital budgets must be approved and funds sought through a separate approval process. This approach is effective because the provincial governments, which are responsible for virtually all medical and hospital funding, have the political legitimacy, the technical expertise, and the financial leverage to offset the influence of care providers.

The Canadian experience is particularly important for the United States because our political and social institutions, as well as the structures of our health-care systems, are very similar: Canadian and American hospitals are largely voluntary and nonprofit; physicians practice mostly under a fee-for-service reimbursement system; physicians care for patients in and out of the hospital; and hospital-based specialists and office-based generalists are not separated, as they are in France, Germany, and Britain.

Next Steps

What does all this have to do with the elderly? Although the Medicare Catastrophic Coverage Act of 1988 included both an expansion of hospital benefits and coverage of out-of-hospital prescription drugs, these benefits will continue to be the focus of federal policy on health-care cost-containment strategies, with increased cost-sharing by the elderly as a key element. The issues raised by the increasing number of uninsured and underinsured, including persons with AIDS, as well as the increasing burden on individuals to pay directly for care out of pocket, will not be dealt with until costs can be controlled and a consensus is reached about the appropriate role of government in health- and long-term care financing. Before a consensus is reached, some steps can be taken to control costs.

Cost Containment

The key to effective cost containment lies in controlling the rapidly rising costs of hospital care, which can be accomplished by reducing utilization of hospital services, reducing the price of services provided, or controlling expenditures. We believe that all three strategies must be used. In the short run, hospital cost increases can best be controlled through prospectively set global budgets. While this can be accomplished most easily through the public financing of national health insurance, rather than through continued reliance on pluralistic financing of health services from public and private sources, it is also possible through state regulation.

The likelihood of implementing publicly funded national health insurance seems slim at the present time, but effective steps can be taken in the absence of a national system of financing. The first priority must be given to hospital cost containment, because equity of access cannot be achieved without it. Although Congress reduced Medicare hospital reimbursement substantially in the Tax Equity and Fiscal Responsibility Act of 1982 and augmented that cost-containment effort in the 1983 Social Security Amendments, these actions are not enough. Even if this approach is effective in reducing Medicare hospital expenditures in the short run, it may result in cost shifting to third parties and in diminished access or quality of care for the elderly unless the Medicare cost-containment policies are part of a comprehensive system of regulation that includes all third-party payers. This approach has proved more effective than separate approaches by Medicare, Medicaid, and private health insurance companies. We support a system of all-payer regulation at the state level that can both control expenditures and provide payment for the care of the uninsured and underinsured.

In addition, nursing home expenditures must be controlled by limiting growth of the supply of nursing home beds, and prospectively setting payments for nursing home care. Prospectively determined global budgets should also be adopted for nursing homes. If global budgeting is not adopted, prospectively determined per diem rates can be established on a regional basis, rather than on an institution-by-institution basis.

Physician fees, which have risen steadily over the past decade, are being addressed by Congress and by the Physician Payment Review Commission, established in 1986 by Congress as an independent agency to advise both Congress and the Department of Health and Human Services. The commission's 1989 report to Congress includes proposals for changing the method used by Medicare to pay physicians and for slowing the rates of increase in expenditures and utilization of services.

Congress should initiate a major study of the experiments in health-care financing, competition, and regulation in the United States, particularly comparative studies across states. Studies examining the experiences of Canada and European countries also should be conducted. These research and analysis efforts should involve the Congressional Budget Office, the Office of Technology Assessment, the General Accounting Office, the Health Care Financing Administration, and the National Center for Health Services Research. The present levels of research funding should be doubled to $100 million annually. The stakes are too high to ignore the multibillion-dollar experiments now under way.

National Commission

Although we strongly advocate publicly funded national health insurance, we recognize that there are widely divergent views on this issue. At the heart of the problem is a lack of consensus on the proper role of government in health care. To address these and other issues, a bipartisan national commission on comprehensive health care has been created to examine the health-care system and to recommend changes, particularly in health-care financing, that will make the system more responsive to the public's needs. Fifty-two years ago the Committee on the Costs of Medical Care, organized and financed by private foundations, issued its final report,[38] which focused on major reforms needed in the system, including financing reforms. Although this report was widely criticized by organized medicine, it formed the foundation for future debate and discussion on issues of health policy and health care, particularly for health-care financing. Thirty-three years ago, the President's Commission on the Health Needs of the Nation issued its report.[39] Although the recommendations of this commission were also opposed vigorously by organized medicine, many of the recommendations found their way into public policy in the 1960s and 1970s. Both commissions, because of the importance and thoroughness of their work, made lasting contributions to the development of health policy in the United States.

Recently, the American Medical Association issued a health policy agenda for the American people,[40] a 195-point program developed by a broad consortium of private and public interests convened under the auspices of the American Medical Association. This report addressed a wide range of problems but failed to generate much public attention or support.

In 1986, another effort was initiated by the private sector to examine the health-care system and to make policy recommendations. The National Leadership Commission on Health Care, which is made up of 34 leaders in health care, business, law, economics, ethics, and public policy, and which is supported by private foundations, corporations, and labor unions, outlined a range of problems and recommendations in its January 1989 report.

The commission addressed three major health care problems—cost, quality, and access. In response to these problems, the commission proposed a new public/private partnership to provide universal access to a basic level of health care services.

There is growing public support for some form of national health insurance, either privately mandated or publicly funded. Most polls on the subject indicate that people are willing to pay higher taxes to ensure some adequate form of health insurance and also some basic long-term care insurance. The time has come for policymakers to turn their attention from a preoccupation with health-care cost containment to the issues of access and quality in order to achieve the goal of equity called for by the President's Commission for the Study of Ethical Problems in Medicine and Biomedical and Behavioral Research in its 1983 report.

References

1. Alford, R. R. 1975. *Health Care Politics: Ideological and Interest Group Barriers to Reform*. Chicago, Ill.: University of Chicago Press.
2. Lee, P. R., Estes, C. L. 1983. New federalism and health policy. *Ann Am Acad Political Soc Sci* 468:88–102.
3. President's Commission for the Study of Ethical Problems in Medicine and Biomedical and Behavioral Research. 1983. *Securing Access to Health Care: The Ethical Implications of Differences in the Availability of Health Services*, Vol. 1, Washington, D.C.: Government Printing Office, 4–5.
4. Enthoven, A. C. 1980. *Health Plan: The Only Practical Solution to the Soaring Cost of Medical Care*. Reading, Mass.: Addison Wesley.
5. Ginzberg, E. (ed.) 1986. *From Physician Shortage to Patient Shortage*, Boulder, Colo.: Westview Press.
6. Graduate Medical Education National Advisory Committee. 1980. *Summary Report to the Secretary, Department of Health and Human Services*. Washington, D.C.: Government Printing Office.
7. Ginzberg, E., Brann, E., Hiestand, D., Ostow, M. 1981. The expanding physician supply and health policy: The clouded outlook. *Milbank Memorial Fund Q* 59(4):508–541.
8. Fuchs, V. 1981. The coming challenge to American physicians. *N Engl J Med* 304(24):1487–1490.
9. Ginzberg, E. 1983. Cost containment—imaginary and real. *N Engl J Med* 308(20):1220–1224.
10. Gibson, R. M., Waldo, D. R. 1982. National health expenditures. *Health Care Financing Rev* 4(1):1–35.
11. Levit, K. R., Freeland, M. S. 1988. National Medical Care Spending. *Health Affairs* 7(5):124–136.

12. Maxwell, R. J. 1981. *Health and Wealth*. Lexington, Mass.: Lexington Books.
13. Haber, S., Henton, D., Melville, J., McCall, N. 1986. *Health Care For The Uninsured and the Underinsured: A San Francisco Challenge*. San Francisco, Calif.: United Way of the Bay Area.
14. Sulvetta, M. B., Swartz, J. 1986. *The Uninsured and Uncompensated Care*. Washington, D.C.: National Health Policy Forum, George Washington University.
15. Blendon, R. J., Aiken, L. N., Freeman, H. E., Kirkmann-Liff, B. L., Murphy, J. A. 1986. Uncompensated care by hospitals or public insurance for the poor. *N Engl J Med* 314:1160–1163.
16. Taylor, A., Wilensky, G. R. 1983. The effect of tax policies on expenditures for private health insurance. In *Market Reforms in Health Care*, ed. A. J. Meyer. Washington, D.C.: American Enterprise Institute.
17. Estes, C. L., Lee, P. R. 1981. Policy shifts and their impacts on health care for elderly persons. *West J Med* 135(6):511–518.
18. Rubin, R. N. 1982. The new federalism for health: shifting responsibilities and reducing costs into the 80s. *JAMA* 247(21):2911–2912.
19. Estes, C. L., Newcomer, R. J., and Associates. 1983. *Fiscal Austerity and Aging. Shifting Government Responsibility for the Elderly*. Beverly Hills, Calif.: Sage Publications.
20. Dowling, W. L., House, P. J., Lehman, J. M., Meade, G. L., Teague, N. T., Vandan, M., Watts, C. A. 1976. *The Impact of the Blue Cross and Medicaid Prospective Reimbursement Systems in Downstate New York*, Final Report. HEW-05-74-248. Washington, D.C.: Government Printing Office.
21. Biles, B., Schramm, C. J., Atkinson, J. G. 1980. Hospital cost inflation under state rate-setting programs. *N Engl J Med* 303(12):664–668.
22. Schwartz, W. B. 1981. The regulation strategy for controlling hospital costs: problems and prospects. *N Engl J Med* 305(21):1249–1255.
23. Coelen, C., Sullivan, D. 1981. An analysis of the effects of prospective reimbursement programs on hospital expenditures. *Health Care Financing Rev* 2(3):1–40.
24. Caper, P., Blumenthal, D. 1983. What price cost control? Massachusetts' new hospital payment law. *N Engl J Med* 308(9):542–544.
25. Melia, E. P., Aucoin, L. M., Duhl, L. J., Kurokawa, P. S. 1983. Competition in the health care marketplace: A beginning in California. *N Engl J Med* 308(13):788–792.
26. Kinzer, D. M. 1983. Massachusetts and California—two kinds of hospital cost control. *N Engl J Med* 308(14):838–841.
27. Trauner, J. B., Luft, H. S., Hunt, S. S. 1986. A lifestyle decision: Facing the reality of physician oversupply in the San Francisco Bay Area. In *From Physician Shortage to Patient Shortage*, ed. E. Ginzberg. Boulder, Colo.: Westview Press.
28. Thurow, L. 1985. Medicine vs. economics. *N Engl J Med* 313:611–614.
29. Levit, K. R. 1982. Personal health care expenditures by state, selected years 1966–1978. *Health Care Financing Rev* 4(2):1–45.
30. Reinhardt, U. E. 1981. Health insurance and cost containment policies: The experience abroad. In *A New Approach to Health Economics*, ed. F. M. Olesen, 151–171. Washington, D.C.: American Enterprise Institute.

31. Marmor, T. R. 1975. Can the U.S. learn from Canada? In *National Health Insurance: Can We Learn from Canada?*, ed. S. Andreopoulos. New York: John Wiley and Sons.

32. Evans, R. G. 1981. *Slouching Toward Chicago: Regulatory Reform as Revealed Religion.* Discussion Paper No. 81–42. Vancouver: Department of Economics, University of British Columbia.

33. Rodwin, V. G. 1981. The marriage of national health insurance and *la medecine liberale* in France: A costly union. *Milbank Memorial Fund Q* 59(1):16–43.

34. Evans, R. G. 1983. Health care in Canada: Patterns of funding and regulation. *J Health Polit Policy Law* 8(1):1–43.

35. Detsky, A. S., Stacy, S. R., and Bombardier, C. 1983. The effectiveness of a regulatory strategy in containing hospital costs: The Ontario experience, 1967–1981. *N Engl J Med* 309(3):151–159.

36. Andreopoulos, S. (ed.) 1975. *National Health Insurance: Can We Learn from Canada?* New York: John Wiley and Sons.

37. Simanis, J. G., Coleman, J. R. 1980. Health care expenditures in nine industrialized countries, 1960–1976. *Soc Secur Bull* 43(1):3–8.

38. United States Department of Health, Education, and Welfare, Committee on the Costs of Medical Care. 1932. *Medical Care for the American People*, Final Report. Washington, D.C.: Government Printing Office.

39. President's Commission on the Health Needs of the Nation. 1951. *Building America's Health. Financing a Health Program for America*, Vol. 4. Washington, D.C.: Government Printing Office.

40. American Medical Association. 1987. Health policy agenda for the American people. *JAMA* 257:1199–1210.

Part Three

Available and Emerging Sources of Care

Health providers in this country offer an unrivaled cornucopia of care to the elderly population through acute-care facilities, nursing homes, community-based long-term programs, and social health maintenance organizations. But fragmentation has long tempered the impressive scope of these services; integrated care has too often taken a backseat to administrative and internecine rivalry. Most providers target their own client population, enforce unique eligibility requirements, report to different administrative and regulatory authorities and receive separate financing. For an aging person who finds it impossible to negotiate the resultant maze, fragmentation has particularly devastating consequences.

Efforts to curtail this hazardous discontinuity represent one of the most hopeful developments in geriatric care today. Case management, in which a team of social service experts and health professionals design an appropriate package of care from a menu of options, is playing a central role in unifying service delivery. No single component of the health-care system analyzed in this section can be expected to meet all the needs of all the elderly all the time. Rather, each is an interdependent contributor to a larger whole, an actor whose individual strengths combine into a successful production.

William A. Read and James L. O'Brien discuss why hospitals are well positioned to extend their reach beyond acute services and begin meeting comprehensive long-term health needs.Structurally equipped to provide vertically integrated care, they are spurred on by an increasingly competitive marketplace, new reimbursement techniques that carry strong incentives to minimize hospitalization, and the recognition that top-shelf hospital care demands a well-coordinated follow-up program.

In their article on the Robert Wood Johnson Foundation's Hospital Initiatives in Long-Term Care Program, authors Cynthia A. Coombs, Carl Eisdorfer, Karyn L. Feiden, and David A. Kessler look at 24 hospital-based demonstration projects around the country that have molded theory into practice by providing comprehensive, case-managed care to a geriatric population. While each program was structured to meet the individual needs of its patients, sponsoring institution and community, the challenges that arose in the course of each design and implementation process proved startlingly similar. One important lesson learned is that the probability of programmatic success jumps markedly when certain key issues are identified and resolved.

Social health maintenance organizations (SHMOs), which offer all the traditional services of health maintenance organizations plus long-term care, have recently caught the eye of forward-looking health providers. Jay N. Greenberg, Walter N. Leutz, and Stuart H. Altman provide a behind-the-scenes tour of the SHMO experiment, launched in 1980 with four demonstration programs. Its strength rests in its unique capacity for consolidation: one provider organization assumes all financial risks and coordinates comprehensive service delivery to an elderly population with a broad spectrum of care needs.

Bashed by the public, vigorously defended by the industry, and earnestly studied by academics, solutions to the problems of nursing homes remain vexingly elusive, write Iris C. Freeman and Bruce C. Vladeck. Particularly plaguing has been the dearth of hard data on nursing home characteristics, the lack of uniform performance standards, and the severe constraints on the public purse. To improve the nursing home system, the authors urge that lines of communication be opened between government regulators and reimbursement agencies, that resident councils be established, and that residents be encouraged to participate in planning their own treatment.

The demands for long-term care divide into two distinct categories, according to experts Stanley J. Brody and Judith S. Magel. Comfortably in place are mechanisms to finance short-term long-term care (STLTC), the hospital-based services that generally accompany a period of recuperation following acute illness. By contrast, long-term long-term care (LTLTC), which is required to maintain those with chronic and progressive disabilities at optimal levels, is in desperately short supply. The authors say that understanding the distinction between the transitory needs of STLTC and the ongoing demands of LTLTC is key to developing appropriate systems of care.

Because family care complements both these prongs of long-term care, Elaine M. Brody and Stanley J. Brody take a compassionate look at the interlocking needs of the elderly and the family members who provide their informal support systems and call for respite care and better day programs. Although financial, managerial, and ethical problems accompany any efforts to integrate formal and informal care, a working partnership clearly has the keenest potential to strengthen both systems.

The potency of cooperative effort is also the theme of this section's final article, where James P. Firman asks how health-care services that are both efficient and equitable can be provided. His bold solution: participatory consumerism. By flexing their economic muscles as effectively as they have tensed their political ones, a well-organized, well-informed elderly population can become an important force in the marketplace. Firman's prototype health-care cooperative would be independent, consumer-financed, and tailored to enhance the way older consumers bargain for, select, and finance appropriate medical and social care.

Nine

The Involved Hospital

William A. Read and James L. O'Brien

Hospitals have long played a central role in providing health-care services to the elderly. No other community institution serves more older people: over 4 million persons, or 20% of those 65 years old or older, use hospital inpatient facilities at least once a year, accounting for approximately 10 million episodes of service.[1] During 1981, costs for hospital care accounted for over two-thirds of the dollars Medicare spent for personal health care.[2] While most elderly are healthy, and only 17.5% of noninstitutionalized elderly report limitations in performing activities of daily living, the elderly are at a higher risk for hospitalization than the overall population.[3] In 1981, the rate of hospitalization for persons age 65 years and older was three times greater than that for the overall population—namely, 4155 acute inpatient days per 1000 persons versus the national average of 1217 days per 1000 persons.[4] The old-old, persons age 75 years and older, not only are the most rapidly growing segment of the elderly population, but also use substantially more health-care resources. While the old-old comprised 4% of the population in 1981, they accounted for 13% of hospital discharges and 21% of all days of care.[4]

The pervasive role of hospitals in caring for the elderly is due mainly to their organizational characteristics. Hospitals are well-suited to meet the contingencies associated with illness of older adults. In particular, they are available 24 hours a day and possess both the facilities and expertise to handle complex medical problems—problems that are often exacerbated by the cognitive impairment, loss of fitness, and functional decline associated with the presenting illness of many older adults.

Faced with the challenge of caring for the growing elderly population, hospitals are expanding their mission to care for the elderly within a framework of services and principles oriented toward maximizing functional independence and autonomy. The renewed interest in long-term care (LTC) has been stimulated by the turbulent changes characterizing the health-care system since the 1970s. In the context of the growing elderly population, five trends have been especially important in modifying the role of the hospital as a service-delivery organization, the relationships between providers, and, ultimately, the future of hospitals as providers of LTC. First, the disproportionate use of health-care resources by the elderly, particularly in the last years of life, has led to questions about the traditional orientation in caring for the elderly in inpatient, acute-care settings. Second, unprecedented inflation during the 1970s led to private and public initiatives to contain spiraling costs by restricting utilization of hospital inpatient services. Third, competition was generated by the entry of new providers offering services that had been delivered previously only by hospitals. Fourth, and by some accounts the most important, health-care corporations grew, bringing with their growth movement toward higher levels of integrated control. Fifth, most recently, practitioners of health care have been adjusting to the implementation of the Medicare prospective payment system.[5]

The Traditional Orientation

Historically, hospital care for the elderly has centered on providing acute inpatient services, supplemented with LTC services following hospitalization. Acute inpatient care, the mainstay of hospital services, consists primarily of highly technical, cure-oriented medical services aimed at the prevention of death and the preservation of life through the diagnosis and treatment of localized injury and illness. Institutional and community-based services for both transitional care and LTC, the traditional domain of other providers, is oriented toward maximizing functional independence or sometimes providing maintenance care, to persons who are chronically ill and often progressively disabled. Hospitals traditionally have been the gateways into the LTC system; roughly 34% of nursing home residents come from the general hospital.[6] Regulations governing Medicare and Medicaid reimbursement for nursing home stays may even require a period of hospitalization in order for a beneficiary to be eligible for the reimbursement of services.

Initial concern with escalating health-care costs centered on the idea that care for the dying was focused too heavily on the highly technical, cure-oriented services provided in hospitals. In 1978, for example, Medicare beneficiaries who died cost an average of $4909 for covered services in their last year of life, or about four times the amount provided to surviving beneficiaries. As a group, decedents comprised 5.9% of the Medicare beneficiaries but accounted for 28% of Medicare expenditures.[7] These findings highlight the dilemmas associated with the traditional orientation of caring for the elderly. The guiding ideal of medical care, to preserve life at all costs, may lead to an over-reliance on costly technology and little concern for the quality of the life maintained. Costs of care can be minimized through the use of less-expensive and less technologically oriented centers, such as hospices.

The characteristics of many elderly patients and the risks associated with hospitalization suggest that the approach described above is limited. In one study (conducted at a 400-bed community hospital) of 279 patients over the age of 70, 19% were considered mildly confused, and 31% were moderately or severely confused. For patients age 85 or older, the proportion who were moderately or severely confused increased to 54%. Psychoactive medications or sedatives were prescribed to 43% of the patients, 34% had impaired hearing, 40% had impaired vision after correction with eyeglasses, and 25% had speech impairments. Overall, the group showed considerable age-correlated disability in the basic activities of daily living, such as moving around and self-care ability (eating and dressing skills), worsened with increasing age.[8]

Furthermore, many elderly patients experience an irreversible decline in their level of functioning that cannot be accounted for by the illness that led to hospitalization.[8] One factor that has been suspected of contributing to the accelerated decline of the elderly's capabilities is hospital-induced (iatrogenic) illness.[9] In a study by Reichel, 146 of 500 patients age 65 or older experienced 193 untoward reactions and complications associated with hospitalization, including 61 accidents and traumas (including falls) and 54 reactions to medications. Thirty-one of the subjects had reactions to diagnostic and therapeutic procedures, 19 experienced hospital-induced major psychologic decompensation, 17 acquired infections, and 11 were affected by other problems.[10]

At a large urban teaching hospital on the Northeastern seaboard, several groups of patients were studied through medical records review and follow-up. One group consisted of frail, elderly women age 75 and older who were admitted to the hospital with hip fractures (one of the 25 most common ailments among the elderly) within a 6-month period. Of the total number in that group, 38% were incontinent of urine following surgery and 20% were incontinent at discharge from the hospital. Moreover, 23% were confused and disoriented on admission, 39% after surgery, and 20% at discharge from the hospital. Of the 20% discharged while confused and disoriented, a significant number were dead in six months. Why did they die? There were no supportive services in the home. They lay abed, suffered poor nutrition, were confused, developed upper respiratory infections, and died of pneumonia.[11] Confusion, disorientation, and incontinence are problems preventable through adequate geriatric acute care and planning for posthospital care.

While there are no uniformly accepted standards that define an appropriate level of service or mandate the choice of intervention during an episode of illness, there is indirect evidence that medical intervention itself is excessive and contributes to the risk of iatrogenic illness. According to Bunker, physicians in general tend to be optimistic about new medical techniques.[12] However, their optimism, reflected in the employment of new techniques, may not be based upon sound evidence about the value of procedures, either in terms of their cost-effectiveness or their efficacy in particular circumstances. Even when the appropriate research on the benefits of new techniques has been conducted, the special contingencies of applying them to older adults are rarely evaluated.[13]

Wennberg has compiled evidence that suggests that physicians may overutilize some surgical procedures. Wide regional variation in the number of procedures performed, even when controlling for various health indicators, suggests that the rate may be based more on normative practices than on the need for surgery or the efficacy of other treatment.[14] If this is the case, it is possible to reduce the number of procedures without adversely affecting the health of patients.

Cost Containment

In response to the unprecedented growth in health-care expenditures, and the recognition that such growth could not go unchecked, the private and public sectors initiated measures to contain costs, most often through limiting utilization of services or providing incentives that essentially restricted utilization. In the public realm, health systems agencies and professional services review organizations, among other federal and local agencies, were formed to review utilization patterns and limit expansion of hospital services through regional control and planning.

The private sector modified employer-paid health insurance packages to encourage more selective health-care consumption by beneficiaries. If deductibles for hospital services were not already a part of a policy, they were introduced; when they were already in place, they were increased. Employees often were required to contribute a larger share of the premium costs or a significant proportion of all medical bills. Second-opinion programs mandated that patients visit a second physician prior to the performance of some highly utilized surgical procedures if they were to be reimbursed.[15,16] According to one survey of corporate benefits managers, restricting payment of benefits for services rendered on an outpatient basis is one of the most popular cost-containment strategies of benefit programs.[17]

Competition

Many changes in health-benefit programs spurred the growth of alternative forms of health-care delivery systems. Physicians, the hospital's traditional source of referrals, entered into direct competition with hospitals for the revenues available in the ambulatory care and diagnostic services market by opening free-standing ambulatory care centers and testing laboratories to take advantage of the changes in reimbursement policies. With the passage of the Health Maintenance Organization (HMO) Act in 1983, and other legislation, competition in the health-care marketplace was further broadened.

HMOs, delivery systems that both insure and provide services, are an important innovation in the financing and delivery of care. While only 7.9% of the population is currently enrolled in HMOs, the growth rate for HMO enrollment, historically 10% per annum, grew to 15% in 1983 and 21% in 1984.[18] The number of Medicare enrollees grew by 38% between 1984 and 1985, compared to a 25% overall growth in HMO enrollees.[19]

The full effect of HMOs on the health-care delivery system, both now and in the future, is not understandable solely in terms of the absolute or relative numbers of enrollees in HMOs. Rather, the effect will depend on changes in consumers' health practices and expectations about the availability of medical services arising from their participation in HMOs. In particular, what sort of service will be expected and demanded in the future from a cohort of consumers with many years of experience as HMO enrollees?

Cost-containment strategies and increased competition have had a pronounced effect on hospitals. Hospital occupancy dropped from 74% in the first quarter of 1983 to 62.1% during the third quarter of 1985. Hospital admissions declined 8.9% from 1981 to 1984, with an additional 3.8% decline during the first nine months of 1985; the number of inpatient days declined a total of 4% during this same period. The rate of decline in admissions was not uniform across age groups: between January 1983 and January 1985, hospital admissions for patients under 65 years of age declined from 6.62 to 5.93 million, while for those 65 years old and older, the admissions during the same period declined from 2.96 to 2.81 million—a 10% decline in the under-65 population versus a 5% decline for the elderly. This change is reflected in the rise in the average cost per case: the rate of growth increased from 7.7% to 9.2% between 1984 and 1985. Not only is the hospital taking care of fewer patients, but the patients it cares for are older and sicker.[20]

Growth of Health-Care Corporations

The rise of hospital corporations has been called "the most important health-care development of the day."[21] Between 1980 and 1985, the number of hospitals belonging to multihospital systems increased from 1797 to 2208, accounting for 341,382 and 396,925 hospital beds, respectively. Together with the increase in number of hospitals belonging to multihospital systems, there has been an overall decline in the number of systems; there were 267 in 1980 and 250 in 1985.[22] Not only is there a trend toward increasing membership in systems, but there is also a trend toward centralization into fewer systems. The changes associated with this development are multifaceted and include:

- a movement toward a higher level of integrated control;
- a change in the type of ownership and control, mostly through the growth of for-profit hospitals;
- horizontal integration, i.e., increased membership in centrally managed multihospital systems and a concomitant decrease in the number of free-standing institutions;
- diversification and corporate restructuring;
- vertical integration, or a shift from single-level-of-care organizations to organizations that provide various levels of care;
- industry concentration of both ownership and control of health services in regional markets.[21,23]

Given the characteristics of the hospital operating environment described previously, it is none too surprising that health-care systems have grown. There are numerous advantages for hospitals participating in multiinstitutional systems:

- the combined size of many institutions permits the savings associated with volume purchasing and makes capital available at lower interest;
- hospitals increase access to specialized corporate services, including planning, marketing, and managerial expertise, centralized computer facilities, and sophisticated cost-accounting capabilities;
- small hospitals, with less-stable occupancy and high excess capacity, have access to funds during times of financial difficulty;

- their combined size may give individual hospitals an advantage in the marketplace and increased influence with legislators;
- limits on new construction have restricted competition, making existing hospitals attractive as an investment. [23,5]

The growth of vertically integrated systems is particularly important for understanding hospital interest in LTC. In purely economic terms, providers are diversifying into new markets offering higher potential for growth and profitability while maintaining their traditional acute-care market. Vertically integrated systems allow hospitals access to revenues generated in other components of the health-care system. Similarly, when patients enter the hospital system through more than one access point, the likelihood is increased that when another service is needed, such as acute care, the clients will return to the hospital, thereby enhancing revenues generated through traditional services. As a growth strategy, diversification makes more sense than continued acquisition of free-standing hospitals. [24]

Hospitals' commitment to vertically integrated systems of institutional and community-based LTC is reflected in the growth of alternative hospital services. Between 1978 and 1983, for example, the number of hospital-based, Medicare-certified home health agencies grew from 319 to 566—a 77% increase. [25] Moreover, an additional 247 hospital-based agencies were certified by Medicare between October 1983 and September 1984. [26] According to the American Hospital Association's 1985 Survey of Hospital Services for the Aged and Chronically Ill, 33.3% of responding hospitals stated that they provided home health services. [27] Similarly, the number of hospitals providing skilled nursing and/or LTC units grew from 681 to 900 between 1978 and 1984. [28] (See discussion of survey results below for further details on typical services provided by hospitals.)

The economics of the situation, of course, only make sense within the broader issue of hospital responsibility and the hospital's role as a community provider. Given its mission, and given the current operating environment, the financial benefits accruing from participation in horizontally and vertically integrated systems in turn enhance the hospital's ability to provide efficient, cost-effective care. These new forms of corporate organizations are especially significant in hospital's planning of LTC programs for the elderly, as they make available many options, discussed below, that may not have been feasible prior to their participation in a system.

Prospective Payment System

Among the most dramatic changes in the hospital's operating environment has been the implementation of the Medicare prospective payment system

(PPS) (Public Law 98-21, Title VI) in 1983 (see Maddox and Manton, Chapter 4). The law has radically restructured the financial incentives involved in caring for a patient. Rather than maximizing revenues by maximizing services or costs, the hospital can now maximize its income by minimizing the utilization of services during a hospital stay, providing the same services at a reduced cost, or discharging patients. The financial risk of caring for the elderly has shifted from the federal government to the hospital and patient. All other factors being equal, the introduction of prospective pricing has resulted in a flurry of hospital interest in developing long-term programs.

In a special survey of all U.S. hospitals conducted by the American Hospital Association's Hospital Research and Educational Trust, respondents were asked to identify changes in the delivery and organization of services to the elderly that their hospitals made since the implementation of PPS in October 1983. The following list summarizes the results:

- Increased emphasis on discharge planning   80.7%

- Installation of new management information systems for diagnosis-related groups or cost accounting   55.8%

- Increased coordination of the delivery of already existing services   54.5%

- Implementation of new programs/services to address a wider range of health needs   49.4%

- Expansion of outreach services to the community   44.8%

- Offering of special programs to increase staff awareness of special needs of the elderly   32.9%

- Revision of hospital mission to incorporate a specific focus on care for the elderly   17.8%

- Conversion of some acute-care beds to LTC beds   12.2%

The incentives for hospitals to develop LTC programs to comply with regulatory pressures are clear. Extending hospitalization beyond what is medically necessary due to a lack of appropriate discharge options, such as a shortage of nursing home beds, is now extremely costly. For example, in Illinois, during an 11-day census, $9 million was spent on hospital days that were potentially nonreimbursable. Patients awaiting alternative levels of care were located in 78% of Illinois hospitals.[29] In those situations where there is no access to postacute services, the incentives to limit inpatient expenditures threatened the provision of high-quality care. Diversified services diffuse the financial risk of providing acute-care services to older adults. In theory, increased access to LTC services, provided either by the hospital itself or within the community, enables the hospital to manage more cost-effectively by providing appropriate care options when discharging a patient, thereby reducing the risk that the patient remains hospitalized longer than the standard length of stay or returns to the hospital because home care was not provided.

Prospective pricing directly links the fiscal viability of the hospital with the practice of physicians, who traditionally have made the decisions about caring for patients. In order to succeed in this environment, hospitals and physicians will be required to recognize and integrate economic considerations when planning hospital treatment. Mechanic has noted that prospective pricing has transformed the traditional relationship between patients, hospitals, and physicians from advocacy for an individual patient to allocation of limited financial resources to a group of patients.[30]

Whatever the outcome, PPS has given hospitals an incentive to provide or procure access to a variety of services, including new types of acute-care services as well as both transitional and chronic LTC services. Hospitals operating under incentives for short lengths of hospital stays must appropriately place their patients in posthospital services. To maintain quality of care, hospitals must ensure continuity of care.

Comprehensive, Coordinated Care: The New Imperative

While physicians and others recognize and often voice the shortcomings of the traditional orientation to medical care for older adults, and on a case-by-case basis design treatment protocols in light of individual probabilities of survival and availability of services, nothing short of a systematic and comprehensive reappraisal of medical care for older adults is required. The success of hospital ventures in LTC for an elderly population characterized by changing levels of functioning and need is predicated on the delivery of appropriate care in response to acute episodes of illness and the financial stability of the acute-care component of hospital care services.

On a conceptual level, the actualization of a philosophy of LTC that preserves health while maintaining functional capacity and personal autonomy requires both a corporate response involving the development of alternative services and a concomitant shift in the ethos underlying the practice of acute care for the elderly. Acceptance, development, and proliferation of services that place a premium on maintaining the elderly in the community mean that our ideas of health have to be expanded to include a broader, more holistic perception of elderly persons and their need for services.

The single most important consequence of integrating these values under the rubric of health care, from a hospital perspective, entails a shift that repositions acute care in the system of care. Acute care is only one element in a continuum of services providing for the health-care needs of

Table 9.1. Long-Term Care Services (percent hospitals reporting, N = 3197)

Services	Hospital-Owned and Operated	Access through Formal Contract	Access through Informal Contract
Inpatient Services			
Hospital-Based Skilled Nursing Facility	19.0	3.5	17.2
Swing Beds	14.2	0.6	5.3
Intermediate Care	12.3	12.0	43.8
Freestanding Skilled Nursing Facility	3.6	15.1	44.5
Psychiatric Long-Term Care	1.4	14.8	44.1
Ambulatory Services			
Day Hospital	12.4	0.8	10.0
Day Rehabilitation	7.5	0.9	13.3
Adult Day Care	5.1	1.7	30.1
Linking and Referral Services			
Emergency Response System	35.8	4.2	20.0
Information and Referral	33.2	2.4	31.2
Phone Contact	16.0	1.7	23.7
Maintenance and Support Services			
Education	54.4	1.6	17.4
Home Health	33.3	21.6	34.8
Durable Medical Equipment	17.3	11.5	55.0
Homemaker	15.8	16.2	47.3
Hospice	13.9	12.0	38.9
Home Meals	12.8	8.6	57.4
Respite	9.1	3.0	31.7
Transportation	8.5	3.2	57.7
Congregate Meals	4.2	3.2	51.8
Home Visitors	3.3	2.6	33.3
Alternative Housing Arrangements			
Senior Apartments	2.3	2.7	55.4
Continuing-Care Retirement Center	0.8	1.5	31.6
Sheltered Housing	0.8	2.1	43.5
Foster Care	0.4	1.8	30.4

Source: Results of 1985 Survey of Hospital Services for the Aged and Chronically Ill

an elderly population. As they expand their mission to incorporate LTC, hospitals will need to fit the acute-care model into a long-term continuum of care that takes into account the special needs of the elderly.

Providing new services, in and of itself, is no guarantee that the services are accessible or utilized to their full advantage. Current reimbursement mechanisms, along with such other factors as physicians' and consumers' inadequate knowledge about the availability, efficacy, or appropriateness of alternative forms of care, hinder the timely development and coordinated delivery of services to the chronically ill. New mechanisms are required to enhance awareness of such services, to ensure that these alternatives are integrated into treatment planning, and, finally, to guarantee that these services are implemented without delay when the need arises.

Faced with the limitations and opportunities brought about by changes in the operating environment, hospitals have begun developing hospital-managed, comprehensive, medical and social service programs for the frail and chronically ill elderly. Current hospital involvement in delivering LTC was demonstrated in the survey of the American Hospital Association's Hospital Research and Educational Trust, which examined 25 different institutional and community-based LTC services. A total of 3529 community hospitals, or 59.7%, responded to the survey, making it the largest study of its kind. The survey results are summarized in Tables 9.1 and 9.2. Table 9.1 shows how many hospitals provide LTC services directly or make them accessible via formal and informal contracts. Table 9.2 breaks down those services into their component parts.

The move toward developing comprehensive services that reflect the shifting ethos of care is being buttressed by new forms of arrangements between providers within a single institution and between multiple institutions. While the future role of the hospital in the delivery of LTC services will in part depend on the reimbursement system, the current changes in relationships among providers, which emphasize the rationalization of service delivery and operational efficiencies, are establishing a framework that ensures continued hospital participation in meeting the LTC needs of the elderly.

Fully 66.1% of the surveyed hospitals reported that their long-range plans included the development or expansion of services for the elderly. As community institutions, hospitals are gearing both their planning and programmatic efforts in cooperation with the elderly and other community agencies. Of hospitals planning services, 43.8% conducted surveys among potential consumers and/or their families detailing such information as patterns of use, satisfaction with existing services, and the need for new services. Moreover, 27.3% of the hospitals involved the community elderly in their planning process, while 16.1% also involved family members. Finally, 34.0% involved other community agencies, 25.8% involved

Table 9.2. Separate Services for Older Adults (N = 3451)

Type of Services	Percent Hospitals Reporting	N
Inpatient Services		
Rehabilitation Inpatient Services	1.9	65
Medical/Surgical, Acute	2.1	71
Psychiatric, Acute	0.8	29
Ambulatory Services		
Organized Outpatient Department	4.5	155
Psychiatric Clinic	0.9	30
Rehabilitation Outpatient Services	1.2	41
Assessment/Linking/Referral Services		
Geriatric Assessment Team	4.4	150
Discharge Planning	3.9	136
Outreach Planning	4.4	150
Geriatric Consultation	3.2	111
Information and Referral	3.4	116
Case Management	2.8	96
Pre-admission Screening Program	2.6	88
Health Maintenance and Support Services		
Patient/Family Education	4.0	123
Health Promotion/Wellness Program	3.3	113
Senior Volunteers	15.7	543
Home Health	4.6	156
Homemaker or Personal Care	1.0	33
Hospice	0.5	17
Home Visitors	0.8	24

other providers, and 13.4% discussed their plans with advocacy groups representing the elderly. These figures represent a significant new hospital interest in, and emphasis on, cooperating with community groups and incorporating sound planning strategies in the development of new programs.

The Hospital Perspective: Positioning for the Future

Incentives for hospitals to mount long-term health-care programs, either on their own or through linkages with other providers, differ from hospital to hospital. Some of the typical reasons offered by hospital trustees, administrators, and planners are enumerated below (personal communications).

First, LTC programs are crucial in fulfilling the mission of a caring institution. The elderly are accustomed to turning to hospitals when they are ill; it is, therefore, the hospital's responsibility to meet their needs appropriately, comprehensively, and efficiently. After identifying gaps in the range of services offered in the community, many hospitals start LTC programs for the chronically ill and elderly to ensure high quality of care and the availability of services that address a continuum of care needs.

Second, diversified, coordinated health-care programs ensure high quality of care by ensuring continuity of care, characterized by comprehensive assessment of the elderly's medical and social needs, monitoring of the changing levels of illness over time, evaluation of the appropriateness of services as the level of illness changes, and following of the patient through the system of providers to ensure immediate access to prescribed services.

Third, hospitals possess sophisticated administrative expertise and quality assurance mechanisms and are well positioned to develop new programs that require management strength. Innovative programs that coordinate a wide range of services to meet complex care needs demand efficient and cost-effective management to ensure the financial viability of the programs.

Fourth, hospital leaders see vertically integrated comprehensive care programs as a competitive strategy to increase market share. Hospitals can advertise to potential clients that "we can coordinate your total care needs and provide you with access to a full range of services." This is effective as a marketing approach for attracting elderly clients to these programs and for increasing the visibility of the hospital as a responsible, full-service community provider for all health-care needs.

Fifth, the most critical component of a capitated payment system is minimizing hospitalization through coordination and provision of alternative services. A hospital that coordinates and delivers alternative services for the elderly better positions itself for the future—a future that many believe will be dominated by HMOs, social health maintenance organizations, and preferred provider organizations.

Finally, and possibly most important in terms of quality of care since the introduction of prospective pricing, hospital provision of a continuum of LTC services buffers the hospital against the risk of inappropriately long lengths of stay by ensuring that elderly patients have appropriate postacute services.

A Multidisciplinary Team Approach to Care

Geriatric Assessment

A growing body of evidence compiled over the last decade indicates that geriatric assessment units are effective in improving the diagnosis and treatment of frail elderly patients as well as in reducing utilization of acute inpatient and nursing home services and the overall costs of health care. Research on the efficacy of geriatric assessment units also highlights the danger of a short-term approach to solving hospital financial problems and evaluating the effectiveness of medical intervention.

Rubenstein has identified four objectives of geriatric assessment programs. They are: 1) improving the accuracy of diagnosis of the elderly by identifying unreported illnesses and making definitive diagnoses of treatable problems; 2) designing rational therapeutic plans that address a full spectrum of needs through multidisciplinary assessment that takes into consideration the psychological state, functional abilities, and social support of the elderly; 3) determining the most appropriate placement upon discharge from the hospital by guarding against inappropriate institutionalization; and 4) enhancing quality of care while making the best use of limited health-care resources.[31]

Geriatric assessment is usually conducted by multidisciplinary teams of professionals that include nurses, physicians, social workers, and other specialists. The practical issues facing hospitals designing a geriatric assessment unit include designing program objectives and admission criteria and deciding upon the program location, the composition of the staff, and the assessment instruments. For example, geriatric assessment can be provided on either an inpatient or an outpatient basis. Adequate funding and a consistent referral pattern need to be established to ensure the success of the program.

In 1979, the Sepulveda Veterans Administration Medical Center established a 15-bed inpatient assessment unit within a 29-bed intermediate care ward.[31] The team includes an attending physician, a geriatric fellow, a physician assistant, a social worker, nurses, and nursing assistants. A clinical psychologist, a dietitian, occupational and physical therapists, an audiologist, a fellow of geriatric dentistry, and a public health nurse consult on a part-time basis. Within 48 hours of being admitted to the assessment unit, the patients are evaluated. Assessments of functional abilities, cognitive abilities, emotional states, and support networks are conducted using standardized and well-researched evaluation tools. At the end of a week, the geriatric assessment team meets to plan hospital treatment, as well as posthospitalization services. The average length of stay in the geriatric assessment unit is between two and three weeks.

In a randomized clinical trial at the Sepulveda Veterans Administration (VA), half of the patients who were eligible were admitted to the geriatric assessment unit (the experimental group), and half received no geriatric assessment services (the control group). The results of the study were dramatic. There was a 50% difference in 1-year mortality. Twenty-four percent of the patients admitted to the assessment unit had died within a year, compared to 48% of the control group. As in other geriatric assessment studies, one to four new diagnoses per patient were discovered upon closer examination, and although the patients were identified as having more illnesses, they were less likely to be receiving prescribed drugs. The latter has meant fewer complications associated with inappropriate medications. Both immediately after hospitalization and at the 1-year follow-up, patients in the experimental group were functioning at a higher level and were capable of conducting more daily activities. Finally, after controlling for mortality, overall hospital utilization and nursing home stays had decreased.[32]

The most interesting results were related to costs. The initial length of stay for patients receiving geriatric assessment services was 2–3 weeks. The total number of hospital and nursing home days, outpatient visits, laboratory tests, and consultative and ancillary services were obtained from the VA in order to estimate total direct costs of the care for both groups. All VA services were available to both groups of patients; follow-up care for the experimental group was provided in a special geriatric outpatient clinic. Not only was the experimental group hospitalized initially for a longer period of time, but because of the intensive assessment and the number of clinical staff involved, its initial costs exceeded the costs for the control group. However, after controlling for mortality, the overall utilization of inpatient services and nursing homes during the year, as well as the overall costs for health-care services, were lower for the experimental group. The full-year direct cost savings offset the initial cost increase; the savings associated with geriatric assessment were more than adequate to cover the costs of the program.

Rubenstein suggests that approximately 5–10% of a hospital's over-65 inpatient population can benefit from geriatric assessment, as can an unidentified number of other patients in the community. In the Sepulveda VA, evidence indicates that some patients are more likely to benefit from geriatric assessment services than others. The program seems to most benefit patients who are perceived to be at risk of institutionalization, who receive inadequate primary medical care, who have poor social support, and who have lower socio-economic status. Assessment of patients with these characteristics also produced the greatest cost savings. Eligibility requirements for admission into the geriatric assessment unit have to be carefully considered and implemented to ensure the success of the program.

The implications of these findings for hospitals operating under the current reimbursement system, for health policy researchers, and for decision makers are numerous. The smooth and effective operation of the geriatric assessment unit, a regular feature of the British health-care system, depends upon the availability and accessibility of a wide range of services. Thus, its efficacy requires a true systems approach to care. As such, it is a model that would most benefit an HMO or other form of capitated payment system, or a "closed" health-care system, such as the VA or the British system. The current fragmentation in reimbursement and service delivery is not amenable to the development of comprehensive geriatric assessment, or so it seems. As hospitals increasingly join health-care systems or alliances, contract with HMOs, and begin to provide multiple levels of care, geriatric assessment may prove to help coordinate the delivery of services and reduce the average length of stay. In spite of the start-up and operational costs associated with geriatric assessment, a long-range view indicates that both patients and institutions can benefit from it. A short-term approach to keeping costs low may in fact be associated with long-term operational inefficiencies and excessive costs.

Case Management

One mechanism that hospitals will employ to improve quality of care as well as to reduce lengths of stay and encourage the use of newly developed services will be some form of case management.

> Case management refers to a system of locating, coordinating and monitoring a defined group of services for a defined group of people. The purpose of case management in continuing care is to make the use of community institutional resources more systematic. The case manager has a dual focus: on meeting the client's individual needs and on making good use of the community's resource.
>
> The components of case management include: case finding, assessment, care planning, service arrangement and monitoring. Ordinarily, case management involves coordination across the services of several agencies and over a prolonged period of time.[33]

The most typical case-management models are the brokerage model and the consolidated direct service model.[34] In the brokerage model a package of care is arranged from existing community resources, while in the consolidated direct service approach, care is delivered through an institution's own services. It is important to note that case management is not discharge planning; instead, it expands upon discharge planning through greater coordination, follow-up, and monitoring.

Physicians, nurses, and mental health professionals participate in assessing the patients' needs and the planning of treatment. Drawing upon the expertise of groups of clinicians, interdisciplinary case-management teams maximize the efficient use of health and social services by integrating acute and long-term care services in a comprehensive program of care and enhance quality of care by addressing the social, psychological, and medical needs of the elderly person over extended periods of time.

The brokerage model of case management is likely to proliferate in the context of the formalization of relations among hospitals and providers of alternate levels of care, such as home health agencies and nursing homes. Case management facilitates smooth transitions between providers and is a natural outgrowth of interinstitutional programs; it is one mechanism that fully capitalizes on the advantages of these arrangements. It ensures a steady stream of clients and immediate access to posthospital services. The conjunction of case management and formal interinstitutional relations is likely to enhance the growth potential of both. Widespread implementation of case management is also likely to further modify working relations among hospital staff and departments in unpredictable ways. The team approach to care will have repercussions on defining professional authority over care for the elderly. Nurses and social workers, among others, will be more involved in planning treatment for the elderly in the new health-care environment.

Geriatric Acute Care

One strategy to minimize the risk of iatrogenic illness, and to meet the special needs of the elderly population during hospitalization for acute episodes of illness, is to care for the elderly within special acute-care units. Geriatric acute care focuses on the restoration or maintenance of functional capacity. Given the characteristics of elderly patients, a typical geriatric acute-care unit emphasizes the following operational goals: increased patient orientation, decreased confusion, increased social interaction among patients and staff, appropriate self-care to maintain and enhance functional ability, and discharge planning started early in the hospital stay.[35] At Durham County General Hospital, the geriatric acute-care unit consists of a small ward rather than private or semi-private rooms, enabling a greater degree of patient observation and socialization. Group dining facilities, patient, family, and staff educational programs, and careful attention to toileting are other aspects of the unit designed to support the goals described above. Physical therapy and rehabilitation services are emphasized, while intensive diagnostic and medical procedures are minimized. Finally, patients are encouraged to dress in their own clothes during the day. The patients who are likely to benefit from the special care on the unit are older than 75 years, have recently experienced a decline in self-care ability, and are experiencing acute confusional states related to dementias or adverse drug reaction. Special geriatric acute-care units are not especially beneficial for patients who are ambulatory, continent, and able to care for themselves or patients who are chronically disabled, with low potential for recovery.[35]

Taken together, geriatric assessment, case management, and geriatric acute-care units represent a new ethos in caring for the elderly during acute phases of illness: hospital care is only a single aspect of the LTC needs of the elderly population. Support services that assist the elderly in maintaining functional abilities and personal autonomy, and as appropriate, ensure death with dignity, will have central places within the emerging hospital role.

Hospital-Medical Staff Relationships

Measures designed to promote new patterns of medical practice and service utilization by the medical staff are being instituted and will grow in importance. Hospitals cannot exist without physicians, and physicians cannot practice medicine without acute-care facilities. Yet, both hospitals and physicians are faced with an inherently contradictory incentive that has heightened with the implementation of the PPS. On the one hand, the hospital's fiscal viability is dependent on continued influx of referrals and the use of services,[5] that is, hospitals depend on physicians to provide them with inpatient referrals, prescribe hospital services, and generate a large share of hospital income. (In some for-profit hospitals, physicians who do not perform adequately in this regard are removed from the staff or are not given the resources they prefer or require.) On the other hand, excessive utilization of inpatient services decreases the profitability of caring for an individual elderly patient, and cumulatively these patients may represent a significant strain on the hospital.

Vertical integration alleviates the contradiction by making available alternative services to recapture revenue potentially lost due to decreased hospitalization and ancillary service utilization. For example, many hospitals form affiliated home health agencies to reduce average length of stay, generate new sources of revenue, and gain a solid patient base. The revenues generated by the use of new, less costly home care services can replace the revenues that previously were generated through ancillary services.

Among the most significant developments associated with the growth of centrally managed, multi-institutional hospital chains and the implementation of PPS is the increased emphasis on centralized and extensive management controls. The burgeoning use of computerized management information systems enables hospital administration to become significantly more involved in managing the clinical activities of the hospital. Administrators can now identify and monitor utilization of ancillary services, provision of services to individual patients, and the practice patterns of physicians.

Undoubtedly, hospital efforts to monitor service utilization and influence physician practices through administrative regulations will only succeed with the cooperation of medical personnel. Hospitals and physicians will work closely together to formulate explicit treatment protocols and practice guidelines. One may expect significant amendments of hospital by-laws to control physicians whose practice patterns jeopardize the hospital's financial security. Such measures, which have already begun to be implemented, include educating physicians about their utilization and encouraging informal peer pressure to modify these patterns. Another option currently under consideration by some hospitals ties physicians' payment to their own financial performance and to the overall performance of the hospital. Some hospitals have offered preferred stock options to physicians to encourage direct interest in the overall performance of the hospital. Finally, one may expect hospitals to establish guidelines that further delimit the conditions under which the hospital can exercise its right to limit or even revoke privileges.

The point of these measures is not to interfere with the physician's right to plan and implement treatment, but to sensitize physicians to the economic implications of medical decisions in treating the elderly. The importance of these measures within the emerging complex of medical and social services provided by hospitals should not be underestimated. As an interim measure, these options heighten physician awareness of alternatives to hospitalization and increase the likelihood that alternative services will become a more regular feature of treatment. In the long run, these measures will ensure that the elderly will be given the most appropriate care in the most appropriate setting.

Interinstitutional Arrangements

Benefits

In practical terms, it is neither feasible nor appropriate for many hospitals to develop and provide new LTC services, particularly when communities are already served by well-established providers. To gain immediate access to available services, hospitals enter partnerships with already existing community providers. Gaining formal access routes to programs or starting new programs with other providers offers many advantages to the participants:

- Hospitals benefit from the expertise of established providers of LTC services who have had experience with the special contingencies of caring for patients and administering these programs. It is most efficient to split the job according to the strengths and weaknesses of existing providers.

- Duplication of services, an inefficient use of limited financial resources, would be avoided.

- For many innovative services, such as parenteral nutrition, the unit costs are high and demand is low. By broadening the consumer base, a regional group of providers jointly offering services may make such previously unfeasible services more successful.

- Alliances between hospitals and other providers represent an active commitment to promote good community relations and a coordinated, unified approach to caring for the community.

LIBRARY ST. MARY'S COLLEGE

- Contractual arrangements may allow for immediate access to services by avoiding the delays associated with certification or implementation of new hospital programs.

- A joint effort to provide a single specialty service expands the referral base for other services of the participating institutions by providing an alternative entryway into the system of care.

- Joint projects allow greater access to financial resources, capital, and planning expertise.

The form of the contractual arrangements, the providers who enter into them, and the specific services provided are as diverse as the hospitals and as unique as the needs of the community each institution services.

Disadvantages

The growing popularity of new forms of institutional collaboration, related to the particular advantages accruing from such arrangements in a competitive and cost-conscious environment, represents the institutional form of the tendency toward increased rationality characterizing systems of action.[36] Institutional collaborations are regarded by hospital administrators as one technique for achieving rationality in the delivery of health care. Along with the benefits discussed, there are both risks and difficulties associated with interinstitutional collaboration. First, it is often difficult for institutions with widely different philosophies of patient care to work closely together: the differing practices in home health agencies and hospitals, for instance, often impede contractual negotiations. Second, while vertical integration and interinstitutional collaboration offers the potential for systemwide integration of care, it also presents the risk that health-care systems develop into unresponsive bureaucracies. To the extent that strictly technical or economic solutions to the problems in the health-care system disregard issues of quality of care and social welfare, they are misguided. Institutional collaboration is an effective strategy so long as the appropriateness of the ends and a commitment to individual and social welfare are kept in mind.

Joint Ventures and Contracting for Services

The specific form of collaboration, the institutions involved, and the services provided are varied. Aside from networks of informal referral patterns among community providers, the simplest arrangements are contracts for the delivery of specific services. The financial benefits and liabilities associated with the purchase and delivery of services accrue to the participating institutions; no new legal entity is involved in the transactions. A more

LIBRARY ST. MARY'S COLLEGE

complex form of collaboration involves the formation of a new corporation to provide specific services, that is, joint ventures.

The two common models for joint ventures are general and limited partnerships. While each raises complex operational, financial, and governance issues, and must be negotiated in light of tax and other laws governing corporations, they differ in terms of liability and management structure. Each of the partners in a general partnership has a role in the management of the new corporate entities and shares in the profits and losses. Limited partnerships are structured so that a group of general partners share the liability and management while a group of limited partners contribute capital but have limited liability and little or no role in management.[37]

According to a recent survey of 400 hospital executives, joint ventures are most often in place for ambulatory care, including surgery centers, urgent care centers, and diagnostic facilities (37% of the respondents), and facilities such as medical office buildings and laboratories (24%). In addition, 16% had joint ventures for alternative delivery systems, such as HMOs and preferred provider organizations, and 13% had joint ventures for the delivery of subacute and long-term care programs, such as nursing homes and home health programs. The hospitals entering joint ventures are likely to be urban and suburban teaching hospitals with more than 200 beds. It is likely that other types of hospitals will enter into joint ventures and that subacute and long-term care will gain in popularity.[38]

At present, 40% of the hospitals surveyed have entered into joint ventures with physician group practices, 24% with individual physicians, 19% with other hospitals, and 9% with corporations.[38] To a lesser extent, hospitals are forming contracts and joint ventures with senior centers, senior housing complexes, Area Agencies on Aging, adult day care centers, and social service providers. As the numbers of both chronically ill and well elderly increase, contracts and joint ventures with these other providers will become increasingly common.

Other than joint ventures for the start-up of new health-care services, two trends in contracting between providers have especially significant consequences. The first pertains to contracts designed to minimize the disruption associated with the transition of patients between providers, and the second, to decentralization of hospital services and expansion into the community through contracts with senior organizations and housing complexes.

The first trend is typified by hospitals contracting with nursing homes and home health agencies. Drawing on the particular strengths of their institutions, for example, hospitals and nursing homes are implementing administrative procedures and standards for transferring patients between institutions. Contracts specifying who has responsibility for transporting patients, admission standards for hospital patients needing specialized nursing home care, nursing home patients needing hospital care, and bed reservations for these special patients are recent developments worth watching. These contracts also include specifications regarding the sharing of medical information, staff, and ancillary services, and often they detail specific responsibilities for prescribing delivery and managing services.

Contracts with home health agencies also specify innovative arrangements for the sharing and training of staff, administrative and ancillary services, and treatment responsibilities. One important feature of many contracts is the degree to which they are responsive to the special care needs of clients. Through closely working together, staff can better understand the characteristics of patients, the services of other providers, and the appropriateness of particular types of services in specific circumstances, thereby reducing inappropriate placement and maximizing the utility of intervention.

The second important consequence associated with contractual arrangements and joint ventures results from the effective decentralization of the hospital function. Contracts are being formed with senior centers, housing complexes, and other social agencies to provide outpatient medical and rehabilitation services, health promotion, education, and community outreach. The hospital function is no longer restricted to centralized campuses. Health-care delivery in alternative settings must conform to the contingencies of the particular circumstances, thereby modifying the traditional patient and institutional roles. Working with senior centers, for instance, improves the hospital's understanding of the well elderly, and better enables educators to plan programs. Caring for the elderly in housing complexes similarly will broaden the scope of understanding of the health needs, living problems, and functional abilities of the elderly. A change in the understanding of the elderly's real health-care needs will serve as a catalyst to modify hospitals' response to these needs, furthering the growth in ambulatory care centers, home care, and health promotion and education.

Capitated Programs and Other Long-Term Care Insurance Models

As multihospital systems have diversified into new enterprises by acquiring and developing alternative services, they have sometimes fallen short when it comes to local-level, regional planning for services. Hospital systems have achieved vertical integration at the corporate organizational level, but have not necessarily developed vertically integrated long-term systems of care at the local level. Developing comprehensive services at the regional level can and ought to be encouraged by corporate systems; from a quality-of-care perspective, vertical integration and joint ventures make sense only to the extent that they enhance local institutions' ability to provide high-quality service.

Prepaid capitated systems that include substantial LTC benefits (HMOs, SHMOs) and LTC insurance are two of the many options available to local providers supported by multihospital health-care systems. (SHMOs are discussed in greater detail by Greenberg et al., Chapter 11.) Developing LTC insurance with the insurance industry is another option gaining serious attention from the leadership of the health-care systems. Historically, hospitals had a role in voluntary acute-care insurance: more than 60 years ago, the problems of overestimating the risk served as the insurance industry's rationale for not developing insurance for hospitalization.[5] Today, faced with similar uncertainty, the insurance industry has yet to develop adequate LTC insurance. (See Feder and Scanlon, Chapter 7, for more information on this subject.) Just as hospitals developed acute-care insurance, hospital systems are in a unique position to develop model LTC insurance. They are involved in the delivery of LTC services and are qualified to control their use, manage the funds, and market the insurance. These elements can be combined in an adequate program of insurance and services. Similarly, hospitals are well positioned to form joint ventures with HMOs to develop LTC insurance to supplement Medicare benefits.

Conclusion

In summary, we have identified five factors reshaping the delivery of hospital services to a growing elderly population: the limitations of the traditional approach to acute-care incentives restricting utilization of inpatient services, competition from new providers, the growth of centrally managed health-care corporations, life-extending new medical technologies, and the implementation of prospective pricing. These factors will have an immediate but lasting effect on hospitals and will give shape to a radically different system of care, both at the level of the structure of the hospital industry and at the level of patient care.

The economic survival of hospitals will most likely be based on a strategy of managed care. In this case, managed care refers to vertically integrated health-care systems in which hospitals, through alliances and negotiated contracts with other providers, participate in managing a risk pool of enrolled clients using preadmission screening, sophisticated management information systems, and case management targeted to patients with high care needs. Such a vertically integrated system can influence health-care choices so that the most cost-effective utilization will take place. Successful vertically integrated systems will include both the provision of insurance and the delivery of comprehensive health-care services. This centralization, along with a large client base, will allow these systems to provide services at a marginal cost, making their profits on insurance premiums. The following changes, which already are occurring, are likely to continue:

1. The principles and practice of hospital care will be modified to limit the utilization of inpatient hospital services and to promote noninvasive, ambulatory care. Acute care, a single aspect of the overall health-care needs of older adults, who are characterized by changing levels of illness and functioning, will be managed by multidisciplinary teams of clinical specialists.

2. The hospital's mission will undergo a radical reorientation in line with the above. The freestanding community acute-care hospital of today is evolving into a full-service health-care center. In this role, hospitals will be both direct providers and brokers of comprehensive health and social services.

3. As leaders in community health networks, hospitals will greatly modify working and financial relations with other providers. Hospitals and other providers, who have often worked informally together in the past, will begin to develop comprehensive contractual and financial arrangements for patient care, service or facility planning and implementation, financial risk sharing, joint staffing and education, and a host of unforeseeable joint ventures. In times of limited resources and a growing elderly population, the health-care system will place great emphasis on rational planning, efficient allocation of resources, and high productivity.

4. Finally, hospital–medical staff relations will become increasingly formalized as representatives from each group begin to work more closely together in the planning, delivery, and financing of new services.

The results from the Survey of Hospital Services for the Aging and Chronically Ill indicate that hospitals already offer many innovative and unique programs compared to those traditionally available to older adults and the chronically ill. Hospitals are directly and indirectly involved in a broad range of LTC and geriatric programs that provide an indication of the typical services of the future. The survey also demonstrates that hospitals have included consumers and other health-care providers in their communities in the planning and implementation of services.

Currently, however, there are hospitals that neither offer any particular LTC or geriatric services nor have access to them through a community provider. The mission of some of these hospitals probably precludes the need for such services. Yet the significant number of hospitals that cannot gain access to these services indicates the difficulties hospitals face in caring for patients in the current payment environment. The Medicare payment system, which provides incentives for hospitals to limit inpatient expenditures, combined with lack of access to postacute services, may threaten the provision of high-quality care. Extending hospital stays beyond what is determined to be medically necessary due to lack of appropriate discharge options is extremely costly. The current Medicare payment system in itself does not threaten quality of care. It is only a problem within a wider context where no other service options are available. Rational policy development and implementation ought to consider the broader system of health-care services and the effects of policies aimed only at one portion of a complex system. Reimbursement policies encouraging the development of alternative, less costly services, together with administration controls encouraging proper utilization and cooperation between providers, need to be explored more fully.

Despite decreasing occupancy and increasing financial constraints, hospitals are adapting to meet the health-care needs of a changing population. The rapid growth in services for the aging and chronically ill, especially prominent since 1983, will continue for the foreseeable future. Hospitals will diversify and become more complex organizations, delivering and arranging for a full range of health and social services.

The hospital industry is moving to establish comprehensive programs characterized by coordination and continuity of LTC services. By limiting high-cost hospital acute care and by making available a broad range of subacute, transitional, and community-based LTC services in conjunction with other providers, hospitals can assure consumers the highest quality of cost-effective care.

References

1. Brody, S. J., Persily, N. A., eds. 1984. *Hospitals and the Aged: The New Old Market.* Rockville, Md: Aspen Systems Corp.
2. United States Senate, Special Committee on Aging, and the American Association of Retired Persons. 1984. *Aging America: Trends and Projections*, PL3377(584). Washington, D.C.: Government Printing Office.
3. Rice, D. P., Estes, C. L. 1984. Health of the elderly: Policy issues and challenges. *Health Aff* 3(Winter):25–49.
4. See Ref. 3, p. 31.
5. Starr, P. 1982. *The Social Transformation of American Medicine.* New York: Basic Books.
6. See Ref. 1, p. 37.
7. Lubitz, J., Prihoda, R. 1984. Use and costs of Medicare services in the last years of life. *Health Care Financing Rev* 5:117–131.

8. Warshaw, G. A., Moore, J. T., Friedman, S. W., Currie, C. T., Kennie, D. C., Kane, W. J., Mears, P. A. 1982. Functional disability in the hospitalized elderly. *JAMA* 248:847–850.
9. Steel, K., Gertman, P., Crescenzi, C., Anderson, J. 1981. Iatrogenic illness on a general medical service at a university hospital. *N Engl J Med* 304:638–642.
10. Reichel, W. 1965. Complications in the care of five hundred elderly hospitalized patients. *J Am Geriatr Soc* 13:973–983.
11. Brody, S. J. 1983. The fractured hip: A multidisciplinary problem. Abstract. *Gerontologist* 23:184.
12. Bunker, J. P. 1985. When doctors disagree. *NY Rev Books* 25(April):7–12.
13. Rowe, J. W. 1985. Health care of elderly. *N Engl J Med* 312:827–835.
14. Wennberg, J. 1984. Dealing with medical practice variations: A proposal for action. *Health Aff* 3(Summer):6–32.
15. United States Bureau of Labor Statistics. 1981. *Employee Benefits in Industry, 1980.* Washington, D.C.: Government Printing Office.
16. United States Bureau of Labor Statistics. 1984. *Employee Benefits in Medium and Large Firms, 1983.* Washington, D.C.: Government Printing Office.
17. Gardner, S. F., Kyzr-Sheeley, B. J., Sabatino, F. 1985. Big business embraces alternative delivery. *Hospitals* 59(March 16):81–84.
18. Interstudy. 1985. *National HMO Census, 1984.* Excelsior, Minn.: Interstudy.
19. Iverson, L. H., Polich, C. L., Dahl, J. R. 1985. *The 1985 Medicare and HMOs Data Book.* Excelsior, Minn.: Interstudy.
20. Hospital Research and Educational Trust. 1986. First nine months of 1985 hospital costs and utilization. *Econ Trends* 1(4):1.
21. Relman, A. S. 1983. The future of medical practice. *Health Aff* 2(Summer):5–19.
22. American Hospital Association. 1985. *1985 Directory of Multihospital Systems, Multi-State Alliances and Networks.* 6th edition. Chicago, Ill.: American Hospital Association.
23. Brown, M. 1979. Systems development: Trends, issues, and implications. *Health Care Manage Rev* 4:23–32.
24. Holt, S. W. 1985. Vertical integration in home care, Part II. *Caring* 4(April):50–52.
25. Christensen, B., Mistarz, J. E., Riffer, J. 1984. Home care wrap up: Rapid growth pattern tracked. *Hospitals* 58(March 1):33.
26. Johnson, K. A. 1985. Exploring home health care opportunities as a result of the prospective payment system. *Caring* 4(April):54–61.
27. Read, W. A., O'Brien, J. L. 1986. *Hospital Survey Series: Emerging Trends in Aging and Long-Term Care Services.* Chicago, Ill.: Hospital Research and Educational Trust.
28. Evashwick, C. J., Read, W. A. 1984. Hospitals and long-term care: Options, alternatives, implications. *Healthcare Financial Man* 38(June):60–66.
29. Tellis-Nayak, V. 1985. *An Emerging Alternate Level of Health Care and the Hospital Role.* Naperville, Ill.: Illinois Hospital Association.
30. Mechanic, D. 1984. The transformation of health providers. *Health Aff* 3(Spring):65–72.

31. Rubenstein, L. Z. 1986. Geriatric assessment programs in the United States: Their growing role and impact. *Clin Geriatr Med* 2:99–112.
32. Rubenstein, L. Z., Josephson, K., Wieland, G., English, P., Sayre, N., Kane, R. 1984. Effectiveness of a geriatric evaluation unit: A randomized clinical trial. *N Engl J Med* 311:1664–1670.
33. Kane, R. A. 1983. *Case Management in Long-Term Care: A Policy Analysis for Hospital Social Work.* Santa Monica, Calif.: Rand Corporation.
34. Zawadski, R. T. 1983. The long-term care demonstration projects: What are they and why they came into being. *Home Health Care Serv Q* 4:5–22.
35. Warshaw, G. A. 1983. Hospital care for elderly patients: Initial findings and future research. *Center Reports on Advances in Research.* Durham, NC: Duke University Center for the Study of Aging and Human Development.
36. Eldridge, J. E. T. 1980. *Max Weber: The Interpretation of Social Reality.* New York: Schocken Books, 65.
37. Rosenfield, R. H. 1984. Market forces set off skyrocketing interest in hospital-doctor ventures. *Modern Healthcare* 16(May 1):70–74.
38. Wolff, S. O. 1985. Joint ventures: The trends and potential pitfalls. *Trustee* 38(October):13–16.

Ten

Lessons from the Program for
Hospital Initiatives in Long-Term Care

*Cynthia A. Coombs, Carl Eisdorfer, Karyn L. Feiden,
and David A. Kessler*

In 1983, 24 hospitals were selected to participate in the Robert Wood Johnson Foundation Program for Hospital Initiatives in Long-Term Care. The program's key objectives were to create demonstration projects that would involve hospitals in the mission of making affordable and more comprehensive health-care programs available to the elderly; to assist other care providers in meeting the long-term health-care needs of at-risk populations, such as those recently discharged from a hospital; and to reduce initial or subsequent admissions to a hospital or other institutional setting. Underlying those objectives were the convictions that society is committed to providing appropriate care to the elderly, that traditional models of acute inpatient and institutionally based long-term care do not adequately meet many of the needs of the elderly, including their preference for independent living, and that hospitals are well suited to play a leadership role in developing new approaches to care. Demographic trends in the United States, which ensure an increase in the elderly population, particularly among those over the age of 75, were also an important catalyst for action.

After a year of planning and four years of program implementation, 24 different models have been created to meet the need for long-term care of an older hospitalized patient group. Robert Wood Johnson Foundation funding for the programs ended early in 1988, but every sponsoring institution has planned to retain all or at least some components of the projects they have developed. One of the key discoveries made during the past four years was that similar strategic and tactical problems arose in the design and implementation of every program. Despite this, no single formula emerged to guarantee the viability of a comprehensive hospital-based geriatric care program. Indeed, each success depended heavily on framing situationally appropriate responses to those predictable challenges.

A respect for the local factors that influenced service availability, modes of financing, and organizational structure was crucial. For example, the existence of social service resources outside the hospital and the nature, needs, and preferences of the local community helped determine whether a project could and should contract for most of its services or develop and provide them directly. The hospital's mission, history, finances, and internal politics, and the nature and extent of other health-care providers within the community similarly influenced appropriate design. By understanding the relevance of such factors and how they can influence a fledgling long-term care project, planners can heighten the probability of effective implementation—and avert an otherwise inevitable mishap.

This article is an outgrowth of a series of focus group meetings held around the country during the fall and winter of 1987. At those meetings, project leaders shared their observations and extracted the lessons learned from four years of operational experience. Our endeavor here is not to promote a particular model for designing a hospital-based long-term care program, but to examine a number of issues raised with considerable frequency and to identify some of the solutions that were found. A formal evaluation, conducted by a Brandeis University-affiliated team and funded by the Robert Wood Johnson Foundation as a separate initiative, is also underway.

The Structure of the Initiative

The Foundation's decision to solicit hospital sponsorship of programs that provide comprehensive and coordinated long-term medical and social services to the elderly was based on several theoretical and practical considerations.

One conviction was that many frail elderly are medically able to avoid or delay institutional care—and the vast majority are eager to do so—if an appropriate array of medical, health, and social services is available to them. The provision and coordination of such services is highly complex, however, and requires the commitment and oversight of a carefully selected institution or agency. Although hospitals have traditionally limited themselves to the provision of short-term acute medical care, they are well positioned to oversee more comprehensive programs, since they are already a major point of entry into the health-care system for many elderly people. Many hospitals, in fact, have begun to expand into multilevel care on their own. This trend is fueled in part by a reimbursement system that rewards early discharge and also reflects the continued need for care of many elderly patients. Given the apparent inevitability of this trend for post-discharge ongoing care, the need for sound models of hospital-integrated long-term care is critical.

It was also perceived that hospitals brought unique strengths to the task. They frequently have the trust and respect of the community and may be the only local institution equipped with the resources, staff, and 24-hour-a-day capabilities necessary to develop and manage a system for long-term support and care. Further, in their capacity as discharge planners, many hospitals are already familiar with the process of making referrals to a wide range of community service agencies, home health care, and long-term care institutions. Indeed, hospitals are among the few institutions in the community to intersect the array of both health and social services on a continuing basis.

From the hospital's standpoint, participation in this national project was attractive for several reasons. Since the enactment of Medicare in 1965, hospitals have come to rely increasingly on revenues generated by elderly patients, and they are sensitive to any trend that could alter that mutually dependent relationship. The changes brought about by new financing mechanisms and an ever more competitive health-care environment have heightened hospital interest in long-term care. Prospective payment, for example, has increased the pressure to reduce lengths of stay and to maximize the appropriate use of acute-care facilities. The result is that transitional care for discharged patients has become a more important concern than ever.

Hospitals also see long-term care programs as a way to increase patient volume and protect market share. At $650,000 per project over a four-year period, the funds—while significant—clearly did not represent the total costs of providing a package of coordinated services to significant numbers of elderly within the community. Those hospitals already examining programs for continuing care to the aged as a logical extension of their traditional mandate saw the grant as support for advancing more rapidly in that direction. When asked specifically why they applied to the Robert Wood Johnson program, most hospitals cited the desire to develop a coordinated system of inpatient, outpatient, and community-based care, to improve existing hospital-based geriatric services, and to respond to increasing community needs. Some of the larger institutions felt that the grant would provide not only financial help but the prestige that could impact positively on program development in geriatric care.

The initiative was deliberately designed as a demonstration program to encourage innovative thinking and experimental approaches. Each of the 24 selected sites was given wide programmatic latitude, although a core of home care and community-based services was expected to be made available to a defined population, in addition to the existing acute-care hospital services. At least two types of long-term care services were to be provided directly; projects could either furnish the rest themselves or contract for them. The Foundation also required that every project provide case management and training programs for patients, family, and staff. The initiative was specifically aimed at keeping patients out of nursing homes and similar facilities and was described as providing "long-term caring," rather than institutionally based long-term care.

Consistent with the project's designation as a demonstration project, the Advisory Committee sought geographic and institutional diversity. Thus sites were located in 20 different states, from Hawaii to Massachusetts. Seven were in rural areas. The smallest hospital had fewer than 50 beds and the largest more than 1200, with the remainder distributed between 200 and 1000 beds. Twelve projects were sponsored by major academic teaching centers, nine by community hospitals, and seven by public facilities—categories that are not mutually exclusive. The communities in which the majority of the projects were located typically had a high proportion of elderly residents and significant numbers of low-income and minority people.

As expected, given the flexible program requirements and the diversity of the institutions selected to participate, the scope and nature of the projects varied dramatically.

Project Design

As a result of the four-year initiative, significant changes were made in the way that each hospital provided services to the elderly. At least one completely restructured its approach to inpatient care of those over 65 by adding functional assessment and detailed hospital and posthospital care planning to traditional acute services. More commonly, efforts were made to bolster the discharge planning functions and to formalize the links between inpatient hospital and outpatient follow-up care. All of the projects provided noninstitutional long-term care services, either by furnishing the services themselves or by coordinating them, usually through a series of contracts with community agencies.

Three of the more ambitious sites developed the groundwork for the establishment of a social health maintenance organization (SHMO) by integrating inpatient, outpatient, and community-based long-term care services for their patients. One of them went a step further by assuming a degree of financial risk in the service delivery system.

One of the more important structural decisions with which each of the programs grappled was whether to begin efforts to integrate long-term care within the hospital at once or to build a more self-contained project, with the hope of eventually weaving it into the hospital fabric. In this context, the physical location of each project has more than symbolic significance—15 were located in the hospital itself, with the remainder in free-standing offices or attached to other health-care institutions. When asked for their own rankings, the majority of projects said they fell somewhere in the middle of the continuum between complete integration into hospital operations and none at all.

Both the integrated and the discrete approach present their own hurdles, and the choice proved to be institutionally specific. At its best, an integrated project could restructure daily hospital routines as it attuned an entire system to the special needs of the elderly. In at least one instance, project personnel were involved in a hospital's daily work rounds as well as with patient discharge plans. However, in the main, the barriers to institutional change proved manyfold. Professional turf battles, a multilayered, hard-to-penetrate bureaucracy, especially at large or university-affiliated hospitals, and the inertia of established practices all delayed program implementation. Foundation grantees who opted for integration were generally slow to position themselves within the hospital, although not unsuccessful in outcome.

Given the freedom to create a project from scratch without the necessity of challenging institutional conventions, self-contained projects, by contrast, got off the ground rapidly. Sequestered from the hospital mainstream, however, they successfully provided services to their clientele but had limited influence on hospitalwide care of the aged patient.

Regardless of how it was initially launched, each project ultimately needed to achieve recognition within the institution if it were to become effective and long-lasting. Significantly, as the Robert Wood Johnson Foundation grant came to an end, integrated projects were the ones most likely to receive hospital support for continuing their operations.

Another crucial design question was the extent to which hospitals opted to provide comprehensive services to the elderly themselves or to contract for those services. Again, the local communities were a prime determinant. In service-rich environments, project sites found that establishing linkages among existing providers was more cost-efficient than duplicating what was already available. In communities where the range of services was more limited, the desire to be comprehensive obliged some of the hospitals to develop new services from scratch.

In determining whether to provide services directly, or to contract for them, the viability of local agencies had to be considered because unanticipated funding cuts could easily disrupt service provision. Conflicting goals and strategies often created tension between projects and community-based service agencies and the issue of control sometimes became a sticky negotiating point. In several instances, contract negotiations took more than a year and ongoing meetings were required to resolve new issues as they arose. The decision to contract out or develop services in house was not an all-or-nothing one, of course, and most Foundation grantees opted to contract with community agencies for certain services while providing others themselves. In a few instances, interpersonal conflicts among agencies created serious problems, as did historical tensions between agencies and hospitals.

With a basic design in place, it then became necessary to target potential clients. Many hospital-based projects initially envisioned serving all the frail elderly within their jurisdictions for an indefinite period of time, but that goal generally proved unrealistic and inappropriate. It soon became clear that not all frail elderly needed a case-managed array of specialized geriatric services—and that financial and staff resources were not available for all who did. Projects began to target the population most in need of services and to develop eligibility criteria most likely to capture that group. Proper targeting and clear definition of the service package proved important to ultimate success.

Age, physical and cognitive disabilities, multiple diagnoses, living alone, and limited or unavailable family support were all good predictors of need. More than two-thirds of the population served by Foundation projects were over 65. Forty percent of the patient population lived alone and more than half were widowed, separated, or divorced. Almost 75% of them were deficient in at least one activity of daily living (such as bathing, dressing, and cooking), with 18% reporting six or more such deficiencies. Predictably, the level of disability was a more meaningful factor in the need for case-management services than was age; age, in fact, was relevant only to the extent that it was linked to increased disability.

Even with a narrowed target population, the limitations of time, staffing, and financial resources invariably excluded appropriate clients. To reach those in greatest need while preserving their own viability, additional restrictions were often added to eligibility criteria. Residency requirements, Medicare and Medicaid eligibility, insurance coverage, and a requirement that primary care be delivered by the sponsoring institution were sometimes imposed.

The Provision of Services

Once the outline of each program was determined, a package of inpatient, outpatient, home-based, and community-based services had to be selected. Like other components of project design, this was not a static decision;

over time and with experience, the offerings were refined.

In response to the mandates of the initiative, which were aimed at countering the historic fragmentation of geriatric care, virtually every project offered some form of service or case management. Case management has been broadly defined as a method by which a trained health professional, social worker, or interdisciplinary team coordinates the delivery of comprehensive health and social services to the elderly. To ensure that proper coordination of care began at the inpatient stage, two projects developed independent geriatric diagnostic and evaluation units for elderly clients, while several others arranged a special physician consultation service for elderly patients admitted to the hospital. Other forms of coordinated care included nurse- or social worker-led inpatient assessment, usually in preparation for discharge; short-term (two months or less) follow-up after discharge; and open-ended, long-term case management.

While the effort to coordinate geriatric services was a major task of each long-term care project, the development of new services did not emerge as a major activity. Indeed, projects devoted less than 20% of their efforts to such efforts; only one dedicated more than half its time to making new services available. If a hospital did not provide a service deemed important to comprehensive geriatric care, contracts with community agencies were usually sought to fill the gap. Most projects provided some form of psychogeriatric services, rehabilitation, and geriatric medical care directly on either an inpatient or outpatient basis. Contracts were most likely to be obtained for transportation and escort services, congregate or home-delivered meals, and homemaker services, and in some cases for adult day care and home health care, skilled nursing, and hospice care.

Projects chose to satisfy the Foundation's training requirement in several different ways. The majority offered some educational programs to the elderly themselves or to their families; in addition, training was often made available to hospital professionals, community service providers, and interns or residents.

The shortage of trained personnel was a problem for many long-term care projects. Although half offered some form of home health care, there was a substantial chronic need for aides to provide homemaker, personal care, chore, and live-in services. Geriatricians were in short supply and projects cited a long list of other services they believed were sorely needed yet could not furnish. Day care, transportation, affordable housing, financial counseling, psychiatric services, respite care and training for primary caregivers, dental care, and physician house calls were frequently mentioned service gaps, although some projects did find ways to provide each of these.

Case Management: The Unifying Force

Under the Hospital Initiatives Program, several models of case management were developed in the context of local conditions, and each one changed significantly over time. After identifying the target population, a point of intake had to be selected, an array of services assembled, and instruments developed to screen and assess clients. Staff who were to evaluate clients at intake, develop a care plan, and monitor its implementation were then carefully chosen. Most projects opted for an interdisciplinary team—including a nurse, social worker, and physician—to carry out the initial assessment and to develop the care plan, and then to assign a nurse or social worker to implement the plan. The final steps in the case-management process involved defining a role for family members, planning and scheduling follow-up and reassessment, and ultimately establishing criteria for program discharge.

One of the most interesting points to emerge from the experience of project hospitals is that two distinct groups of elderly people benefit from case management. The majority of clients needed only "short-term long-term care" as a way to make the transition between the hospital and fully independent living. The bulk of case-managed clients were likely to cycle through a project within about six months; their need for follow-up care was continually reassessed, with the goal being the phased withdrawal of services. They quickly became inactive clients, monitored only by infrequent telephone calls, if at all. A very few of the frailest elderly, however, required case-management services indefinitely. This "long-term long-term care," or chronic care, was highly labor-intensive and time-consuming, depleting a substantial, arguably disproportionate, share of program resources.

The distinction between these two groups, however unexpected, was significant. One implication is that in collecting data about case management, figures regarding average duration and intensity of service use must distinguish between the two categories of this bimodal distribution or the numbers become meaningless. Planners and managers of a hospital-based long-term care program also need to be clear about this finding because it affects resource consumption levels. Budgeting, staffing, and service provision are all directly affected by the ratio of transitional to chronic care patients.

By facilitating a smooth transition from the hospital to the community, case management is of measurable value to a hospital genuinely committed to ensuring continuity of care for the elderly. Reports from the individual projects were somewhat unexpected in that case management seemed to increase hospital readmissions but reduced emergency room visits and admissions from the ER, indicating that hospitalization was more likely to be planned and appropriate. Lengths of stay for subsequent hospital admissions also appeared to have been reduced, possibly because such complications as malnourishment were less likely with the case-managed elderly.

As has been shown elsewhere, there is scant data to suggest that case management reduces the costs of care to the elderly or extends life. The value of a case-managed, comprehensive care system is difficult to calculate yet of great subjective importance—all evidence points to its use as a highly effective tool for improving the quality of life for elderly patients and their caring families.

Implementation Issues

The implementation of hospital-based long-term care involved a commitment to systemwide change on the part of a broad spectrum of individuals. Board members, administrators, physicians, and other hospital personnel, patients and their families, and service providers within the community all play a role in this most complex of undertakings. Support from each of these groups of players was repeatedly cited as key to achieving project goals. Not surprisingly, sound management skills, political savvy, and personal persuasiveness on the part of the project's chief proponent—most often the CEO, COO, or the Chief of Medicine, but sometimes a senior hospital administrator, department head, or a health-care planner—were critical to garnering institutional commitment. Clarity of vision, strategic timing, credit sharing, close links to other hospital departments, and an ability to convey enthusiasm and devote appropriate energy to the project also played pivotal roles in the successful achievement of program goals.

Administrative commitment to a long-term care project depended heavily on the perception of its value. Data that documented cost savings and evidence that it furthered the hospital's mission or improved its market share were particularly crucial. If the elderly represented a hospital's major constituency or a constituency it was most eager to attract, then a project perceived to enhance its reputation for caring, to expand the availability of geriatric services, or to position it as a leader in the field of aging was welcomed. The prospects of filling beds, obtaining fuller reimbursement for the use of acute-care facilities, improving the facility as a teaching model with enhanced prestige, and/or bringing a new patient population into the hospital sphere were also powerful weapons in strengthening the hospital's support of a project.

Physician support for hospital-based long-term care projects was slow to build. A traditional lack of interest in the nonmedical components of care, a reluctance to alter familiar decision-making patterns, and the perception that case management would threaten their role as primary caretakers combined to make many physicians wary of the initiative. However, most institutions had some initial physician support and the pace of referrals was likely to quicken once a physician had a single satisfactory experience with a long-term program or realized that it could ease workload while improving patient care. Peer support and enthusiasm from leaders among the hospital staff also proved of great value.

An alliance between the medical and business sides of a hospital was highly advantageous to project success; support from at least one faction was imperative. Upper-echelon administrators and influential physicians were more likely to welcome a long-term care initiative where positive working relationships and informal ties with its proponents already existed. Their commitment often attracted adequate physician referrals, supplemental funding, and public praise. Benign neglect or open hostility by the leadership, in contrast, consigned projects to relative obscurity. In a number of instances, however, when a project was stagnating because middle management personnel could not move it along, the CEO or COO intervened and the project rapidly progressed, typically with a change in leadership.

Community support was best obtained by responding to local needs and concerns and was also an important measure of success. Projects created in isolation or without regard to their potential effect outside the hospital stood little chance of gaining backing from influential local leaders. Of even greater consequence, they were unlikely to attract the patient populations they sought. The overall image of the hospital played an important role in community acceptance: hospitals with good reputations in their community were significantly more likely to win acceptance for a long-term care project.

Successful affiliations between the hospital and community agencies demanded a clear definition of the roles of each, a process for ensuring a smooth transition from one service provider to another, equitable financial terms, and mutually agreed-upon goals. At their best, such arrangements created new opportunities for networking, enabling hospitals to become more familiar with existing community services, while local agencies learned more about the functioning of the hospitals. Unfortunately, differences in philosophy of care, hostility toward the "medical model," and issues of turf and patient (or client) control challenged a number of alliances and forced the abrogation of several contracts between community providers and the hospital-based long-term care projects. Indeed, issues of control and perceived power played as important a role in interagency relationships as financial factors.

Project leaders identified several other issues relevant to implementation. The ability to market services proved important to the achievement of project goals; failure to get information to the targeted population was a significant obstacle and often slowed the pace of enrollment. An unanticipated problem was the frailty of many family caregivers, such as spouses and elderly children, which added to the burden borne by case managers and service providers. The time required for the acceptance of innovation was greater than expected—coordinated geriatric care has been institutionalized very slowly, and communication gaps remain between the long-term care projects and some hospital departments. Finally, the organization of the program in relation to hospital departments was a relatively frequent source of initial conflict. The relations between the departments of social work or discharge planning and the new project required resolution, particularly when differing professional players—such as social workers and nurses—were included.

Financing the Project

Today's competitive health-care climate inextricably links the broad goal of improving care to the elderly with harsh economic realities. However, even in the absence of national health-policy initiatives that refine financing mechanisms for long-term caring, the ethical obligation to serve the elderly cannot be ignored. Even without the guarantee of full reimbursement, hospitals may at times have to use their own discretionary funds to help meet chronic care needs.

Staff at the most successful of the initiative sites were able to attract additional support from a patchwork of available public and private funding for inpatient, outpatient, and home care geriatric services. They recognized that one aspect of care management was to stay attuned to the changing mandates of a range of funding sources. As needs and available revenue sources changed, they interpreted funding guidelines creatively and lobbied for income-generating services and sometimes new corporate structures through which to provide services.

Even the most creative of entrepreneurs eventually ran into the problem of resource limitations. Over and over again the projects cited lack of money as a debilitating obstacle. They recognized that the fragmented and confusing Medicare and Medicaid reimbursement systems are heavily weighted toward acute care, leaving significant gaps in funding for long-term care and social services. Third-party reimbursement was virtually unavailable for needed case management, and private sector funds for low-income clients ineligible for public programs were hard to obtain. Heavy administrative and paperwork burdens were also cited as a problem.

During the course of the project, federal and state policies changed. As a result, several anticipated sources of revenue did not materialize. One avenue of creativity for projects was cut off when federal waivers—which allowed hospitals to reapportion their Medicare dollars between acute and long-term care services—were barred, although project sites in Massachusetts and North Carolina did receive Medicaid waivers. The numbers of private pay patients and the availability of other private sector support did not grow as quickly as expected, which also disrupted financial planning. Finally, limited federal dollars for social services forced cutbacks in some of the community agencies working with project clients.

The extent to which the elderly themselves were able to pay directly for services was an issue of concern to many project sites. While the discretionary income of the elderly averages almost twice that of people under 35, some project directors detected a reluctance to use those funds to pay for health services. In particular, the elderly are less willing to pay for case management and assessment, which may seem somewhat amorphous, than for tangible medical services. Fee-for-service charges for case management were tried by several sites but with only limited success.

As the projects begin their first year without Foundation grant dollars, reimbursement considerations are certain to dominate planning efforts. Expanding their fee-for-service components, charging consultation fees to guide other hospitals in developing geriatrics programs, and exploring the feasibility of linking to a health maintenance organization or a SHMO are among the approaches under consideration.

The Changing Role of the Hospital and the Future of Geriatric Care

While the absence of coordinated funding for long-term care still obstructs programmatic development, hospitals are likely to continue expanding beyond the acute-care arena. Many of the forces propelling the move into long-term care have already been cited. The restructuring of Medicare reimbursement via the prospective payment system is only the most visible evidence of intensified cost concerns. The policy, which provides hospitals the incentive to move patients out as quickly as medically feasible, has been widely criticized for encouraging "quicker and sicker" discharges. It has also made the availability of appropriate outpatient and community-based services critical. The demographic imperative and a recognition of the historical inadequacy of transitional and chronic care services are also highly influential factors in the growing attention hospitals are paying to long-term care.

Further, there is a mounting recognition that the acute care and hospital bias of health-care financing has led to high resource consumption without necessarily providing the most appropriate care to the elderly population. If research and clinical experience continue to show that the elderly are best served by a well-coordinated program of care, in which acute-care hospitals play an important but not necessarily dominant role, then hospitals will have only two choices. Either they will have to accept a reduced role in geriatric care, with its concomitant loss of revenue, or they will have to position themselves in a system of health care that also includes social, psychological, and personal supports.

Given their economic dependence on the elderly, the former is not likely to be an option selected voluntarily. Should hospitals choose the latter alternative, as the most successful initiative projects have done, opportunity and challenge lie ahead. Structuring a viable system of long-term supportive care to maximize adaptive capacity when full recuperation is not a realistic alternative is a sensitive task. Careful attention must be paid to functional assessment of the patient and appropriate services must be prescribed. This strategy requires a detailed knowledge of the patient's physical and social environment as well as access to supportive care both in and out of the home. From the programmatic perspective, shifting finance mechanisms, expansion into new service areas, and an ability to respond quickly to the changing demands of the marketplace are also requisite. If those who pay for much of the health care of the aged—federal and state governments and third-party payers—ultimately develop a prospective, capitated system of reimbursement for long-term care, as seems likely, hospitals with a strategy for providing a continuum of comprehensive, well-coordinated services are the ones most likely to remain fiscally sound.

As the limitations of our society's health-care resources become increasingly apparent, questions of equity and efficiency dominate the policy debate and those hospitals involved in geriatric services will inevitably become embroiled in such discussions. These issues reflect only a subset of the concern over the hospital's role in health care in the future.

For the past four years, the 24 Robert Wood Johnson Foundation sites have grappled with one compelling question: How can we improve care to the elderly in a way that serves the interests of the elderly population, the health-care system, and society? The separate strands of clinical needs and demographic, financial, and social change appear to be converging on one answer: hospital-managed transitional and long-term care services. Such services complement the hospital's traditional acute-care focus and offer multiple benefits, but they also require careful development and gradual implementation.

In short, the hospital as a major component in an organized system of managed and financed care seems an emerging trend. The isolated acute-care hospital, unless it is unique in its qualities and it has a well-developed market share, seems at considerable risk—and indeed in terms of its role in our future society, perhaps this form of social Darwinism is entirely appropriate.

Eleven

The Social Health Maintenance Organization

Jay N. Greenberg, Walter N. Leutz,
and Stuart H. Altman

In the spring of 1980, the Office of Research and Demonstrations of the Health Care Financing Administration (HCFA) awarded a 3-year planning grant to the University Health Policy Consortium at Brandeis University to develop the prepaid, vertically integrated system of care for the elderly that has come to be known as the social health maintenance organization (SHMO). In this model, a single provider organization assumes responsibility for a full range of ambulatory, acute inpatient, rehabilitative, nursing home, home health, and personal care services under a prospectively determined fixed budget. Elderly persons who reside in the target marketing area enroll voluntarily in response to the marketing efforts of the SHMO.

Four SHMO demonstration sites were selected and operations began in March 1985. Initially slated to run for three years, the SHMO program has been extended by Congressional mandate until 1992.

The major innovative features of the model are:

- Comprehensive health care and long-term care (LTC) benefits

- Consolidation of health care and LTC under case management in one organized delivery system

Work on this chapter was partially supported by grants from the Robert Wood Johnson Foundation and the Health Care Financing Administration, DHHS.

- A provider organization at financial risk for both medical care and LTC
- Voluntary enrollment of an elderly population who have a broad spectrum of care needs
- Active participation of both Medicaid-eligible and non-Medicaid-eligible Medicare enrollees
- Pooled private and public financing of health care and LTC services
- Extension of insurance principles to LTC

In short, the SHMO consolidates the system at all levels: provider, population, finance, and risk. Full consolidation gives the SHMO the potential to be an extremely powerful intervention. It was hypothesized that consolidation of services would make it possible to redefine and coordinate provider roles and relationships and to do so without some of the regulatory and reimbursement constraints that have historically shaped relationships. The membership concept gives providers authority to manage care of individuals across the full spectrum of services. The balanced membership has an important financial function in that the premium creates an insurance mechanism for LTC. It was hypothesized that prepayment and pooling of funds would remove financial barriers to innovation. Finally, giving financial risk to the SHMO was designed to make cost-effectiveness an important criterion for decision making.

During an initial planning stage, each of the four demonstration sites developed its systems and negotiated contracts with HCFA and state Medicaid agencies. Site planning and development were financed by eighteen foundations and the sponsoring organizations themselves. Initial target membership for the first year of operations was approximately 4000 members per site. Actual figures were much lower: Kaiser-Permanente had 3174 enrollees; SCAN had 1140; Elderplan had 776; and Seniors Plus had 433. Enrollment, however, has increased steadily and by December 1987, almost 15,000 Medicare patients had been accepted into SHMOs.

While this fully consolidated model represents a powerful intervention, the SHMO presents difficult challenges to the professionals and organizations that are attempting to develop and run it. Brandeis and the first four SHMOs faced issues and problems in selection of partners and organizational arrangements, recruitment of a "balanced" enrollee population, selection of benefits and benefit structure, development of financing and reimbursement methods, and timely identification and correction of operational problems.

The development of the SHMO can best be described as a balancing act. At both the organizational and professional levels, the SHMO must balance autonomy with control, interdependencies with division of labor, and the ability to act quickly with the need to communicate with all partners. It must balance risks to the developers with risks to payers. Indeed, the project as a whole must balance the desire for major system change with the dual realities of limited knowledge and limited abilities of all parties to take risks.

The Four Sites: Basic Characteristics and Provider Arrangements

The four organizations sponsoring demonstration projects are the Metropolitan Jewish Geriatric Center (MJGC, Brooklyn, N.Y.), Kaiser-Permanente Medical Care Program (Portland, Ore.), Ebenezer Society (Minneapolis, Minn.), and Senior Care Action Network (SCAN, Long Beach, Calif.). These providers were selected because each has demonstrated a capacity for providing high-quality services and because they represent a variety of organizational configurations and diverse experience in providing acute and chronic care to elderly populations. This diversity required each sponsor to take a different route to developing a fully integrated system.

Organizational and Risk Relationships: Some Basic Issues

Even in a fully integrated system there are limits to interdependencies and consolidation. The need for integration must be tempered by the need of the constituent parts to maintain professional and organizational autonomy. In part this is true because it is obviously unreasonable to expect that agencies and professionals with a history of independence would be willing, at least initially, to cede a great deal of that control. But, perhaps more importantly, consolidation must be limited because caring for the elderly requires skilled professionals with a certain amount of autonomy to exercise their trained judgment. Concern for quality of care, therefore, sparks the need both to integrate the system (to have continuity and case management) and to limit the extent of that integration.

Thus, the overriding task of organizational design for the SHMO was to find a workable balance between integration and autonomy of the parts. Because in varying circumstances different balances might prove appropriate, and various organizational structures may prove equally acceptable, planners had to define a reasonable set of choices and approaches and to recognize the advantages and disadvantages of each, given the particular circumstances of the site. When analyzing options for organizational design, we found it useful to focus on three basic parameters: the nature of the partner(s), the nature of the partnership, and the nature of the risk-sharing relationship among the partners.

It soon became clear that most SHMO sponsors (except perhaps large health maintenance organizations [HMOs]) need partners to complete the system of care required in the model. It was also clear that partners would be chosen on the basis of such factors as their ability to provide the rest of the services, their resources (e.g., financial, experiential, political), and their willingness to adapt their operating procedures and systems to the SHMO effort.

One particular question that arises in the selection of partner providers is relative size. While picking a large partner (e.g., an HMO) may appear attractive to a small sponsor in terms of acquiring access to funds, market, experience, and other benefits, it may be more difficult to influence a large partner to conform to SHMO system goals. A large agency may be less willing to adapt to the needs of a small one; or, more simply, if the SHMO is a small part of an agency's business, it may not make sense to make significant modifications in its predominant operations to accommodate an experimental program. Size also affects the number of partners needed to generate a complete delivery system. Small partners, especially if their participation is on a contract basis or if there is competition among them, may be more easily influenced by the sponsor. However, a large number of providers increases coordination problems at least proportionately.

The second aspect of organizational structure is the formal relationships among the sponsor and the partners. The structuring of these relationships must take into account the need to see the system through the planning and development phase to orient the providers toward the mutually accepted goals of the SHMO, and to retain sufficient autonomy for provider agencies and professionals to allow them to maintain high-quality care and to take care of their corporate interests. There is no "best" way to structure these relationships. The relationships at each site must fit the nature of the sponsors and other participants. Solutions must also be sensitive to the legal, financial, and policy constraints of critical outside actors, most notably the government and the local market. While there is probably a limited range of distinct legal relationships (e.g., partnerships, independent corporations, subsidiary corporations, contractual service agreements), these basic forms can be modified and shaped to fit particular needs and circumstances.

The third component of the organizational structure is the method by which the partners share financial risk and reward. Three basic principles were used in establishing these risk relationships in the SHMO. First, those who have control should take financial responsibility, and where control is shared, responsibility should also be shared. A major recurring task in designing internal risk-sharing arrangements in the SHMO is defining where control begins and ends, and in turn, where a provider's risk should begin and end. Second, the risk-sharing arrangements should provide incentives that encourage cost-effective outcomes *for the system over all*, and the financial incentives of each individual provider should not conflict with these system incentives. Realizing this principle in an SHMO is more difficult than in an HMO because the SHMO has a wider range of services and providers. Moreover, risk related to control must be balanced with risk related to proper incentives. Third, the internal risk-sharing agreement should not be complex.

The most difficult challenge in SHMO internal risk sharing is deciding how to allocate risk for acute and long-term care. In the HMO model, physicians control the use of ambulatory and inpatient services. Thus, it is easy to capitate physicians for the former and to put them at some kind of joint risk for the latter, giving the decision-makers incentives to economize across the entire system. The SHMO has a broader system span, but systemwide incentives still make sense. For example, physicians obviously have some control over the use of LTC services in the SHMO. It can be argued that they should therefore share some risk for these services. Conversely, the LTC providers should probably share some risk for hospital costs. If they do not, and physicians do not share risk for LTC, why should the LTC providers make their best effort to get patients out of the hospital?

These issues would be much easier to work out if known, acceptable standards of performance were available for each of the various providers, but since there are no such standards and since a major aim of the demonstration has been to change current patterns, tying a great deal of risk to a target performance level for any individual provider would have been dangerous. To get around this problem Brandeis recommended that the sites use a bottom-line* approach to internal risk sharing. All sites considered the approach, and some accepted it, as outlined below.

Organizational and Risk Relationships at the Four Sites

Table 11.1 presents a summary of the basic characteristics of each site and their respective organizational and risk arrangements.

MJGC owns two large nursing homes and operates a variety of community-based programs. It saw the SHMO as a way to extend and consolidate its services to the elderly. [2] For medical services, MJGC created a new geriatric medical group in conjunction with Cornell University Medical College. Hospital services are purchased from two community hospitals, and LTC is obtained through MJGC. To pull the participants together, MJGC formed a closely controlled nonprofit corporation called Elderplan, Inc., which is licensed in New York State as an HMO. Elderplan makes incentive payments to the medical group for meeting performance targets in the medical and hospital areas, but the two also share risk for bottom-line

---

*Bottom line refers to the sharing of risk across all services by all partners.

Table 11.1. Overview of SHMO Demonstration Sites

Site Sponsor	Type of Sponsor	Relationships to Partner(s)	Key Opportunities and Obstacles
Metropolitan Jewish Geriatric Center (MJGC, Brooklyn, N.Y.)—Elderplan, Inc.	Comprehensive chronic care agency	Capitation contract and bottom-line risk sharing with small affiliated medical group Community hospital contracted on modified per diem basis	*Opportunity:* A large untapped market *Obstacles:* Creating an HMO and medical group
Kaiser-Permanente Medical Care Program (Portland, Ore.)—Medicare Plus II	Large, established HMO	No partners— SHMO added to existing Kaiser system	*Opportunity:* Use experience and reputation *Obstacles:* Creating LTC services
Ebenezer Society (Minneapolis, Minn.)—Seniors Plus	Comprehensive chronic care agency	Partnership with large, established HMO for all acute medical care Bottom-line risk sharing	*Opportunity:* Expertise and images of partners *Obstacles:* Competitive HMO market
Senior Care Action Network (SCAN, Long Beach, Calif.)	Case management/ brokerage	Separate contracts with medical center hospital and new hospital-affiliated IPA medical group Both on capitation/risk basis	*Opportunity:* Large untapped market *Obstacles:* Management and incentives in the system

Source: Ref. 1.

(total system) profits and losses. Since MJGC's development effort has required the formation of several new entities, it has been expensive. However, the focus of all parties toward the SHMO and the substantial changes in its delivery of acute care have made this a very powerful model.

Kaiser-Permanente-Portland is a large, established HMO that was an original site in the HMO Medicare demonstration.[3,4] Participation in that demonstration and the SHMO were motivated in part by the Kaiser system's large and growing elderly membership and the attractions of prepaid Medicare reimbursement. Given Kaiser's size and experience, the company decided to develop the SHMO's LTC services on its own, rather than to take on a formal partner. Issues of internal control were more difficult to work out than structural issues. Since the SHMO, known as Medicare Plus

II, has a small, new program grafted onto the large and established Kaiser system, it was not possible to use direct incentive systems to motivate staff to cooperate with the SHMO effort. In contrast to MJGC, the key issue at Kaiser was trying to convince staff to cooperate with SHMO goals and practices.

Ebenezer Society is a comprehensive LTC provider with a range of services very similar to MJGC's. However, because Ebenezer had more limited corporate goals for expansion and faced an already competitive HMO market in the Twin Cities, it was favorably disposed to follow the model of an LTC agency affiliating with an existing HMO, rather than starting its own. It chose as its partner the Group Health Plan, Inc. (since renamed Group Health, Inc.), the largest and oldest HMO in the area to form the Seniors Plus SHMO. The partners solved incentive and service-delivery issues early in the effort. Between them they already controlled all the services required in the model, and they decided to share financial risk on the bottom line: each would be reimbursed for its cost and then divide remaining profits or losses. They had more difficulty structuring their relationship to allow integration around SHMO business while still allowing each partner's other business to remain independent. The solution was a formal partnership with a series of written understandings concerning limits of liability and restraints on associated behavior.

SCAN is very different from MJGC or Ebenezer. A brokerage-model case-management agency, it provides no direct services of its own, but relies on an extensive network of referral relationships with existing community providers in the long-term and acute-care sectors. Still, SCAN's corporate goal for the SHMO was not unlike MJGC's, and it made the same key decision to establish a new HMO (SCAN Health Plan, Inc.) that the parent agency would closely control. Due to its limited resource base and close working relationships with some large providers, SCAN decided to involve existing community providers closely in the SHMO. SCAN uses a hospital-based IPA (independent practitioner association) for medical services and St. Mary's Medical Center for hospital services and pays both partners on a capitation basis, with relatively strong risk-incentive provisions, especially in the case of the hospital. Whether these internal controls will be more or less effective than the total system performance rewards used at the other LTC sites is an interesting question that continues to be followed in the demonstration.

As shown in Table 11.1, each of these sites faced a different set of internal and external opportunities and obstacles in development, which can only be highlighted here. Although Elderplan could draw on MJGC's chronic care experience, it faced the major tasks of building an HMO and a medical group from the ground up. Its major opportunity was a market that was large and basically untapped. Kaiser could rely on experience, image, and an established major market share. Its challenges were to test the viability of adding LTC benefits to an established HMO, to serve an aging membership, and to sell the community on its capacity to deliver LTC. Ebenezer and Group Health had a positive image and expertise in their respective areas. They faced the external challenge of establishing a place in an extremely competitive HMO market that included several senior plans, and the internal challenge of making the partnership work. SCAN's major problem was establishing some control over and proper incentives within a delivery system consisting of chronic care and medical services that were all contracted rather than internally produced. Like Elderplan, it had an opportunity in a large, relatively untapped market.

Of course, other models for organizing SHMOs are possible. A hospital-sponsored model is an obvious one, and in fact, the first SHMO site designated was Mercy Hospital in Springfield, Massachusetts. Mercy withdrew early in the planning phase, however, when questions arose about financial feasibility, the size of its market, and support from physicians. Currently, several hospitals around the country are developing SHMO-like systems. In some instances the hospital itself is forming a wholly owned subsidiary, and in other cases the hospital is forming a joint venture with its medical staff. This sudden interest in the SHMO model by hospitals is not surprising given recent changes in the methods by which Medicare reimburses hospitals, the rapid vertical integration of the health-care industry, and the likelihood that most payers might ultimately turn to capitation as their primary method of payment.

Obtaining a Balanced Membership

An essential feature of the SHMO model is a balanced membership. That is, the membership should roughly reflect the local community population in terms of health status, especially chronic impairment status. The demonstration placed some additional requirements in the membership area in order to test the model's potential in the competitive open market. Sites enrolled members voluntarily through conventional marketing techniques and enrolled both Medicare-only and Medicare-Medicaid elderly.

The general rationales for the balanced membership were the need to create an insurance mechanism through the premium and the need to demonstrate how the care of the entire population can be managed. The overriding issue that was faced in actually obtaining the balanced population was selection bias, that is, how to attract and enroll a population that was neither "sicker" nor "healthier" than the desired population. Obviously, the potential for selection bias was enhanced by the open-market model. If for the sake of argument the program had been set up to serve the entire elderly population in a community or if members were randomly assigned to the program and compelled to join, the potential for adverse selection would not have arisen except in a statistical sense.

One approach to avoiding unfavorable selection is found in the insurance industry, where applicants are commonly screened for preexisting health conditions and are excluded if such conditions are found. This screening is a legitimate basis of premium assumptions, but the method of determining Medicare premiums assumes that health status will be controlled by age, sex, and whether an individual is on welfare or resides in a nursing home. Screening on factors outside the formula "cheats the system."

The SHMO demonstration was prohibited from using such "pure" health screens to restrict membership, but it has devised a "queuing" method through which applicants are accepted or put on a waiting list according to their level of physical impairment. All of the sites except Kaiser have queued the severely impaired elderly at least some of the time in order to obtain a balanced membership. Except in the earliest days of the demonstration project, none have queued the moderately impaired elderly. Queuing is not health screening, in that a representative community sample of high-risk types will be allowed to join. In fact, the programs were required to enroll their "fair share" of high-risk applications. Thus, the queuing mechanism protects not only the SHMO from adverse selection but also the government from favorable selection.

Queuing has proven effective in obtaining a case mix that fairly closely reflects the characteristics of the Medicare population as a whole. At least 80% of SHMO members at the sites that employ queuing are able-bodied or mildly disabled; between 7% and 14% are moderately disabled and from 5% to 8% are severely disabled. The impact of queuing is most startling at Elderplan. In 1986, it was estimated that if all the queued elderly were actually enrolled in the SHMO, the percentage of the membership that is severely impaired would jump from 6.3% to 16.5%.

Benefit Coverage

The SHMO model calls for a broad benefit package because one of its underlying assumptions is that substantial downward substitution of services is more likely when the financial incentives of prepaid capitation combine with a vehicle to act on these incentives—namely, an array of lower-cost alternatives. In addition, market surveys suggest that potential enrollees prefer an array of home- and community-based services.

As shown in Table 11.2, each site provided all Medicare Part A and Part B services without the copayments and deductibles associated with these services. This discussion of the SHMO benefit package and service limits refers to the package offered to non-Medicaid eligibles. Dual (Medicare

Table 11.2. SHMO Benefits Package (for Non-Medicaid Eligibles) Compared with Medicare Parts A and B Coverage

Service	Medicare Benefit	SHMO Benefit
Institutional Services		
Acute Hospital	90 days each benefit period plus 60-day lifetime reserve. $356 deductible per spell of illness on Part A benefits required. Copays noted below are 1984 figures and assume deductible has been paid. For each day from 61st to 90th day, the beneficiary pays $89. For each reserve day, the payment is $178.	Unlimited number of days for prescribed hospitalization at hospital approved by SHMO. Complete hospital services (inpatient and outpatient), including all physicians' and surgeons' services. No deductibles, no charges.
Psychiatric Hospital	190 days lifetime. Copayments same as inpatient hospital.	190 days lifetime. No copays, no charges.
Skilled Nursing Facility Care Meeting Medicare Criteria	After 3 consecutive days in hospital and then transfer to SNF: first 20 days, no charge; 21st through 100th day, $44.50 per day.	No prior hospitalization requirement. No deductibles, no charges. Kaiser and SCAN: 100 days. Elderplan: 365 days. Medicare Partners: unlimited days.
Skilled and Intermediate Nursing Facility Care of a Custodial Nature	Not covered.	Covered up to limits of chronic care benefit. Kaiser: 100 days. Elderplan and Medicare Partners: $6500. SCAN: $7500. Co-insurance and benefit periods vary (see Table 11.3).
Medical and Related Services		
Physician's Services	Medicare pays 80% of allowable charges after $75 annual deductible on part B benefits is paid. Includes ambulatory (outpatient) surgery. Physicals and preventive care not covered.	Covers Medicare deductible and co-insurance. Ambulatory surgery, routine physician exams, preventive care included. Kaiser: $2 per visit. Elderplan includes authorized house calls by physician or physician extender.
Nurse Practitioner and Physician's Assistant Services	80% of allowable charges when provided incident to physician services.	Covered in full. Kaiser: $2 per visit.
Mental Health OP Visits	80% of physician charges up to $250 maximum (after $75 deductible). 80% of other professional charges.	Kaiser: 6 visits/year to psychiatrist; no limit to other professionals. Other sites: 20 visits per year. Copay per visit: Kaiser, $2; Elderplan, $5; Medicare Partners, $10; SCAN, no

Service		
Foot care	...when performed as necessary part of a covered medical service. Medicare pays 80% of allowable charges.	...other sites no charges. Elderplan in addition provides routine foot care at $2 per visit.
Blood and Blood Products	First three pints not covered; then 80% of allowable.	Covered in full.
Medical Equipment and Supplies	80% of allowable charges on durable medical equipment, prosthetic devices, and supplies.	Durable medical equipment, prosthetic devices, and supplies covered in full when ordered and provided by plan.
Lab and X-ray	Part B Services—80% of allowable charges	Covered in full.
Dentistry	80% of allowable charges *only* if it involves *surgery of the jaw*, setting fractures of the jaw and facial bones, treatment of oral infection, dental procedures that are integral part of medical procedures. Routine dental services not covered.	Medicare benefits covered in full, no charges. In addition, all sites cover dentures under the chronic-care benefit limits, with copays (Kaiser, 10%; Medicare Partners, 20%; Elderplan and Medicare Partners, 20%; SCAN, $50). SCAN also covers routine care; Medicare Partners covers diagnostic and preventive care; Elderplan covers erupted tooth extractions and denture repair ($15 copay).
Outpatient Physical Therapy and Speech Pathology Services	Part B Services—80% of allowable charges.	Medicare outpatient physical therapy and speech pathology services covered in full by sites. No charges except Kaiser, $2 regular fee.
Out-of-Plan Services	Emergency and nonemergency services covered anywhere in the U.S.	Approved emergency services covered anywhere in the world. Kaiser and SCAN, no charges; Elderplan and Medicare Partners: 80% coverage of first $500, then same coverage as hospital and medical services described above.
Pharmacy	Not covered.	Prescription drugs covered at all sites. Copay range $1–$3.50.
Optometry	Only covered if related to treatment of aphakia or if part of a covered medical service.	Covered in full. Kaiser: $2 copay. Elderplan specifies one exam per year.

(continued)

207

Table 11.2. (Continued)

Service	Medicare Benefit	SHMO Benefit
Audiometry	Not covered.	Covered in full. Elderplan and Medicare Partners specify one exam per year. Kaiser: $2 copay.
Eyeglasses	Not covered (contact lenses for post-cataract surgery patients: approx. 80/20 per part B).	Covers one pair glasses in each 24-month period. Kaiser and SCAN: no charge. Elderplan: $10 copay, Medicare Partners: 50% copay.
Hearing Aids	Not covered.	Covers one hearing aid in each 24-month period. Kaiser: no charge. Copays: Elderplan, $40; SCAN, $50; Medicare Partners, 50%.
Home Health and Other Community-Based Services		
Medicare Home Health Services (includes visiting nurse; home health aide; occupational, speech and physical therapies; and social work services)	100% of allowable costs, skilled care criteria and home-bound.	Medicare home health covered in full. Coverage expanded beyond skilled care and home-bound criteria when approved for long-term care plan.
In-home Support Services (such as homemaker, personal health aide, medical transportation, medical day treatment, respite care; and arranging and coordination of other services, such as home-delivered meals, chore services, additional transportation, electronic monitoring)	Not covered.	Covered with limits, copays, and renewability conditions as specified in Table 11.3 (varies by site).
Hospice Services (includes home health care, inpatient treatment for acute and chronic symptom control, family respite, outpatient drugs, counseling and volunteer services for terminal cancer patients)	5% copay or $5 per prescription for outpatient drugs, whichever is less. 5% copay for inpatient respite costs, up to a maximum of $304. All other hospice services are fully covered.	Covered in full (no copays).

Source: Ref. 5.

and Medicaid) eligibles are entitled to all services in the state Medicaid plan and those SHMO benefits not already included in the state Medicaid plan. In addition, acute-care benefits include dentures, prescription drugs, optometry, audiometry, eyeglasses, hearing aids, and preventive visits. Some of these have copays, as shown in Table 11.2. All sites offer unlimited hospital days, and two sites have significantly extended "Medicare-type" skilled nursing facility (SNF) benefits.

The expanded-care benefit package at each site includes case management, home nursing and therapies, personal care and homemaker services, adult day care, medical transportation, hospice and respite care, and chronic care in an SNF or intermediate care facility (ICF). Sites also include or arrange for home-delivered meals, electronic response systems, chore and escort services, and other necessary transportation.

While the service package is similar across sites, the depth and structural characteristics of the expanded care benefit vary substantially among the sites. The key structural features are summarized in Table 11.3. Elderplan is offering a gross benefit of $6500 per year that is "intertwined"; that is, it can be applied to either institutional or noninstitutional care or some combination thereof. Co-insurance is $10 per visit for home- and community-based services up to a maximum of $100 per month and 20% of costs for nursing home care up to a maximum of $200 per month. The benefit is fully renewable in either setting for each new "benefit year." That is, the annual term of the benefit begins from the point when the member first obtains an LTC plan, not from the point the member first joins the program.

The Elderplan benefit structure puts some specific constraints on resource allocation for case managers. Defining the benefit on the basis of a 12-month benefit period with monthly copay limits makes it possible if not probable that heavy users (more than five visits per week) will exceed the benefit well before the year is up. Members then need to go to self-pay or Medicaid spend-down status until the benefit is renewable. The monthly copay limit causes a somewhat faster use of benefits than an open-ended per-visit or percentage charge and thus restricts the case manager's ability to stretch benefits across the full year through higher monthly cost sharing. These limits impose pressure on case managers to find ways of monitoring and stretching out available resources for members who do not easily qualify for spend-down eligibility. Finally, with the renewable nursing home benefit, the plan does not have any financial incentives for encouraging institutionalization of costly home-care cases.

Like Elderplan, Seniors Plus limits the non-Medicaid expanded-care benefit to $7500 per year, with 20% copayment (see Table 11.3). There is no monthly benefit limit, so that, as at Elderplan, case managers are under pressure to impose some limits in cases where the benefit is likely to run out before the year is up. Unlike Elderplan, Seniors Plus has no stated monthly

Table 11.3. Structure of Long-Term Care Benefits at the Demonstration Sites

Structural Characteristic	MJCC's Elderplan	Ebenezer's Senior Plus	Kaiser's Medicare Plus II	SCAN
Annual Benefit Maximum (gross)				
Institutional	$6500	$7500	100 nursing home days per spell of illness	$7500
Home- and Community-Based	$6500	$7500	$12,000	$7500
Maximum Possible Total Annual Value	$6500	$7500	$12,000	$7500
Renewability of Institutional Benefit	Fully renewable	$8000 lifetime limit	Only for a new "spell of illness"	Fully renewable
Benefit period				
Institutional	By benefit year	By contract year	By contract year	By benefit year
Home- and Community-Based	By benefit year	By contract year	By month ($1000)	By benefit year
Cost Sharing				
Institutional	20% of costs to maximum of $200 per month	20% of costs	10% of costs	15% copayment
Home and Community	$10 per visit to maximum of $100 per month	20% of costs	10% of costs	$5 per visit to a maximum of $100 per month

Source: Ref. 6.

limit on copays, so that Seniors Plus cannot pay more than 80% of expanded-care costs at any time. This reduces the pressure on case managers somewhat. Also, Seniors Plus uses the "contract year" rather than "benefit year," so that it is possible for an enrollee to exceed the expanded-care benefit within a 12-month period.

For SNF or ICF care, Seniors Plus imposes a lifetime limit of $8000 (with 20% copay) for Medicare-only clients, which contrasts to Elderplan's renewable benefit. This lifetime limit could encourage expensive chronic-care clients to enter nursing homes. On the other hand, the requirement for admission review and ongoing review at regular intervals of all SHMO nursing home residents may encourage movement back to community services wherever possible. It will be important to monitor this throughout the demonstration.

Table 11.3 shows that Kaiser's Medicare Plus II has by far the deepest expanded-care benefit of the four sites and that the benefit is structured differently. A $12,000 annual benefit is allocated to $1000 monthly maximums for home- and community-based services. Thus the resource coordinators do not need to worry about benefits lasting the whole year, they have more to offer than at other sites, and the small 10% copay reduces the effect of the member's resources on decision making. All of these factors decrease the likelihood of members' spending-down in the community. Also, the monthly versus annual definition of benefits makes the distinction between benefit year and contract year less important. Kaiser made the same choice that Seniors Plus made in enhancing the value of home care by making its institutional LTC benefit basically nonrenewable (and in Kaiser's case, considerably less valuable).

SCAN's expanded-care benefit is $7500 per benefit year and is fully renewable in both institutional and noninstitutional settings. Co-insurance is 15% of costs for nursing home care and $5 per visit for home care (with a $100 per month co-insurance cap on home care). Thus, the benefit structure constraints on providing expanded care are similar to constraints at Elderplan (see Table 11.3).

In summary, there are some important differences in the sites' expanded-care benefits, and these differences reflect site-specific assumptions regarding demand, the effect of local competition on adverse selection, and the plan's ability to control the utilization of expanded-care benefits. For Medicare enrollees not eligible for Medicaid, all LTC benefits must be financed out of acute-care savings and private premiums. Therefore, variations in LTC benefit packages also reflect different assumptions regarding expected acute-care savings and the magnitude of the private premium.

In addition, given the limited resources available for expanded-care services, all of the SHMO sites faced decisions about the most cost-effective targeting of these services. Two of the sites—Kaiser-Permanente and Elderplan—decided to provide expanded-care benefits only to members who qualify as nursing home certifiable (NHC). NHC status is not measured uniformly; rather, each state sets its own preadmission screening criteria that weighs a variety of disabilities and medical treatments. A third site, Seniors Plus, officially provides expanded care only to NHC-eligible members but in practice makes frequent exceptions and allows case managers broad decision-making authority. At SCAN, seniors who are classified as moderately or severely disabled are generally eligible for expanded-care benefits. Moderately disabled seniors are assigned to inactive status when their needs are met through informal sources of care.

Each site also has criteria for monitoring disabled members who are not receiving expanded care. Typically, monitoring is conducted by telephone anywhere from once a month to once every six months. Elderplan has a more elaborate system in place: eligible members are called twice a month and a case manager usually visits the home as well. Such monitoring allows for ongoing assessment and keeps a case manager aware of a patient's changing health status.

Financing and Reimbursement

The SHMO is financed by a pooling of public and private dollars. More specifically, for non-Medicaid eligibles, the SHMO receives a monthly capitation payment or premium from Medicare and a monthly premium from the enrollees themselves. In addition, the enrollee is required to pay various copayments for LTC services (see Table 11.3). For Medicaid eligibles, the SHMO receives monthly capitation payments from both Medicare and the state Medicaid program. At Seniors Plus, the county also provides financing for Title XX eligible enrollees.

Translating this rather elegant concept into actual rates turned out to be a formidable task. First, the current method that Medicare uses to reimburse HMOs has some perverse incentives built into it. Second, state Medicaid programs have little or no experience in setting capitation rates for elderly recipients. Finally, since funds are pooled, each payer was concerned about cost shifting. For a complete treatment of these points, the reader is referred to Leutz et al.,[6] especially Chapter 6.

Medicare Rate Setting

The concept and basic elements of prospective, capitated Medicare reimbursement were established prior to the SHMO demonstration.[7] Under the established methodology, called the Adjusted Average Per Capita Costs (AAPCC), a program is reimbursed according to what it would have cost Medicare to serve the enrolled population in the fee-for-service sector.

More specifically, it includes Medicare's share for Part A and B acute-care services, that is, allowable costs less beneficiary payments for copays, deductibles, and expenses after benefits are exhausted. Medicare pays the SHMOs 100% of AAPCC.

The current AAPCC methodology begins with the estimate of Medicare's national per capita costs for the next year.

Second, the method estimates Medicare's per capita costs for the next year in the program's target county. This is called the Area Prevailing Costs (APC) and is obtained by multiplying the national figure by a 5-year unweighted average of the ratio of national to county costs. Third, the formula estimates how expensive the enrolled population is relative to the county population according to a table of underwriting factors. The current underwriting factors (Table 11.4) are based on a statistical analysis of Medicare's fee-for-service costs in relation to beneficiary characteristics, as reported in the 1974–76 Current Medicare Surveys. The factors adjust reimbursement according to sex, age, a person's Medicaid eligibility, and

Table 11.4. AAPCC Aged Underwriting Factors

Sex/Age	Institutional	Community	
		Welfare	Non-Welfare
Part A			
Male			
65–69	2.00	1.35	.70
70–74	2.25	1.65	.85
75–79	2.25	2.00	1.05
80–84	2.25	2.25	1.15
85 and over	2.25	2.30	1.20
Female			
65–69	1.70	.90	.60
70–74	1.90	1.15	.70
75–79	2.01	1.45	.85
80–84	2.00	1.70	1.05
85 and over	2.00	1.85	1.10
Part B			
Male			
65–69	1.75	1.25	.85
70–74	1.80	1.45	1.00
75–79	1.80	1.55	1.10
80–84	1.80	1.60	1.10
85 and over	1.80	1.60	1.10
Female			
65–69	1.55	1.10	.70
70–74	1.60	1.15	.85
75–79	1.60	1.20	.95
80–84	1.60	1.20	.95
85 and over	1.60	1.20	.95

whether a person resides in an LTC institution. The formula adjusts the APC by multiplying it by the ratio of the program membership's weighting of the underwriting factors to the county population's weighting. Thus, if the members are more frequently in the high-cost cells than county residents, the AAPCC will be higher than the APC, and vice versa. HCFA has been reviewing alternatives to the current formula for many years but has made no changes to it. In any event, the current SHMO demonstration will not be affected by an alteration in the formula, since negotiations have been conducted on the basis of the current formula but future SHMO sponsors should determine early which formula applies to them. It is important to reiterate that these factors represent differentials in acute medical costs and to understand that Medicare payments are meant to be sufficient to cover these acute costs, rather than LTC costs as well.

The current formula poses serious problems for the SHMO. This problem refers to the institutional underwriting factors, whereby reimbursement for an individual increases approximately twofold when the individual enters an LTC institution. Since it is a major goal of the SHMO to increase the proportion of seriously impaired individuals who can be maintained in community settings, a perverse incentive is created for the SHMO: a seriously impaired individual who is maintained in the community is reimbursed at the low community resident rate. Assuming that community-based and institutional benefits are about equal in value and thus equal in cost to the plan, it would make financial sense for the SHMO to encourage the individual member to enter an institution.

Because of this undesirable incentive, and because analysis of 1977 Current Medicare Survey data shows that extremely impaired beneficiaries who reside in the community are just as costly to Medicare as are nursing home residents,[8] alternatives to the current AAPCC formula were explored, and an alteration in the application of the current formula was requested. Under this modification, SHMO programs are reimbursed according to the institutional underwriting factors for enrollees who are assessed to meet state certification requirements for placement in nursing homes but who remain in the community. It is hoped that this nursing home certifiable (NHC) formula will give SHMOs incentives to maintain their impaired enrollees in community settings.

In order to incorporate a factor for NHC in the AAPCC, it was necessary to modify the current AAPCC underwriting factors for community residents. This is because the expensive NHC group's costs are included in the community-resident group's costs in the calculation of the current AAPCC underwriting factors. The modification of the factors was calculated by Brandeis using the 1977 Current Medicare Survey. The Medicare costs of community beneficiaries who were in bed or at home most or all of the time due to a disability or who needed the help of another person in

Table 11.5. NHC-Revised Underwriting Factors for the Aged (Based on AAPCC Underwriting Factors Received November 1984)

Sex/Age	Institutional	Welfare	Non-Welfare
	Part A		
Male			
65–69	2.00	1.32	.67
70–74	2.25	1.61	.81
75–79	2.25	1.98	1.00
80–84	2.25	2.25	1.09
85 and over	2.25	2.31	1.13
Female			
65–69	1.70	.85	.58
70–74	1.90	1.07	.65
75–79	2.00	1.36	.77
80–84	2.00	1.64	.96
85 and over	2.00	1.81	.97
	Part B		
Male			
65–69	1.75	1.23	.83
70–74	1.80	1.43	.98
75–79	1.80	1.53	1.06
80–84	1.80	1.58	1.07
85 and over	1.80	1.58	1.07
Female			
65–69	1.55	1.07	.69
70–74	1.60	1.10	.82
75–79	1.60	1.12	.89
80–84	1.60	1.12	.89
85 and over	1.60	1.12	.89

getting around in the community (about 5% of the community sample) were removed from the community groups, and the factors were recalculated. The modified community factors displayed in Table 11.5 are on the average about 5% lower than the community factors in Table 11.4. This is consistent with the fact that the NHC beneficiaries who were removed are about twice as costly as the average. That is, 95% of the community beneficiaries are reimbursed at 95% of current AAPCC factors, and 5% are reimbursed at 200% of current factors: $.95 \times .95 + .05 \times 2 = 1$. The underwriting factors in Table 11.5 are used to reimburse SHMOs. (The institutional factors are the same as Table 11.4.)

Medicaid Rate Setting

The majority of the other third-party payers—the four state Medicaid agencies—have little or no experience with prospective reimbursement mechanisms, and development has been different in each state. Only the

California Medicaid program has ever prepaid health costs for the elderly. While California was able to establish separate rates according to Medicaid eligibility category and nursing home certifiability status, it did not have the data necessary to take a full rate-book approach. In Minnesota the site and state agreed in advance to base the premium on a rate-book formula derived from state spending data. In New York the site and the state negotiated the rates for separate service components and used a limited set of Medicaid spending data and the site's initial finance estimates as points of reference. The site in Oregon used national data to devise Medicaid adjustments in its SHMO community premium rate buildup. However, the state had difficulty determining the potential cost effect of the LTC part of the site's offer, and currently pays only acute care for Medicaid enrollees.

Private Premiums

The cost of LTC services must be covered entirely from acute-care savings, private premiums, and copayments. The sites estimate acute-care savings to be somewhere between 20% and 30% of fee-for-service hospital costs, but these expected savings cover only a fraction of the cost of LTC. The sites feared that a private premium high enough to cover the balance of expected costs of LTC would result in substantial adverse selection. Thus, in the demonstration, setting the private premiums was based more on marketing analyses than service cost calculations, and all sites decided to set private premiums marginally above the cost of private Medicare supplemental policies. As a result, the private LTC benefit is below the level needed to insure for full LTC coverage.

Table 11.6 presents a summary of estimated monthly per-member premiums by payer and by site.

Table 11.6.   Estimated 1984 Monthly Premiums by Source and Site

	Source			
Site	Private Premium	Medicare	Medicaid	Other Public Payers
Kaiser	$47.00	$207.84[a]	$ 18.54[b]	No
Elderplan	$29.89	$274.51[a]	$340.00[c]	No
SCAN	$40.00	$288.53[a]	$ 91.44[c]	No
Senior Plus	$29.50	$233.97[a]	$573.00[c]	Yes[d]

[a]Based upon assumptions regarding enrollee distributions regarding age, sex, Medicaid status, nursing home residence, and impairment levels.
[b]Does not include cost of LTC. LTC was purchased on a fee-for-service basis in the first year.
[c]Based upon assumptions regarding proportions of enrollees who are nursing home certifiable or nursing home residents and Medicaid eligibility category. For Medicare Partners, it is also based upon assumptions regarding the age distribution of Medicaid enrollees.
[d]Maximum of $175,000 for first year will be available for Title XX eligible enrollees for chore and homemaker services.

Public Payer Risk Sharing

Public payer risk sharing in the early years of the program was one of the most difficult and important development issues faced by this project. While all parties agreed that ultimately SHMOs would be required to assume full financial risk (or find nongovernment entities to share the risk), Brandeis and the sites felt that the federal government and state governments should initially share financial risk with the sponsoring organizations. Not only prudent management but also important policy issues justify this position.

Providers in the SHMO face several different types of risks. Fifty years ago, Knight made the distinction between the concepts of "risk" and "uncertainty" in business ventures. The term "risk" applies to possible future events that can be predicted statistically; that is, the possible outcomes are known, and one can assign probabilities to each. In contrast, with "uncertainties" there is not enough information to assign probabilities to outcomes, and the range of outcomes may not even be known.[9] Although much has been learned, the SHMO remains full of uncertainties, including effectiveness in integrating the service system, appeal in the market, structure of new benefits, accuracy of cost estimates, effects of the aging of the membership, and the long-run adequacy of reimbursement arrangements with third parties.

Because of the magnitude of these risks and uncertainties in the demonstration, sponsors cannot be expected to have a great degree of control initially over these various systems or the overall financial outcomes. Following the policy that financial responsibility should flow from control,[10,11] since the SHMO cannot expect to have a predictable level of control, it may be bad policy to put the SHMO at full risk initially for service costs. Too much risk for providers can likely lead to extremely conservative, protective, and possibly dysfunctional behavior—certainly in the areas of cost estimates and benefit levels and possibly in caregiving decisions. Even with conservative strategies, the possibility of bankruptcy for sponsors cannot be ruled out.

In recognition of these potential adverse effects of full risk, and because of the unavailability of conventional private reinsurance for this type of experimental program, Medicare and most Medicaid agencies agreed to "share" risk with the demonstration sites in the initial years of the project. That is, SHMOs still were put in the position of standing to earn or lose money for their efforts, but third parties stepped in to limit losses (or gains) under conditions agreed upon in advance. Such risk sharing was designed to maintain efficiency incentives but at the same time protect against the dysfunctional effects of excessive risk. At least three models for reinsurance and risk sharing currently exist. HMOs commonly obtain reinsurance against potentially catastrophic cost overruns. The two most common models are "individual stop loss," through which the third party takes over responsibility for costs after an individual member's costs pass a set dollar threshold; and "aggregate stop loss," through which the third party takes responsibility for the costs of the entire membership after a set threshold is passed. Both individual and aggregate stop-loss coverage are usually obtained on an individual service, particularly by hospitals. [12] In HMOs these are typically reinsurance arrangements—that is, a premium is paid for the coverage—as distinguished from risk sharing, where no premium is paid but where gains as well as losses can be shared. One important approach to risk sharing, at least according to the literature, [10] is a risk-sharing "corridor." Through this mechanism, the provider and the third party can share set proportions of a particular risk over set ranges of loss (or gain) rather than simply handing the full risk from one to the other at the threshold.

All of these models and features are important precedents, but their use could create problems in the SHMO. Most important, the practice of insuring against costs only in a particular service area is problematic because of the substitutability of services within the consolidated system. If, for example, an SHMO followed the common practice of insuring only against hospital costs, in the context of hospital cost overruns, it might be cheaper for the program to keep a patient in the hospital than it would be to pay for more appropriate nursing home care that is not protected by risk sharing. The same might be said for chronic nursing home care and home care. Thus, the SHMO calls for risk-sharing models that not only protect against major costs, such as hospital care, but also are sensitive to the full range of service costs for which the program is responsible.

A second problem with insuring against particular areas of service costs applies even if a range of cost areas is covered. Aggregate stop-loss arrangements (and to a lesser extent individual stop loss as well) rely on setting a threshold or performance goal as a trigger for coverage. This reliance makes sense in an HMO (especially an experienced one) where performance standards have been established. However, until the performance potential of the SHMO is more clearly established, setting a priori standards can easily distort outcomes. Performance targets for various service areas can acquire a life of their own, whether or not they represent the most efficient and effective mix of services for the membership. Thus, risk-sharing arrangements that treat internal decisions neutrally are the most desirable. Aggregate stop-loss coverage on total plan losses and gains does this most effectively. This "bottom-line" risk sharing gives generalized incentives toward efficiency without specifying what "efficiency" means in each particular service area.

Bottom-line risk-sharing arrangements were recommended for the demonstration by Brandeis and they form the basic structure of risk sharing at most sites. Ultimately, Medicare and Medicaid agreed to share risks with SHMO sponsors during the first two contract years. * Maximum allowable sponsor losses in the first year of operations were limited to amounts ranging from $150,000 to $400,000. In the following year, allowable loss figures were doubled, with Medicare and Medicaid picking up the remainder of the deficit.

Without such a risk-sharing strategy, all the sites but Kaiser would have suffered potentially ruinous losses. In its first 18 months of operation, Elderplan reported a $4 million loss; SCAN was $2 million in the red and Seniors Plus lost $1 million. Kaiser ran in the black by some $675,000. During the following year, Seniors Plus showed a surplus but Elderplan and SCAN continued to show substantial deficits.

The programmatic goal to increase provider risk substantially over time was realized, with all sites reaching full risk by Year 3. Kaiser assumed full risk after its first year; the other three sites took on full financial risk for their SHMOs in the summer of 1987. In general, full risk is an appropriate goal for the SHMO, but it must be approached with caution. Until a provider has proven its ability to control the service costs of the membership at a level consistent with reimbursement levels and high-quality care, and until standards for quality and benefits are established, the strength of risk incentives should probably be limited to levels that can be absorbed without disaster.

Timely Identification and Correction of Operational Problems

While all of the organizations associated with the development of the SHMO believed it to be a sound concept, only limited knowledge was available when they launched the project. In all areas of the program, basic design, policy decisions, and seemingly endless decisions on details were made with very little data and experience. Indeed, many planning assumptions were bound to prove incorrect. Thus, an important development task was the creation of a system of information and inquiry to detect problems early, make timely mid-course corrections, and improve the model. Brandeis and the four sites recognized that there is much to learn about these complex health-care systems and very little time for learning, and so they have created a consortium of SHMOs to share data, experiences, and learning systematically among the five partners. Furthermore, they unanimously agreed to focus a major part of the consortium's effort on understanding and improving caregiving decisions and the decision-making process.

*The first "year" of the SHMO program was actually 18 months to allow sufficient experience for establishing second-year capitation rates.

Perhaps the most important consequence of the SHMO's consolidated strategy is to open up the caregiving decision-making process for examination. Caregiving is a very broad concept and is essentially a process of resource allocation, that is, deciding which clients receive which services from the program, including how much they receive. (The corollary to the process is, of course, deciding which clients and services are excluded.)

Caregiving decisions can be studied as three separate but related decision-making processes: 1) The benefits decision—Which benefits will be covered and how well will they be covered? 2) The eligibility decision—Which members will be eligible or targeted to receive particular services and how will they be identified? 3) The prescription decision—What types and quantities of services should members receive?

The first decision set involves the allocation of resources among various benefit alternatives and the approach to structuring those benefits. Each site made choices about the best ways to structure its limited funds into the most meaningful benefits through devices such as deductibles, copayments, benefit periods, renewability limitations, and different coverage of home care. The effects of each structure on case manager decision making and on member satisfaction, utilization, spend-down, and other areas is an interesting and useful area for comparative studies.

By combining acute and expanded care in the same prepaid system, the SHMO could theoretically shift significant benefit dollars from the former to the latter, thus compensating for current gaps in LTC benefits. However, unless acute coverage is deliberately diluted to compensate for current gaps in LTC benefits—which none of the sites chose to do—only a reduction in hospital utilization rates could achieve such a shift. Reduced hospital use is therefore important to the long-range viability of the SHMO.

Early data (1986) suggest hospital utilization rates for SHMO members are significantly lower than for the Medicare population as a whole. At the low end of the spectrum, actual days of hospital care (annually, per thousand persons) at Seniors Plus numbered 1424; in the larger community, that figure was estimated at 1883. At the high end, actual days of hospital care at Elderplan totalled 2087, in contrast with an estimate of 3742 for all Medicare patients in the community. Ongoing analysis of hospitalization rates will be essential to accurate cost projections and to determining available resources for LTC benefits.

The second decision set involves determining when a member is eligible to receive services. Once again, the freedom within the consolidated SHMO model makes it possible to devise and test a variety of targeting and eligibility models. Because the SHMO enrolls a microcosm of the entire elderly population, it must decide who among the membership should be targeted to receive particular types of services, and it then must decide if and how to go about identifying them. Again the most difficult decisions come in the expanded-care area, which, unlike acute care, has not had a powerful professional making the decisions. Expanded-care targeting schemes can be shaped to reflect provider attitudes toward prevention, the role of informal versus formal care, and the level and types of need that trigger formal intervention, as well as other factors. Along with spelling out criteria for expanded-care eligibility, each site must decide how strictly to enforce its criteria. At Kaiser-Permanente, for example, NHC status is used as the sole determinant despite the fact that it has sometimes shut out individuals who need care while entitling others who do not need it. Revisions in state NHC criteria implemented in January 1987 are likely to ease that paradox. The choices made at each site allow for comparative studies of impact and outcome.

Assessment is an essential component of the targeting/eligibility process and one which warrants in-depth analysis. In the SHMO demonstration, a basic flow chart was established and then modified by each of the sites. New members complete a 43-item Health Status Form (HSF) in which basic background information about social connections, health, and disabilities is collected. At-risk individuals are further screened with a telephone call. If deemed potentially eligible for expanded-care services, a more comprehensive assessment takes place and an expanded-care plan may be developed. At-risk individuals are monitored over time.

The use of the case manager as gatekeeper to eligibility for expanded-care benefits and the allocator of resources for prescribed benefits is an important part of the SHMOs and another area of ongoing study. Every member who receives expanded care is under supervision of a case manager, although not everyone requiring case management also requires expanded services. The way in which the case manager works with the member's family and friends may significantly affect the amount of informal care they provide and hence the amount of formal care the plan must give. A potential hazard of case management, however, is inefficiency and unnecessary dependency.

Further studies on the nature and consequences of the case manager's decisions are needed, as is better criteria for determining the use of the case manager's time in caregiving decision making. The different case-management staffing patterns and service responsibilities in the sites have led to useful comparative case studies. As more assessment and utilization data across sites becomes available, it will enrich the examination of targeting and eligibility issues.

A third decision-making process is the actual prescription of care to members. Once again the SHMO's consolidated approach under service waivers creates flexibility, and the challenges for structuring flexibility are felt most in the expanded-care area. Expanded-care practice has not had the time or the opportunity to devise a recognized and reliable set of decision rules for allocating service resources, and none of the sites devised more than rough rules for initial operations. Rather, resource allocation through prescription is bound by a combination of eligibility limitations and LTC benefit caps.

The goal of research in this area is to describe and analyze how case managers and other professionals, in the context of their particular program environments, allocate services to members. A concomitant task will be to describe and analyze how characteristics of members (including health status and social demographic status) vary across the four sites and to examine how these variations affect use. One possible approach to these analyses is to think of each enrollee residing in a particular "state" at any given time. For example, each could be in a nursing home or a hospital, at home without LTC services, or at home with LTC services; each could leave the plan, or die. It would be very useful to be able to describe these patterns of transition between the "states" for each site and to compare them across sites. Knowing about differences in stay-movement patterns for similar enrollees across sites would yield valuable information regarding differences in styles of practice and would facilitate cross-site learning.

These differences in stay-movement patterns have implications for the quality and the cost of care. For example, if one or more sites use posthospital home care more aggressively than others, these pathway models can be used to estimate the effect of home care (postacute) on the future of nursing home and hospital care, thus testing the degree to which certain services are substitutes for other services. Stay-movement patterns help to estimate service use in a particular state and to estimate the cost of serving a particular type of enrollee, and they permit comparisons of cost and use among different styles of practice.

In addition to comparisons to each other, the four sites currently service other elderly populations that can serve as additional comparison groups. For example, the Kaiser-Portland site can compare the acute-care utilization experience of a SHMO population with the experience of a population enrolled in a similar experiment, Seniors Plus, without LTC benefits. Both of these populations can then be compared to a control population from the general aged membership of the Kaiser Foundation Health Plan. The findings from comparing these three groups could be extremely useful to HMOs in attempting to develop the most cost-effective approaches to serving the elderly population. This research and analysis would fulfill one of the main functions of the SHMO demonstration project: to provide policymakers and caregivers with new bodies of knowledge.

References

1. Greenberg, J. N., Leutz, W. N. 1984. The social/health maintenance organization and its role in reforming the long-term care system. In *Long-Term Care Financing and Delivery Systems*. ed. P. Feinstein, M. Gornick, and J. Greenberg. Washington, D.C.: Health Care Financing Administration, 59.
2. Kodner, D. 1981. Who's S/HMO? *Home Health Services Q* 2:4.
3. Galblum, J., Trieger, S. 1982. Demonstrations of alternative delivery systems under Medicare and Medicaid. *Health Care Financing Rev* 3:3.
4. Greenlick, M., Lamb, S., Carpenter, T., Fischer, T., Marks, S., Cooper, W. 1983. A successful Medicare prospective payment demonstration. *Health Care Financing Rev.* 4:4.
5. Leutz, W., Greenberg, J., Abrahams, R., Prottas, J., Diamond, L., Gruenberg, L. 1985. *Changing Health Care for an Aging Society*, pp. 62–64. Lexington, Mass.: Lexington Books.
6. See Ref. 5, pp. 179–216.
7. Trieger, S., Galblum, T., Riley, G. 1981. *HMOs: Issues and Alternatives for Medicare and Medicaid*. Pub. No. 03107. Washington, D.C.: Health Care Financing Administration.
8. Gruenberg, L., Stuart, H. 1982. A health status based AAPCC: The disability level approach. University Health Policy Center Working Paper. Waltham, Mass.: Brandeis University.
9. Knight, F. 1971. *Risk, Uncertainty and Profit*. Chicago: University of Chicago Press.
10. Leighton, R. 1979. Selective risk sharing: A new reimbursement alternative. In *Perspectives on Medicare Management*. Baltimore, Md.: Health Care Financing Administration.
11. Zelten, R. 1981. Provider reimbursement alternatives and the placement of financial risk: A framework for analysis. *Top Health Care Financing* 8(2):61–72.
12. Miller, S. K. 1981. Reinsurance in an S/HMO environment. University Health Policy Center Working Paper. Waltham, Mass.: Brandeis University.

Twelve

The Nursing Home Conundrum

Iris C. Freeman and Bruce C. Vladeck

Nursing homes have been the subject of so much public obloquy, so much industry defensiveness, and so much earnest scholarship in the last decade or so that the truth ought to be quite clear by now. It is not. Whatever else can be said about nursing homes, the consensus is that they present an obstinate jumble of problems that have to be solved very soon, because there are more and more old people and less and less (or about the same, but that is tantamount to less) money.

In 1985, somewhere around one and a half million people were housed in about 16,000 nursing homes, at an annual total expense exceeding $30 billion. Since 1975, expenditures for nursing homes have grown preeminently among the other rapidly growing components of national health expenditures, and that fact constitutes *the* nursing home problem for some observers. More than half of all nursing home payments arise directly from public programs, and those expenditures have increased so much faster than other budget items that a policy preoccupation with refactoring eligibility and reimbursement systems has, to some degree, eclipsed the equally critical problem of ensuring that people receive services of value equal to the payment.

The risk factors for entering a nursing home have also become increasingly clear. The older the old, the greater is the risk. An estimated 2% of those age 65–75 reside in nursing homes, while the percentage grows to

7% for those age 75–84, and to 16% for those 85 and over.[1] Residents are disproportionately from the single, widowed, childless, and poor subpopulations of the elderly.[2] Incontinence and/or mental impairment are often the distinguishing factors between nursing home residents and those with otherwise comparable disabilities receiving care in their own homes. All projections predict substantial growth in the population at greatest risk of needing 24-hour institutional care.

Despite the commonalities of risk factors, on other dimensions nursing home residents are significantly heterogeneous. Their problems range from those of the short-term resident with intense rehabilitative needs to the physically robust with dementing illness and the severely disabled younger person. It is little wonder that any home attempting to serve this diversity would be hard-pressed to supply the treatment services, environmental comforts, and social activities that are optimal for each client.

Some assertions about the genesis of the nursing home problem ought to be addressed. One misconception is that families abandon elders. A growing body of research reaffirms the conclusion that most disabled elderly persons in need of regular and continuing assistance are getting it at home, largely from spouses, daughters, and daughters-in-law. Incidents of families "dumping" elderly relatives are the minority; many nursing home residents have no immediate family members.

Another assertion is that nursing homes have dominated the long-term care service terrain since the mid-sixties because of the institutional bias in Medicare and Medicaid reimbursement. It would be foolish to argue otherwise, given the consistently minuscule (although now rapidly growing) percentage of those budgets spent for community alternatives.[3] But perceptions of home care are changing, too. A decade ago, the conventional point of view was that care outside the nursing home was always cheaper and always more satisfactory. As time went on, discussion veered toward the notion that costs can go either way, depending on circumstances, but that home care is qualitatively more satisfactory. Currently, there are vexing economic questions about whether the alternatives have demonstrable benefits,[4] vexing social concerns that noninstitutionalization is creating a class of isolates who see no human being other than their twice-a-week homemaker, and no end of worry that a comparatively unregulated home-care industry will eclipse the nursing home scandals of the seventies.

Ironically, there is a subset of long-term care consumers eager for nursing home care, for whom getting in and staying in are the desired but unattainable objectives. Although there is wide variation across states in the number of nursing home beds per elderly person, nursing home occupancy is well over 90% in every state but Texas, with waiting lists typical at the more popular facilities. Over the last decade, bed supply has not kept pace with the growth of the population at risk. This stagnation in capacity growth is largely the result of conscious policy choices at the state level, implemented through certificate-of-need programs, construction moratoria, and tightening of Medicaid reimbursement policies. Whether these will eventually spur the development of alternative care and financing programs, as intended, or will, along with changes in hospital utilization and demography, bifurcate the system between rich and poor, is a pressing policy question.

The suppliers' market meshes with efforts initiated by state Medicaid agencies, particularly since 1981, to reduce nursing home admissions in order to help control expenditures. Preadmission screening, the Janus of long-term care policy, can work both to save the somewhat more able from a trap and as a devious sham that abandons a portion of the needy. With considerably less ambiguity, during one or another state budget crisis, some states have chosen to eliminate Medicaid coverage from lower levels of care and then to reclassify residents into those care levels. The risk that this order of eviction poses to a nursing home resident is no less when it originates in a state budget mark-up than when it results from a nursing home operator's decision to spurn lower-paying or higher-service clientele.

In terms of access to nursing home care, however, scattered state initiatives of this kind have far less effect than basic business logic. Because Medicaid rates are almost invariably lower than private rates, and by law may not be any higher, nursing home operators can maximize net income by favoring the private-pay client. It is, however, fascinating that in Minnesota, discrimination against Medicaid recipients persisted long after Medicaid and private rates were equalized by state law, and had to be subdued by subsequent specific legal prohibition. The varieties of Medicaid discrimination include quotas, requiring a period (characteristically one year) of private payment, eviction when private funds are exhausted, and distinct part certification. In some urban areas, Medicaid discrimination pairs with racial and ethnic bias. [5] Furthermore, lest anyone categorize this a sin of the profitmakers, the practice is at least as prevalent in nonproprietary homes.

Another way nursing home operators optimize income is the preferential admission of easier-to-care-for residents. There is no question that people with specialized medical needs and/or severe mental problems are costlier to nurse and to supervise, and they can create operational and staffing stresses as well as higher expense. Reimbursement systems that are sensitive to case mix constitute the currently popular solution to this sort of discrimination, although one suspects that such systems may just encourage sophisticated operators to discriminate in a more complex fashion.

From all these stubborn characteristics, one might conclude that nursing homes are a dubious invention made precious by scarcity. To make matters worse, the methods we have for quality assurance and financing have evolved with very little qualitative information about the experiences of nursing home residents and their families. The remainder of this chapter describes in greater detail the information we have and do not have, the variability of the terrain, and the types of problems and their causes. It also suggests some transformation at both the public regulatory and professional practice levels. We conclude, however, with cautions about the prospects for progress in nursing home reform, given the current turbulence of the larger health and welfare environment.

Facts and Counterfacts

In theory, policy and practice ought to be based on sound qualitative and quantitative data; for nursing homes, such data do not even begin to exist. A 2½-year study of nursing home regulation, released in March of 1986, confirmed that accurate, complete, and current information on the characteristics of nursing homes (their number, size, ownership, certification, status, age) is not readily available. Information on the outcomes of inspection and enforcement actions was found to be neither complete nor reliable at either the state or national levels.[6]

There is, nonetheless, no dearth of written records, spoken narratives, or strong opinions about nursing homes. Each state health agency has miles of survey data, each page a snapshot in time. Some are tainted by "company manners" and other greater or lesser deceits. Complaint office data, while responding to exigencies of the moment, do not account for all the unblown whistles. Despite the comparative immediacy of complaint investigations over annual or even less-frequent full surveys, documentation still depends on the quality of the evidence and the skills of the investigator. Similar deficits attend the volumes of ombudsman complaint records, although because the ombudsman service involves more personal counsel with the complainant(s), there is greater likelihood of a textured qualitative record. For balance, the most propitious format is the nursing home profile developed by community service organizations, because these are geared to assessing both the strengths and weaknesses in a nursing home's environment and program.[7]

That these records exist is not to say that there is public awareness of them. Unless one works in or around nursing homes or has a family crisis concerning a nursing home admission or problem during residence, there is little likelihood of knowing about the records. Policymakers and the general public do, however, tend to have durable opinions about nursing homes, mostly aversion, but some applause, all reinforced with considerable misinformation and misconception.

Nursing homes most often reach the short agenda of public attention as the result of highly visible scandals. New York and Texas may vie for the most disgraceful instance of the decade, but no state is innocent of comparable stain. To the considerable extent that they constitute the sum of public knowledge about nursing homes, however, such scandals have led to other kinds of distortions, as the public and its representatives have sought to make the worst cases impossible and thereby may have frustrated efforts at the best.

A further impediment to uncomplicated policy discussion is the conspicuous variability among those entities that are legally entitled to operate as nursing homes. As limited illustration, consider the following portraits, one from a nursing home surveyor's finding, the second describing another facility not too far from the first.

A patient who is diagnosed with cerebral palsy and has no functional use of his hands eats his meals with his face in his food. The meat is ground, but he eats whole such items as buttered bread, jello, and canned peaches. The nursing staff was observed to offer no assistance beyond pushing the milk glass and straw forward when his head pushed it beyond his reach. . . . Three times, urine puddles were noted on the dining floor area during the passing of the noon meal trays. The urine was noted to stand 5–15 minutes before being cleaned up. Staff were also seen walking around the urine to pass out trays. . . . In addition to the patient assignments previously mentioned, the director of nurses pulls 2–3 nursing assistants off the floor to staff a daycare program. No additional staffing is provided to cover the nursing needs of the patients of the assistants assigned to the daycare program. When questioned about this, one nursing assistant answered that most sleep in the afternoon anyway. When asked if anyone makes rounds in her absence, she replied no.[8]

[X] is a nondenominational, nonprofit home governed by a 24-member board. Its residents average 87 years of age. Four-fifths receive public assistance. Five years ago, in response to multi-faceted dispirit, the administrator, staff, and residents began to develop a new philosophy and program aimed at physical, intellectual, and spiritual well-being. A notable portion of this soft revolution was the on-site addition of an infant day care center, called the Oak and Acorn. "While the center has its own staff, residents are free to rock, feed, cuddle, and walk the babies. This addition has proven to be a great source of pleasure and satisfaction to the residents, staff, and the parents of the infants. Providing an arena to practice the natural role of nurturing serves to strengthen the self-esteem of the residents." The program, in totality, demonstrates a compatability of give and take with some rather dramatic, objective results. After its first full year, hospital days had been reduced by 50%. The percentage of residents maintaining or decreasing their level of care showed similar gain. Staff turnover rates decreased markedly. One would need to be cautionary about these findings, had the stage been primed for success. Instead, the experiment began at a time when the state Department of Health had recorded one of the highest medication ratios in the state at this time.[9]

These homes, described in 1984, were fewer than five miles apart. They were both licensed as nursing homes by the state health department. They were both certified to receive Medicaid reimbursement by the federal government. Their per diem Medicaid rates for 1985, predicated in part on the prior year's expenses and set by the state human services department, differed, on average, by 50 cents.[10]

For all their compelling differences (disregarding for a moment that they may not even be the most extreme the jurisdiction has to offer), these facilities are accorded some valuable common denominators by agencies obligated to protect the public health and welfare. All this equity looks unfair.

Traditional Problems and Promising Trends

The things that can and do go wrong in nursing homes are, categorically, as familiar as the headlines that announce them. Personal hygiene, dental care, and special diets may be ignored; unappetizing food may be served, even in stingy portions; the staff may be discourteous, may violate privacy, and may deny residents information about medical choices; overbilling and misuse of personal fund accounts can occur; and the environment can be unsafe and unsanitary. These possibilities are too often reality—the stuff of which scandals have been made. There are so many domains of risk that rules for certification or licensure and ombudsman complaint codes typically define more than one hundred kinds of violation or harm.

Conversely, there is no comparable and generally accepted code of all the things that can go right, although both the long-term care professions and quality assurance practices have progressed enough to describe good care as something more than defense against bad outcomes. Good care, such as that in the second vignette above, is an affirmative program—and is, we should add, being delivered by meritorious practitioners, too often without recognition, to a sometimes less than amiable clientele.

While progress heartens, problems have been the pressing and public issue, and these problems are real, even if we do not know precisely how prevalent they are. Knowledgeable people state that the most deplorable conditions have substantially ebbed; however, the offenses have not been eradicated.[11] In public meetings and hearings conducted during the 1983–85 Institute of Medicine study of nursing home regulation, the reasons suggested for the persistence of ill-treatment pointed both at knavish operators and inept public inspectors. Regardless of whys and wherefores, there are regulatory improvements that, if instituted, could vastly improve nursing home accountability.

First, clearer standards are needed. Without specific criteria, consumers do not know their entitlements, facilities do not see their obligations, and legal enforcement is stymied. Second, the frequency and timing of surveys should maximize the element of surprise and should be tied to each facility's performance history. Residents should, to the degree possible, have ample opportunities to participate in interviews. Surveyor training and survey agency resources should be upgraded. Third, state and federal governments must be staunch in the application of sanctions where violations persist or are repeated.

Among the Institute of Medicine recommendations elaborating these guidelines are principles by which regulations should be revised: criteria that focus on resident needs and facility performance, rather than policies and "capabilities"; criteria that reflect a decade's improvement in professional standards; clear, logical, internally consistent expectations that include the whole spectrum of clinical care and personal comforts.

Because of the refined focus of the regulations and the resident-interview skills required for these changes, the report recommends that federal training efforts and financial support of state-level training programs be increased, especially during the period of transition. How this order of recommendations can fare in an era of deficit reduction, when the reduction is occurring on the human service side of the equation, is indeed problematic. It may be that the nearer reach of quality assurance will be in the enforcement of such standards as now exist. Sanctions to be encouraged toward this end are bans on admissions, civil fines, receivership, and emergency authority to close facilities and transfer residents. The last, it is noted, would apply only in life-threatening situations. [12]

Furthermore, close connections need to be forged between the typically separate survey agencies and Medicaid payment agencies. This two-way street ought to ensure that when the survey agency discovers serious care violations, the Medicaid agency is alerted to determine whether the state has paid for services that were not provided. Similarly, if Medicaid auditors find discrepancies in a nursing home's finances, the survey agency ought to be called in to determine whether the financial lapses have affected resident care. There are a variety of formal and informal ways in which this coordination can occur, but experience suggests that health and welfare authorities are mutually leery.

Although the enforcement of standards and the imposition of penalties for malfeasance head the agenda for improving nursing home quality, the bulk of the problems residents have is more subtle than the violation of rules. These problems are the natural hazards of living in a large group and depending on others for daily and intimate care. In this regard, regulation is an incomplete solution. Although great strides have been made in accounting for satisfaction or life quality in a regulatory scheme, conflicts between resident preference and regulatory perspectives are inescapable—

more tasty food and gifts of food versus therapeutic diets, homestyle meal service versus sanitation, religious candles versus the fire marshal's orders. Given individual residents' different values, preferences, and mental capacities, the goal of individualizing quality so as to abate the hazards of group life must necessarily take some nonregulatory turns.

Two strategies are evolving in long-term care facilities to achieve this end: the resident council and residents' rights to participate in planning treatment. Both are mechanisms for creating choices, for inculcating personal responsibility, and for rewarding assertion. At root they contradict the perception of the institution as a juggernaut.

Resident councils take several forms. Town meetings and delegate assemblies are the most likely, with monthly meetings the most popular schedule. Generally, staff are involved in organizing the council, providing clerical assistance and space for meetings, and serving as the conduit for residents' recommendations to the administration. The actual meeting, however, should be private, with staff or guests attending only upon the council's invitation.

Council organization and maintenance rarely happen easily. Not only is facility administration sometimes ill-disposed to the potential for compounded grievances, but staff and family members may be awfully skeptical that governance and self-help are conceivable among so fragile a population. Moreover, residents themselves are often resistant to encouragement to schedule meetings to discuss dissatisfaction openly and to create alternatives.

Whereas resident councils are a means for change in a group, residents' rights to participate in planning treatment are ways to bargain for the individual. Again, they are ways of defining autonomy in making decisions about choices, not a promise (or threat) of independence. More than three-fourths of the states now have nursing home residents' rights statutes or regulations that address some or all of the following:

- The resident's right to discuss treatment and alternatives with individual caregivers

- The resident's right to request and participate in informal care conferences

- The resident's right to include a family member or other chosen representative in the care conference or delegate one of these people to attend in his/her stead

- The resident's right to refuse treatment, medication, or dietary restrictions with prior information about the likely medical or psychological results of the refusal

- The resident's right to refuse participation in experimental research.

Rights also include the less medical matters of personal privacy, communication privacy, and association with people outside the facility.

Few enumerated rights are absolutes, except (at least by intent) the right to be free from abuse. The right to refuse a bath will be tempered to preserve the rights of one's roommate. The right to refuse medication will occasion discharge from the facility if the results of refusal jeopardize the physical safety of staff or other residents. Rights are, at their least, however, currency in negotiated decision making. Contrary to total dependence on the benevolence of experts, and a step short of firearms, bargaining offers opportunities for bilateral gain.

Just as literal assets cannot always be managed and spent by their owner, residents' rights may have to be expressed by a delegate, a surrogate, or an advocate. The integrity of individuals' rights has to be built with the flexibility that admits to the uniqueness and limitations of individual situations. This conceptual elasticity would preserve some basic notion of protection and the opportunity to assert desirable changes, whatever the disability level or cause of confinement.

It would be a manifest pleasure to turn all of our creative energies to these refinements in quality, to girding enforcement, and to compiling, at long last, the comprehensive documentation of the fruits of that progress. Pleasure notwithstanding, such an agenda is myopic.

Conclusion

Improvements to what happens in nursing homes and about nursing homes are ultimately internal to the more fundamental questions of health and social services for the frail elderly. The connection that cannot be ignored is that between long-term care needs and services on the one hand, and income support for the frail elderly on the other, or between public policy in those areas and long-term care policy. Changes in Social Security policy have had an enormous ripple effect on long-term care since 1935; yet the highly charged and highly visible debate over the future of Social Security has been conducted largely without reference to the similarly intense if less visible discussion of long-term care, and vice versa.

Contemporary public spending reductions will doubtless affect the need for, if not the availability of, long-term care services. As calculated by one recent study:

> spending on the aged was cut by a cumulative $26.5 billion for the first four Reagan fiscal years. This reduction amounts to a 3% cut in pre-Reagan spending on aged benefits. Most of the dollar reductions fall on Medicare ($12 billion) and Social Security ($9 billion) but the smaller grant programs that fund locally provided health and social services received the largest proportional cuts (from 22–39%). . . . The cuts had a particularly severe effect on low-income elderly

who depend on multiple benefits. For example, a food stamp recipient who lived in subsidized housing may have experienced all of the following reductions in benefits and services over a span of one–two years: a rent increase, a reduced food stamp allotment, a decline in public transportation, fewer social services, and reduced access to free medical care.[13]

State governments, simultaneously pressured to cut taxes, repair deficits, and repave highways, are by no means thirsty for inherited financial responsibility. On the contrary, they are making their own cuts in provider reimbursement, regulatory agency staffs, homemaker and nutrition programs, and Medicaid eligibility, and in some areas are reducing even nursing home residents' personal needs allowances, which are hardly ever more than a dollar a day and constitute the total discretionary income for Medicaid-eligible residents.

The fiscal conflict between federal and state governments features a hotter-than-ever potato. Which level of government will get stuck with the bill has been a major axis around which long-term care policy has revolved for some time. The questions of where nursing homes belong in a health-care system increasingly dominated by geriatric patients, and what kind of institutions they should be, are largely unaddressed at the national policy level, except as fodder in the conflicts about the appropriate roles of government, individuals, and families.

Meanwhile, the population needing services continues to grow at an alarming rate. Under the best of circumstances, it would take a heroic and largely unprecedented effort to direct public commitment to provide first-rate long-term care services for those who will come to need them. The best of circumstances are not likely to prevail.

References

1. United States Senate, Special Committee on Aging. 1985. *Aging America: Trends and Projections.* 1985–86 ed. Washington, D.C.: Government Printing Office.
2. Institute of Medicine. 1986. *Improving the Quality of Care in Nursing Homes.* Washington, D.C.: National Academy Press.
3. Somers, A. R. 1985. Financing long-term care for the elderly: Institutions, incentives, issues. In *America's Aging: Health in an Older Society.* Washington, D.C.: National Academy Press.
4. Weissert, W. G. 1985. Seven reasons why it is so difficult to make community-based long-term care cost-effective. *Health Serv Res* 20(4):423–432.
5. Sullivan, R. 1984. Study charges bias in admissions to nursing homes. *New York Times* Jan. 23.

6. See Ref. 2, pp. 9–10.
7. Ewig, C., Griggs, J. 1985. *Public Concerns, Community Initiatives: The Successful Management of Nursing Home Consumer Information Programs.* New York: United Hospital Fund.
8. Minnesota Department of Health, Division of Health Systems. 1984. Correction Order, February 18.
9. Freeman, I. 1985. Twice-bound: Several views of women in institutions. Pre-Conference Symposium, Council on Social Work Education, Washington, D.C., February 17. Internal quotations from Rachel Rustad, Stevens Square: Holistic wellness model. Conference Paper: Institute of Medicine Study of Nursing Home Regulation, Washington, D.C., December 4, 1984.
10. Minnesota Department of Human Services. 1985. Printout of Medicaid rates (September).
11. See Ref. 2, p. 3.
12. See Ref. 2, ch. 3–5.
13. Storey, J. R. 1986. Policy changes affecting older Americans during the first Reagan Administration. *Gerontologist* 26(1):28–29.

Thirteen

Long-Term Care: The Long and Short of It

Stanley J. Brody and Judith S. Magel

Policy development and planning for long-term care (LTC) has been distorted by the perception that all old people are indigent, sick, and unable to manage their own affairs. Binstock has characterized this attitude as the scapegoating of the elderly.[1] In fact, a majority of old people are not sick, indigent, or incompetent, and any LTC program should be based on a balanced perspective of the elderly as a heterogeneous population with a wide spectrum of resources and needs.[2]

The appropriate strategy in designing LTC programs is to respond to the diverse needs and disparate resources of the aged through a systems approach. Needs vary in level and intensity, and service resources vary according to the provider and the individual's capacity to mobilize available resources. Similarly, private and public fiscal resources vary, depending on the fixed assets and income of the older people themselves. The challenge is to develop, through management and financing mechanisms, a humane system of LTC that matches the multiple needs and resources of the elderly.

The current organization and financing of LTC for the elderly are inadequate and represent an unacceptable drain on public and personal resources. Despite improved access, advances in medical science and technology, and increased services, the LTC system has been only partially successful in meeting the needs of the growing elderly population. As an outcome of the separate financial and professional lineages of medicine, social work, and other health disciplines, the LTC system has evolved into a collection of poorly related, multiple, parallel, overlapping, and noncontinuous services. Poor definition of goals and a lack of accountability have compromised the quality and continuity of services and burdened financing resources unduly. Continuity of care, which is a sine qua non of effective health-service delivery, is rarely achieved. Services are funded inadequately at the federal, state, and local levels, and are administered at these different levels in a bewildering arrangement of eligibilities and benefits. There is little adequate private insurance available for LTC.

The increase in the elderly population and the aging of that population have contributed to the growing demand for LTC. Growth in services, however, has been restricted by cost-containment measures and an apparent public and private policy of setting an 11% GNP ceiling for medical care. The threat of the anticipated bankruptcy of Medicare contributes to the shrinking base of support. At the same time, public expenditures for health and social services have been decreasing. Even if additional funds were made available, it is unclear whether an expansion of existing services would be the best strategy to meet current and future LTC demands. In an environment in which public expenditures are capped, a reapportionment of existing resources is more probable. This requires a reallocation of existing health-care funds between acute and LTC services based on a reevaluation of the dimensions of need.[3]

Need identification begins with an understanding of the target population. Both the public-policy scapegoating of the elderly and viewing skilled nursing facility (SNF) care as an extension of acute, hospital-based care have contributed to the tendency for financing LTC services that are focused on institutionally based care rather than on identified need. Nonmedical social and health-care support services have been undervalued and underfinanced. Because of the lack of private insurance coverage for the LTC market, public financing, rather than market demand, prescribes the nature of service. In 1980, 57% of nursing home care was supported by public sources, but home-based services received meager public reimbursement.[4] Although public coverage for home health care has expanded, it still represents only a small fraction (1.4%) of Medicare payments.[5]

The failure of the market to provide an unregulated, private mechanism for financing nonmedical support services outside of an institutional setting often means that elderly persons needing these services have to either go without care or purchase institutional care. Limiting public support to institutional services encourages the inappropriate use of those services by elderly persons requiring nonmedical support. The institutional bias of current public LTC financing leads to a "market-basket moral hazard" in which people are encouraged to overconsume formal services in order to acquire the portion of the support care they do need.[6]

Thus, scapegoating the elderly as poor and in need of a high level of service encourages the use of high-cost care over potentially lower-cost options and distorts public perception of the cost of providing care to older persons.[7]

The Heterogeneity of the Elderly

The heterogeneity of the elderly as health-care consumers is reflected in their use of health-care facilities and their expenditures for care. Age, although not in itself a determinant of health status, increases an individual's vulnerability to illness and disabling conditions. Increased longevity has accentuated the diversity of support needs within the older population. For example, there is great disparity in the level and duration of acute care consumed by persons who are between the ages of 65 and 74 and those who are 75 and over. The old-old (age 75 and up) have average lengths of stay of 11.4 days and use 6062 acute-care hospital days per 1000. The old (65–74) have fewer episodes of care; they average 10.1 days of care per episode and experience 3124 hospital days per 1000.[8]

Added years of life also have affected the generational structure of families and the availability of family support. Despite the presence of formal social and medical-care services, the family remains the primary caregiver for the aged. According to Congressional Budget Office estimates, between 3.0 and 6.7 million disabled people received LTC services from family or friends (only half of the disabled population are elderly.)[9] Most (90%) of the approximately 1.3 million persons who reside in LTC institutions are over 65 years.[10] The vast majority of LTC services are not purchased in the market but are provided informally by family and friends.[11,12]

Most older people live independently and have no desire to burden their children with caregiving responsibilities. A small proportion, the home bound, rely on their adult children for support in activities of daily living (ADL). For a growing number of families, the ability of adult children to care for aging parents and relatives is complicated by long distances between residences, smaller family size, inadequate community-based support services, inadequate LTC networks, and the fact that the children themselves are aging. Nursing home placement often is the only alternative for families no longer able to provide personal care or to contract for that care through community agencies. For most of the disabled elderly, the lack or loss of available family support is a principal determinant of nursing home use. It is estimated that 10–20% of people in SNFs and 20–40% of residents in intermediate-care facilities may receive levels of health care that exceed their needs.[9]

Estimates of the level of need for LTC support tend to be exaggerated. Recent Medicaid statistics indicate that, at any given time, on the average, only 3.5% of persons age 65 and over are in nursing homes and extended-care facilities for a stay of more than 90 days. An older person has a 23–38% chance of entering a nursing home for a short-term or a long-term stay at some point during a lifetime,[13] thus encouraging the exaggerated perception of need for SNF beds and financing by planners who may not differentiate between short-term and long-term SNF users.

There is considerable variability within the elderly population in the use of formal or institutional services and in the amount of dollars spent for medical care.[14] At any given time, most elderly persons do not require high-cost acute care or LTC. Although virtually all persons age 65 and over are eligible for Medicare, only 62% of enrollees in Medicare Parts A and B actually used their coverage during 1980. The remaining 38.2% of qualified Medicare enrollees received no reimbursement because they did not require Medicare-covered services, did not meet initial program deductibles, or did not file a claim, or because they received covered services without charge. Of those Medicare enrollees who were beneficiaries, more than half (65.5%) received less than $200 in Medicare reimbursements. The average per-person health-care expenditure for Medicare enrollees during 1980 was $1971; Medicare covered $1005, or 56%, of this expense, and $328 (18%) was covered out of pocket.[15]

The 14% of Medicare enrollees in 1980 who received $2000 or more in reimbursements accounted for 83.7% of all Medicare payments made that year.[15] A disproportionate amount of Medicare expenditures were consumed by the small percentage of enrollees who were in their last year of life or who were in poor health, immobile, or unable to perform their usual activities.[16–18] Kovar observes that the 59% of elderly persons who either moved from community living to institutional care or died during 1980[19] accounted for 22% of total annual medical-care expenditures for the aged. Elderly persons who lived in the community throughout 1980 (23 million) experienced relatively modest medical-care expenditures: 62% had expenditures of less than $500 and 76% had expenditures of less than $1000. The median expenditure for people age 65 and over living in the community was $647 if they were in poor health, but only $200 if their perceived health status was excellent.[20]

Most elderly persons consider themselves healthy. In 1981, 80% of persons age 65 and over perceived their health status as good or excellent, 53% experienced no limitation in their activities, and 74% had no limitation on their mobility.[21] The vast majority (96%) of the elderly live in the general community. This mostly positive outlook on personal health status is consonant with the fact that only a very small percentage of elderly account for the high medical costs of the total aged population.

Efforts are being initiated to describe objectively the decline in function and the corresponding needs for services in the eighth stage of life. One of the earliest efforts was a matrix that compared levels of disability with the coordinate of levels of service. This matrix, prepared as part of a planning program by the Veterans Administration and based on clinical experience, reflected the ambiguity of need caused by the heterogeneity of resources of the aged veteran.[22] More recently, Katz has developed the concept of "active life expectancy," which describes the expected duration of functional well-being as distinguished from life expectancy. An objective longitudinal study of the Massachusetts elderly population, the Katz report demonstrates the feasibility of producing forecasts of functional health expectancy for the elderly, using life-table methods and a measure of functional well-being (index of ADL) as end point.[23] Yet another recent study describes the use of both in-home/community services and institutional care over a 3-year period. During this time, almost half of the target population who had entered either system of care at the minimum level of services died or were discharged. More than 80% of clients who entered at a high level of services in these two systems were no longer being cared for, for the same reasons.[24] Thus, it is clear that data are being accumulated that both support the thesis of limited exposure to LTC and begin to provide a basis upon which service needs may be estimated.

Age-related physical, social, and economic decrements contribute to the need for a range of medical and nonmedical support services.[2] The increase in the elderly population and the distorted projections of the demand on the LTC system have tended to overwhelm policy discussions and instill a general sense of despair. Knowledge of the diversity and growth of this population indicates the solution to the LTC problem. The market for LTC services involves two different client groups: those who require temporary support and those in need of permanent or extended support. The dual nature of the market is suggested, in part, by the elderly's use of SNFs. Among the elderly persons who experienced SNF stays in 1977, 53.7% stayed fewer than 90 days, while 46.3% stayed 90 days or more. The first group, "the temporarily needy, frail elderly" are sent home (39.8%), die (21.2%), or are admitted to the hospital (23.5%).[10] Their transitory support needs may be met through an array of short-term (less than 90 days) institutional, community, and home-care services that can be characterized as *short-term long-term care* (STLTC). The second group are the "permanently disabled, frail elderly." They are not likely to return home from the SNF, but if they do return to the community, they are likely to require continuous long-term service that can be called *long-term long-term care* (LTLTC).[25]

Short-Term Long-Term Care

At least 1.5 million elderly persons already receive STLTC. Invariably, STLTC (or step-down services) follow an acute-care hospital discharge and are needed only for a short period of time (i.e., less than 90 days). STLTC may include inpatient and outpatient rehabilitation services, convalescent care provided through SNFs, rehabilitation hospital day care, hospice care, home health care, and community outreach services (e.g., Meals on Wheels). A model STLTC system is depicted in Figure 13.1.

The elderly are an important and growing market for hospital services. Currently older people account for 25% of all admissions and 38% of all patient-days of care.[26] Hospitals are able to provide a full range of professional and technical resources, emergency care, and specialty services and are experienced in the management of multispecialty, multilevel care. Accordingly, they have the potential capability for managing a STLTC system,[27] and they are an appropriate auspice for STLTC service.

Furthermore, not only do hospitals have a long history of providing acute-care services to the elderly, but also they participate in LTC service through discharge planning. Nationally, nearly one-third of all admissions to nursing homes are from general or short-stay hospitals.[10] Hospital-based or related STLTC care revolves around step-down services designed to

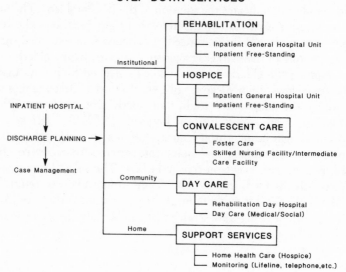

Figure 13.1. A model of a hospital-based system of short-term long-term care. *Source:* Ref. 25.

meet the transitory medical and health needs of older persons. The goal of care is the timely restoration of the individual to community living through improvement of the level of patient functioning and/or of personal and environmental resources. Patient care may be financed by Medicare, private health insurance, out-of-pocket payments, or the trade-off dollars recovered by hospitals under diagnosis-related group (DRG) reimbursement because STLTC services made possible early acute-care discharge.

Development of step-down services fosters the verticalization of hospital care. Traditional boundaries are crossed when services and service settings are organized through service (case) management to respond to the hierarchy of patient-care needs. This organization and monitoring of services can afford continuity of care and timely discharge from the acute-care setting. The many resources required for patient care should be identified through assessment, and the system of care (STLTC services) should include community as well as hospital-based services. The prominence of any one service in the course of treatment may change as the patient progresses through levels of function and stages of care. As the center of community health-care resources, the verticalized hospital may act as a catalyst for system development and organization.[28]

Many hospitals already are actively involved in LTC services.[29-31,27] They have developed step-down services and acquired or built SNF and rehabilitation facilities. In many areas, hospitals are the principal community agency addressing the needs of the elderly. They assume a pivotal position because they service more elderly people (5 million inpatients with 10 million admissions; 10 million outpatients) than any other community agency.[27]

The capacity of the hospital to provide STLTC is determined by the ability of the market to finance service. Medicare, through DRG-based prospective reimbursement, supports the growth of hospital-based LTC services. Nearly all persons age 65 and over are eligible for health-insurance coverage under Medicare and benefit significantly from the program. DRG-based prospective reimbursement addresses the structure of health-care delivery and provides a means of reallocating acute-care resources to alternative-care delivery systems.[32] (See Maddox and Manton, Chapter 4.)

As step-down services develop, discharge options expand, and hospitals can accelerate the movement of patients out of hospital beds in a responsible manner. Revenues realized by minimizing inpatient stays may then be channeled into the development and support of step-down services. By providing a less intense, less restrictive level of care than acute care, step-down services answer the short-term support needs of the recovering elderly patient. For the hospital, these services represent a source of revenue independent of inpatient admissions and outside of DRG review. Medicare may pay for many services, such as inpatient rehabilitation beds, day rehabilitation hospital care, home health services, and possibly short-term SNF stays. Foster-home care may be supported through Social Security Title XX (Social Services) or through Supplemental Security Income (SSI, Title XVI of the Social Security Act).

Moreover, hospital-sponsored step-down services would reinforce the patient's bond to the parent facility, encourage the attending physician's continued involvement with the patient after the acute hospital stay, and promote continuity of care. Properly managed, acute care and STLTC services would be linked in a relationship based on shared goals, resources, referrals, and discharge opportunities. It is also possible that the timely rehabilitation inherent in step-down services and more sensitive inpatient care would result in a higher level of patient functioning at discharge from STLTC services. Consequently, fewer patients would need LTLTC upon hospital discharge.

Although DRGs present an opportunity for hospitals to expand their market and increase the diversity of their services, some hospitals may elect a very different strategy. Apart from the values involved, restricting admissions to "low-risk" younger patients and discharging elderly persons with little regard for follow-up care is a short-sighted means of containing hospital costs associated with long lengths of stay and case severity. Despite these actions, concentrated demand by hospital patients for the limited number of available SNF beds because of the premium on early or timely discharge could result in a backup. In addition, hospitals that opt to ignore the development of step-down services, that rely on SNFs as the method of choice for dealing with older patients under DRGs, or that inappropriately discharge the elderly patient are likely to encounter community disapproval, competitive disadvantage, and political intervention. Congress and the Health Care Financing Administration (HCFA) can be expected to react negatively to that kind of institutional behavior and to intervene with regulations to correct the situation.

Case Management

Those hospitals choosing to pursue the development of STLTC services need to monitor and direct the flow of patients within the acute-care hospital, between the inpatient hospital and STLTC services, and within the STLTC system. Case (or service) management is a mechanism that increasingly is being used by some hospitals to ensure this continuity of care. (It is also discussed in some detail in Read and O'Brien, Chapter 9.) Case management draws on the skills of a team of providers that may include the attending physician, nurses, social workers, therapists, and other relevant health-care professionals, as well as the patient and the patient's family. After team members consult the patient and family, the case manager coordinates the recommendations of team members and tailors a program of care to the individual needs of the patient.

Case management should be distinguished from the discharge planning that is already in place in most hospitals. Discharge planning has tended to reflect medical regulatory concerns, emphasizing the securing of medically related services and limited by the availability of third-party reimbursement through Medicare, Medicaid, Social Security Title XX, Title III of the Older Americans Act, and the Veterans Administration. Because of inadequate insurance coverage and poor communication between institution-based medical-care providers and community-service agencies, the responsibility for obtaining nonacute support services, such as rehabilitation care, home health care, homemakers, social work, and transportation, often is left to the patient or the patient's family.

Problems of "turf" also compromise hospital discharge-planning efforts. Continuity of care is lost when rivalries, indifference, or a lack of communication between community-based service providers and physicians constrains patient care. Recent HCFA-sponsored studies of discharge planning found that "actors involved in a discharge decision are not a team working toward a common goal but a strained coalition."[33] High staff turnover and the lack of shared goals in the delivery of service sabotage effective discharge planning. Physicians may view the health and social services provided by community-based agencies as an inappropriate infringement on medical care or so alien to their training and practice as to make them uncomfortable in making referrals. Under such conditions hospital-based discharge planning is relegated to little more than securing SNF placements.[34]

Utilization review and reimbursement concerns also distort discharge planning. Medicare's requirement of medical necessity biases posthospital care toward the use of covered, but not necessarily needed, services. In the absence of adequate discharge options, the utilization review time-clock has allowed for the misuse of hospital services to "buy" time until an appropriate discharge placement can be arranged. Prospective payment mechanisms, such as DRGs, will no longer allow this luxury of "administrative days" (i.e., inpatient days beyond those justified by the need for acute care).

Case management is an alternative to discharge planning for those patients who are likely to overstay DRG inpatient time constraints. Not all patients are candidates for case management, however. Case management is appropriate for those patients who are at high risk of not being able to arrange for continuing care and whose care may involve several different services and settings.[35] Responsibly guiding patients through the STLTC system, case management is "a method of providing comprehensive, unified, coordinated, and timely services to people in need of them through the efforts of a primary agent who, together with the client (and the client's family), takes responsibility for providing or procuring the services needed."[36]

Hospitals have established criteria for an initial referral to the case-management service and subsequent consideration for admission to the caseload. Essentially indicators of the potential risk of an extended inpatient stay (i.e., a stay exceeding DRG reimbursement limits), these criteria may include:

- Being age 75 or over and living alone

- Lacking the capacity to provide information at the time of admission

- Being likely to become eligible for transfer to a rehabilitation unit

- Having conditions likely to cause increasing disability, such as stroke, heart attacks, or amputations

- Being unable to care for oneself

- Being likely to need special equipment at home

- Having conditions that might affect one's ability to return home

- Having no known family or adequate social and financial support systems

- Having a history of frequent readmissions

- Being admitted from nursing homes, boarding homes, or other LTC facilities.[37]

Under case management, a single professional or agent formally assumes responsibility for obtaining, organizing, and purchasing services to meet the multiple needs of a client. However, the case manager shares this responsibility with the client and the client's family, who are recognized as active caregivers. Including the patient and the patient's family in planning helps to ensure that service goals are properly defined and that the services mesh with the client's and the caring family's needs.

The duration of hospital-based case-management service should be carefully contained. Operationally, the service should end when the patient returns to community living and no longer needs temporary services or enters the LTLTC system (usually within 90 days of discharge from the acute-care facility). Entering into the LTLTC system should include a mechanism for timely referral to the parallel LTLTC case-management system. Without criteria that limit the time that hospital-based case management is responsible, the service may be overwhelmed, losing its capacity for effective help.

Published reports of case-management systems have usually been of the

LTLTC variety. These include the Project Open Health Plan of Mount Zion Hospital and Medical Center (San Francisco), the South Carolina Community Long-Term Care Program (CLTC), and Connecticut Community Care, Inc. (CCCI). The key features of these programs should be examined. 1) Case-management services are targeted to select groups of *high-risk* elderly clients identified through assessment. Risk assessment includes a consideration of living arrangements, family support, medical problems, functional disabilities, and income. 2) The duration and intensity of service are carefully monitored and controlled. The CLTC program requires a follow-up assessment after 90 days of service. At that point, a determination is made about the adequacy of service goals and the efficacy of further service management for a particular client. The CCCI program makes an assessment after the first 60 days of service, and the average duration of service under the Project Open program is 2–3 months. 3) Along with medical, nursing, social work, and therapy professionals, patients and their families are considered active care providers and participate in the development of therapy goals, care plans, and assessment. 4) The per-patient cost of care is identified. (An out-of-pocket fee-for-service option is available to clients in at least one program, CCCI).[38,39]

Case management in LTLTC systems may be successful in minimizing the need for inpatient hospital and nursing home care for elderly clients. A recent study of the utilization experiences of frail elderly clients participating in a case-managed LTC program found that they experienced lower rates of institutionalization and shorter hospital and nursing home stays, and were more quickly placed when nursing home care was required than their peers who negotiated the existing LTC system without case-management services. On the average, case-management clients were estimated to have saved 2.1 days of hospital care and 3.9 days of nursing home residence per year, with no loss in the efficacy of care as measured by mortality and overall rates of institutionalization.[40] Other studies do not show such significant changes in institutional use.[41]

Evaluations of those and other case-management efforts have been restricted to LTLTC systems. It is suggested that case management of STLTC services could promote access to services while minimizing the need for institutional care, but there is little experience with the case-management approach from within a hospital. On the one hand, the attending physician might support the hospital-based program because of the shared service setting. On the other hand, the physician's anxiety about the loss of control over patient care and perceived diminution of his or her role and economic reward might cause concern. In addition, existing service departments responsible for discharge planning may be uncomfortable with the overriding control of a case-management service that may be superimposed on them.[42,43]

Comparison of STLTC and LTLTC

For some patients, the appropriate discharge from a STLTC program is to a system that provides permanent care. Entry to a permanent care (LTLTC) system may be either from the hospital or from the community. While a STLTC system may be appropriately within the orbit of the hospital and may be medically oriented, LTLTC systems involve social, health, and residential care. Within the LTLTC system, medical services are necessary but assume a subsidiary role. The distinction between STLTC services and LTLTC services is based on the goals, length, and nature of care. STLTC services help the convalescing patient return to active, independent, community living. Posthospital services that go beyond 90 days provide maintenance and residential care and are appropriate to the LTLTC model. Moreover, the array of services necessary within the LTLTC system[44] is more comprehensive (Fig. 13.2) than that represented by STLTC (see Fig. 13.1).

The services and the goals of LTLTC are social and require the auspices of a socially oriented agency rather than those of a medically oriented hospital.[2] (A comparison of the two systems is presented in Figure 13.3.) Finally, the fiscal supports that are appropriate to STLTC are neither available to nor appropriate for LTLTC.

Sponsorship of STLTC services increasingly is being assumed by hospitals that envision themselves as community health centers.[31] Diversification of hospital services into nonacute areas is encouraged by competitive markets and organizational resources. A relatively well-developed system of private and public reimbursement provides additional incentives. In contrast, LTLTC services suffer from a lack of adequate formal financing sources and a fragmented system of service delivery (see Fig. 13.4). While STLTC is supported by multiple private and public third-party payment mechanisms, LTLTC has no such support. Only one major funding resource, Medicaid, reimburses one major service modality, the skilled nursing facility (SNF). To the extent that financing defines the scope of service, the organizational and financial difficulties of the LTLTC system are self-reinforcing.

A consistent body of research has established that the family gives most LTLTC support.[12,45–47] Because the family plays such a large role in providing care, the extent of LTC community support services is understated in Medicare and Medicaid statistics. Patients and their families also support almost half of all nursing home costs. Medicaid is the primary public source of payment for nursing home care of over 90 days' duration (but it is supplemented, in part, by the Veterans Administration). Community-care programs for the elderly poor are supported by Title XX of the Social Security Act and Title III of the Older Americans Act. Only a

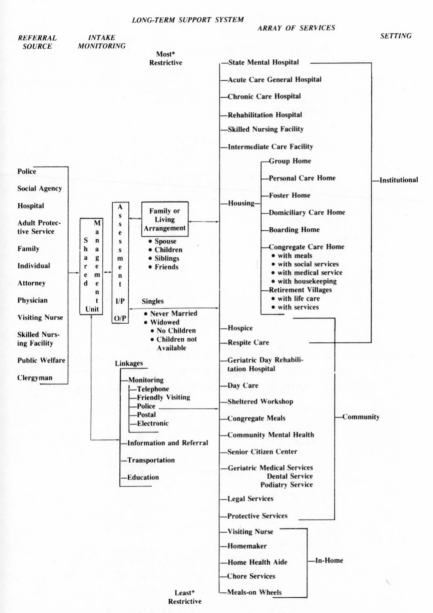

Figure 13.2. The long-term support system: an inventory of recommended services appropriate to long-term care. (*The classification from most to least restrictive is a general view of services and may vary within each service.) *Source:* Ref. 44.

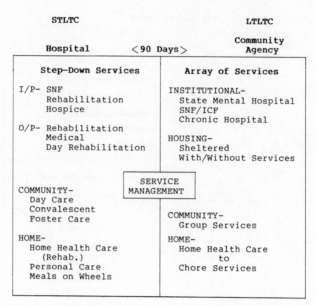

Figure 13.3.   The long-term care service system.

fraction of the demand for LTLTC is covered by these programs. Income eligibility requirements, particularly for those elderly persons whose incomes are above poverty levels, further restrict the availability of LTLTC services.

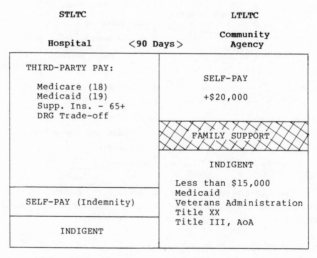

Figure 13.4.   Long-term care reimbursement systems.

The largest share of Medicaid payments (73%) goes for institutional care, including hospitals, nursing homes, intermediate care facilities, and mental health facilities. In 1980, approximately 39% of Medicaid payments were for nursing home care, while only 17.5% were for outpatient, clinic, and home health care.[48,49] Unlike Medicare, Medicaid eligibility is tied to financial need. Beyond a certain minimum level of income and assets, individuals must exhaust personal resources to become eligible for Medicaid coverage.

The cost of a nursing home stay for the LTLTC recipient varies, depending on the length of stay and the patient's eligibility for Medicaid coverage. The average length of a long-term (over 90 days) stay in nursing homes is 2½ years.[10] Persons who enter a facility under a private payment plan are fully responsible for the cost of care until they have exhausted private assets and income. Of those who convert from private payment to Medicaid, 40% do so within the first year of admission.[50] Beyond a certain length of stay, the probability increases that patients will become eligible for Medicaid.[51] Converting from private pay to Medicaid coverage significantly reduces the cost of extended nursing home care for the individual.

The lack of a private insurance system to complement public funding has contributed to the crisis in Medicaid financing. In the absence of private insurance, the current system encourages financially secure elderly nursing home residents to "prematurely" divest themselves of their assets, often through intergenerational transfers. This early divestiture may enable them to quality for public coverage (Medicaid) intended for the indigent. As a result, the economic support for care in SNFs breaks down, because the assumption of a significant contribution by private resources is not realized. Furthermore, the intergenerational divestiture places a demand on Medicaid that hinders its capacity to adequately address the needs of the truly indigent.

Planners' focus on the chronically infirm elderly Medicaid beneficiary exaggerates the perception of risk for LTLTC services. First, the LTLTC population receiving care in an SNF at a given time is 3.5% of the total elderly population, rather than the 5% generally cited.[52] Second, while a period of disability during the latter stages of life is highly probable, it may be of relatively short duration.[23,24] At any given time, 20% of the aged population need some kind of support, and, of that group, many receive adequate service from the informal support system. Furthermore, at the same time that needs have been exaggerated, often for legitimate advocacy reasons, individual and family resources may have been understated; the constructive use of these resources has never been positively exploited to provide for LTLTC through educational and financial incentives.[53]

Almost 60 years ago, acute-care hospitals also overestimated the risk of, and underestimated the resources available for, acute-care costs. At that time, an attempt by Baylor Hospital in Houston, Texas, to insure against acute-care costs received little support from the insurance industry. It wasn't until 8 years later that Blue Cross was established, institutionalizing insurance for acute-care service. The private insurance industry was a follower, not entering the acute-care hospital insurance market until a decade had elapsed and voluntary service-sponsored initiatives had demonstrated the feasibility.[54]

The field of LTC is in danger of repeating historical mistakes. Just as with acute care, the issue is still protection against catastrophic risk, and the same spreading-the-risk approach that Blue Cross and commercial insurers have applied to acute care applies to LTC. Similarly, the same mechanisms of deductions, copayments, and financial incentives can limit demand for LTC.[55–59] The high-cost, low-probability nature of LTC suggests that it is an insurable risk beyond the acute-care episodes now covered by Medicare and existing private insurance vehicles. Paradoxically, the risk of high-cost acute care is similar to some of the risks for LTC. A private LTC insurance option would enable financially secure persons to "save" for future catastrophic LTC support needs. To the extent that private financing systems are able to relieve the burden now carried by Medicaid, by limiting inappropriate use of that program by the middle class, the Medicaid program will be in a better position to meet its legislated goal of service to the elderly poor.

Financing LTC

An extended nursing home stay is expensive, and few individuals can afford to pay their own way in full. The same observation might be made about a variety of other risks in our society. The expensive cost of hospitalization is already covered through insurance. Other high-cost risks are provided for through a combination of savings and insurance mechanisms (e.g., home mortgage and home mortgage insurance and higher-education loan programs). Fortunately, the risk of needing catastrophic LTC services is small. It is appropriate for society to assume responsibility for the coverage of catastrophic care when the recipient needs institutionalization and cannot afford to pay. It is inappropriate to burden public financing systems with the cost of care when less costly alternatives exist and when the recipient of care can assume financial responsibility.

The elderly do not want to be a burden on their children or on society. Many are capable of paying their own way and are willing to do so if they can be assured that they will not end up financially destitute or unable to leave a modest legacy, usually in the form of home ownership. The growing purchasing power of the elderly population means they can make a significant contribution to LTLTC services. Home equity and reverse annuity mortgages have also been much discussed as important sources for financing LTC services.[60] (See Feder and Scanlon, Chapter 7.)

Adult children have a major stake in ensuring the availability of catastrophic LTLTC services for their parents. They, as well as their parents, are at risk should the latter need formal support in their later years. Emerging data show that families continue their informal support activities despite the availability of supplemental formal services. Thus, some adult children could be available to supplement the fiscal resources of parents, if necessary, in purchasing insurance protection for LTLTC.

Private financing for LTC services provides a monetary basis for developing a wide range of support services. Negotiated through a designated LTLTC system and provided through a case-management model, the resulting continuity of care could provide a life-care community without walls. This arrangement would ensure economic feasibility by supplying the right service at the right time and at the right place.

The case-management arrangement for LTLTC uses the same management model that the physician provides in acute care.[61,62] Professional guidance and "gatekeeping" ensure that the beneficiary receives appropriate, quality care. In addition, fostering the appropriate use of services maintains the fiscal integrity of the system. As an alternative to using case-management services, beneficiaries might be offered an indemnity option, which would provide them with a per diem reimbursement for a limited period of time. The advantage to beneficiaries of subscribing to the case-management approach would be the guarantee that all services prescribed would be covered. The critical ingredient of this proposal would be the use of an experienced LTC provider with a proven track record of delivering multiple high-quality services to this population.

Such an arrangement also would help to preserve older people's ties to their own physicians. It should be noted that what is being proposed does not cover any medical reimbursement and assumes that those risks will be met by existing structures. Keeping the medical entitlements separate from the LTLTC system will avoid competition with current physician relationships. Physicians would therefore be encouraged to refer their patients to the designated LTLTC system for care. Similarly, professional case managers would consult with and reinforce the informal support network.

The community hospital, too, would benefit from an insured designated LTLTC system by having a referral source for those patients who need care beyond the STLTC system. Other community social agencies might also look to the designated LTLTC system for fiscally sound purchase-of-service contractual relationships.

The major problem confronting the marketing of LTLTC insurance is to convince the population at risk that disability is a high-probability aspect of aging. Frequently, families participating in discharge planning for an elderly relative recovering from an acute-care trauma are surprised by and unprepared for the patient's poor functional status and dependency. Brody describes the total effect on the family:

> By contrast with the initial phase of the aged patient's treatment, which is supported by third party payment and reinforced by media propaganda, the second stage of care is given short shift by the formal support system. Medicare, Medicaid, Blue Cross, and commercial insurance carriers afford little financial support for long-term care services. The visiting nurse or social worker rarely is dramatized on television. Newspapers do not highlight their role or efforts. It is not surprising that families are not prepared for this aspect of the natural history of disease, particularly with older relatives.[63]

Nevertheless, considering the success that the insurance industry has enjoyed with providing $8 billion per year Medigap insurance, its marketing skill should be equal to the task of educating the at-risk population for LTLTC.

Community-based LTLTC systems can be expanded to form a national network of support, enabling adult children to participate in the care of aging parents when direct personal care by family members is impractical. Increasingly, adult children find themselves residing in different communities than their parents, and a professional intermediary is needed to help them arrange for care of their aging parents. Under this arrangement, local LTLTC agencies would mediate between children in one city and an LTLTC agency in the parent's community that will act as the surrogate family. The goal would be to establish a sound LTC system, based on voluntary agencies providing case management and, either directly or through purchase, the appropriate services. Services would be funded through private insurance paid for by the client or the client's family. A ready market for a national LTLTC system already exists among children now engaged in the long-distance care of elderly relatives.[64]

Summary

Although LTC providers agree that health care for the elderly depends on the continuity of health and social services, the existing delivery system rarely realizes this goal. Part of the problem is the failure of service providers to assume a leadership role in arranging financing of LTC. Establishing an adequate, comprehensive financial structure for LTLTC services is key to the development of a system that ensures continuity of care and access to a broad range of services.

In an era of public expenditure caps, new sources of public financing for LTLTC are unlikely. Nevertheless, the market for LTLTC services is expanding. Increases in population size, life expectancy, personal financial resources, and health-insurance coverage have contributed to a growth in the demand for service and the purchasing power of the older consumer. Despite encouraging market features, the existing LTLTC system has failed to address the needs and economic realities of the elderly population.

For a growing number of elderly persons, private resources are available to purchase personal care services. Increasingly, the market for nonmedical support services extends beyond the elderly to include adult children concerned with the well-being of aging parents living in other parts of the country. Home equity, savings, and other personal resources from the aged and their children may provide alternative financing sources for LTLTC services that are inadequately covered by existing insurance programs. The demand for more comprehensive LTC coverage and the availability of private resources is evidenced by the growth of continuing care, retirement, and life-care communities, and by the rise of private health insurance policies designed to supplement Medicare coverage.

The unprecedented growth of the elderly population has tended to mask its diversity as a market. From a systems perspective, the LTC market is composed of two patient groups served by two sets of LTC services. The largest consumer segment consists of elderly patients who require STLTC services. These patients experience SNF stays of less than 90 days and usually enter the SNF after a hospital discharge. Other STLTC patients are those who receive home care for a similar length of time (i.e., less than 90 days). The second group of service recipients are the LTLTC patients, who experience SNF stays of 90 days or more or need further services to stay in the community. These permanent LTC consumers enter the SNF from either the community or the hospital and are less likely to return to community living following care. The two markets are differentiated by the level and duration of care and discharge status.

The STLTC system is composed of step-down services, including inpatient rehabilitation, convalescent care, and in-home support services. STLTC services meet the established medical requirements of older persons and are supported by Medicare coverage, private health insurance, out-of-pocket payments, and trade-offs within the DRG system. The goal of care is the restoration of the individual to community living or, for some, compassionate terminal care.

Fiscally viable because of trade-offs within DRG Medicare reimbursement, STLTC services may be appropriately provided within the orbit of the general hospital. Hospitals have a long history of service to the elderly and can provide the professional and technical expertise necessary to treat medically oriented needs of the temporarily infirm and disabled elderly. A growing number of hospitals already provide or are actively developing step-down services.

The LTLTC system addresses a different patient group, those who are chronically and often progressively disabled. The service goals, too, are different, involving rehabilitation and maintenance. Because social needs, rather than acute medical problems, are addressed, the services are best organized under a social service system. The institutional or organizational sponsor of LTLTC services will vary depending on the ecology of social services in a given community. Many voluntary organizations already provide an array of LTLTC services and can build on this capacity.

Unlike STLTC services, LTLTC services are characterized by a lack of formal financing sources. Medicaid is the primary source of financing for nursing home care, but cutbacks and limitations on this program have threatened the financial well-being of LTLTC providers and the provision of their services to the elderly poor. Increasingly, providers are finding that they can no longer survive on a Medicaid base alone. Furthermore, a growing population of financially secure elderly are also in need of service. LTLTC providers have a responsibility to reposition themselves in the market and to develop alternative financing options.

The opportunity to develop a well-organized, well-financed LTLTC system requires the use of private as well as public financing options. The insurance principle has already enabled people to meet the catastrophic costs of acute care. It is suggested that the same principle be applied to LTLTC service to meet catastrophic LTLTC financing requirements. The aggressive development of alternate forms of LTLTC financing would improve access to services, promote continuity of care, and allow providers to diversify revenue sources.

Many people believe that the LTC system in this country is fast approaching a crisis. Inadequate and faltering reimbursement systems and the growing demand for services point to the need for an overhaul of the system.

STLTC service needs can be addressed through a hospital-based system whose development requires that the hospital administration, board, and staff be educated on the needs of elderly patients and that they understand how to reapportion DRG funds between acute and STLTC services. The LTLTC problem is more difficult primarily because an adequate financing vehicle still needs to be developed. The creation of appropriate savings and insurance mechanisms for those elderly persons who can afford to pay for services is the major challenge facing health policy. Marketing protection against the disabilities that often accompany aging is a task that private industry has already demonstrated its entrepreneurial capacity to accomplish. The "short" of the solution to LTC is already in hand. It remains for the private provider and the insurance industry to work together to resolve the LTC problem through developing a viable solution for the "long of it."

References

1. Binstock, R. H. 1983. The aged as scapegoat. *Gerontologist* 23(2):136.
2. Brody, S. J. 1973. Comprehensive health care for the elderly: An analysis. *Gerontologist* 13(4):412–418.
3. Brody, S. J. 1979. The thirty-to-one paradox: Health needs and medical solutions. *Aging: Agenda for the Eighties NATL J* 11(44):1869–1873.
4. Gibson, R. M., Waldo, D. R. 1981. National health expenditures, 1980. *Health Care Financing Rev* 3(1):1–59.
5. Grannemann, T. W., Pauly, M. V. 1983. *Controlling Medicaid Costs: Federalism, Competition and Choice*. Washington, D.C.: American Enterprise Institute.
6. Paringer, L. 1983. Economic incentives in the provision of long term care. In *Market Reforms in Health Care*, ed. J. A. Meyers. Washington, D.C.: American Enterprise Institute.
7. Callahan, J. J. 1982. A perspective on home care, cited in Trager, B. 1984. Of interest. *Home Health Care Serv Q* 5(1):108.
8. National Center for Health Statistics. 1980. Utilization of short stay hospitals, annual summary for the United States, 1979. *Vital and Health Statistics* 13(60):20.
9. Congressional Budget Office. 1977. *Long Term Care for the Elderly and Disabled*, 4. Washington, D.C.: Government Printing Office.
10. National Center for Health Statistics. 1979. National nursing home survey: 1977 summary of the United States. *Vital Health Statistics* 13(43):29.
11. Brody, S. J., Poulshock, S. W., Masciocchi, C. 1978. The family caring unit: A major consideration in the long-term support system. *Gerontologist* 18(6): 555–561.
12. Brody, E. M. 1981. "Women in the middle" and family help to older people. *Gerontologist* 21(5):471–480.
13. Liu, K., Palesch, Y. 1981. The nursing home population: Different perspectives and implications for policy. *Health Care Financing Rev* 3(2):19.
14. Lubitz, J., Prihoda, R. 1983. Use and cost of Medicare services in the last years of life. *Health, United States, 1983*. DHHS Pub. No. (PHS) 84-1232. Washington, D.C.: Government Printing Office.
15. Gornick, M., Beebe, J., Prihoda, R. 1983. Options for change under Medicare: Impact of a cap on catastrophic illness expense. *Health Care Financing Rev* 5(1):34.
16. Timmer, E. J., Kovar, M. G. 1971. Expenses for hospital and institutional care during the last years of life for adults who died in 1964 or 1965, United States. *Vital and Health Statistics* PHS Pub. No. 10000. Washington, D.C.: Government Printing Office.
17. Gibbs, J., Newmann, J. 1982. *Study of Health Services Used and Costs Incurred During the Last Six Months of a Terminal Illness*. Chicago, Ill.: Blue Cross and Blue Shield Association, Research and Development Department.
18. Kovar, M. G. 1983. Expenditures for the medical care of elderly people living in the community throughout 1980. *National Medical Care Utilization and Expenditure Survey*, Data Report HHS Pub. No. 4, 1–9. Washington, D.C.: Government Printing Office.

19. McCall, N. 1984. Utilization and costs of Medicare services by beneficiaries in their last year of life. *Med Care* 22(4):329–342.
20. See Ref. 18, pp. 2–3.
21. United States Senate, Special Committee on Aging, and the American Association of Retired People. 1984. *Aging America: Trends and Projections*, PL 3377(584), 53, 61, 63. Washington, D.C.: Government Printing Office.
22. Veterans Administration. 1977. *The Aging Veteran: Present and Future Medical Needs*. Washington, D.C.: Veterans Administration.
23. Katz, S., Branch, L. G., Branson, M., Papsidero, J. A., Beck, J. C., Greer, D. S. 1983. Active life expectancy. *N Engl J Med* 309(20):1218–1224.
24. Stark, A. J., Kliewer, E., Gutman, G., McCashin, B. 1984. Placement changes in long-term care: Three years' experience. *Am J Public Health* 74(5):459–463.
25. Brody, S. J., Magel, J. S. 1984. DRG: The second revolution in health care for the elderly. *J Am Geriatr Soc* 32(9):676–679.
26. National Center for Health Statistics. 1982. Utilization of short stay hospitals: Annual summary for the United States, 1980. *Vital and Health Statistics* 13(64).
27. Brody, S. J., Persily, N. A. (eds.) 1984. *Hospitals and the Aged: The New Old Market*. Rockville, Md.: Aspen Systems Corp.
28. Owen, J. W. 1983. A hospital professional looks at efforts to curb health care costs. *Health Care Commentary*. Washington, D.C.: Health Insurance Association of America.
29. Rocheleau, B. 1983. *Hospitals and Community-Oriented Programs for the Elderly*. Ann Arbor, Mich.: Health Administration Press.
30. Vogel, R. J., Palmer, H. C. (eds.) 1983. *Long-Term Care. Perspectives from Research and Demonstrations*. Health Care Financing Administration (391-955). Washington, D.C.: Government Printing Office.
31. Jette, A. 1983. Meeting the needs of an aging population. *Health Soc Work* 8(4):326.
32. Brody, S. J., Magel, J. S. 1983. Diagnosis related groups: One view. University of Pennsylvania Center for the Study of Aging *Newsletter* 6(2):6–8.
33. Pelham, A. O., Clark, W. F. 1983. When do you go home: Hospital discharge placement decisions for the elderly and implications for community based long-term care agencies, cited in Kleyman, P. 1983. Discharge planning studies. *The Coordinator*, 36–38. Los Angeles, Calif.: Coordinator Publication.
34. Kleyman, P. 1983. Discharge planning studies. *The Coordinator*, 37. Los Angeles, Calif.: Coordinator Publication.
35. Jette, A. M., Branch, L. G. 1983. Targeting community services to high-risk elders: Toward preventing long-term care institutionalization. *Aging Prev* 3(1):53–69.
36. Kemp, B. J. 1981. The case management model of human service delivery. In *Annual Review of Rehabilitation*, Vol. 2, ed. E. L. Pan, T. E. Backer, and C. L. Vash, 213. New York: Springer-Verlag.
37. LeCompte, R. B., Flood, J. F., Rabson, B. 1984. Hospital-based case management: A cost-effective community service for high-risk elderly. In *Hospitals and the Aged*, ed. S. J. Brody and N. A. Persily, 211–212. Rockville, Md.: Aspen Systems Corp.

38. Weiss, L. J., Sklar, B. 1983. Project OPEN: A hospital-based long-term care demonstration program for the chronically ill elderly. *Home Health Care Serv Q* 4(3/4):23–90.
39. Brown, T. E., Learner, R. M. 1983. The South Carolina community long term care project. *Home Health Care Serv Q* 4(3/4):127–145.
40. Miller, L. S., Walter, L. 1983. Estimating the savings created by a case managed long term care system. Paper presented at the 111th Annual Meeting of the American Public Health Association, Dallas, Tex., November.
41. Weissert, W. G. 1985. Seven reasons why it is so difficult to make community based long-term care cost effective. *Health Serv Res* 20(4):424–433.
42. Austin, C. A. 1983. Case management in long-term care: Options and opportunities. *Health Soc Work* 8(1):16–30.
43. Berkman, B. 1984. Social work and the challenge of DRGs. *Health Soc Work* 9(1):2–3.
44. Brody, S. J., Masciocchi, C. 1980. Data for long-term care planning by health systems agencies. *Am J Public Health* 70(11):1194–1198.
45. Branch, L. G., Jette, A. M. 1983. Elders' use of informal long-term care assistance. *Gerontologist* 23(1):51–56.
46. Kohen, J. A. 1983. Old but not alone: Informal social supports among the elderly by marital status and sex. *Gerontologist* 23(1):57–63.
47. Moon, M. 1983. The role of the family in the economic well being of the elderly. *Gerontologist* 23(1):45–50.
48. See Ref. 5, p. 3.
49. United States Health Care Financing Administration. 1983. *The Medicare and Medicaid Data Book. 1983. Health Care Financing Program Statistics,* 25. Baltimore, Md.: Health Care Financing Administration.
50. United States General Accounting Office. 1979. Entering A Nursing Home— Costly Implications for Medicaid and the Elderly, *Report to the Congress by the Comptroller General.* PAD-80-12. Washington, D.C.: Government Printing Office, 16.
51. Meiners, M. R. 1983. The case for long-term care insurance. *Health Aff* 2(2):75.
52. Kastenbaum, R., Candy, S. E. 1973. The 4% fallacy: A methodological and empirical critique of extended care facility population statistics. *Int J Aging Hum Dev* 4(1):15–21.
53. Comptroller General of the United States. 1977. *The Well-Being of Older People in Cleveland, Ohio.* HRD-77-70. Washington, D.C.: Government Printing Office.
54. Starr, P. 1982. *The Social Transformation of American Medicine,* 295–306. New York: Basic Books.
55. Feldstein, M. 1977. The high cost of hospitals—What to do about it. *Public Interest* 48:40–54.
56. Havighurst, C. C. 1977. Controlling health care costs: Strengthening the private sector's hand. *J Health Political Policy Law* 1:471–498.
57. Havighurst, C. C. 1979. Private cost containment medical practice under competition. In *Socioeconomic Issues of Health: 1979,* ed. G. I. Misek, 41–65.

Chicago, Ill.: American Medical Association, Center for Health Services Research and Development.

58. Enthoven, A. C. 1979. Health care cost control through incentives and competition: Consumer-choice health plan. In *Socioeconomic Issues of Health: 1979*, ed. G. I. Misek, 23–39. Chicago, Ill.: American Medical Association, Center for Health Services Research and Development.

59. Stano, M. 1981. Individual health accounts. An alternative health care financing approach. *Health Care Financing Rev* 3(1):117–125.

60. Jacobs, B., Weissert, W. 1983. Home equity financing of long-term care for the elderly. Paper prepared for the Fifth Annual Research Conference of the Association for Public Policy, Analysis and Management, Philadelphia, Pa., October.

61. Gillick, M. R. 1984. Is the care of the chronically ill a medical prerogative? *N Engl J Med* 310(3):190–193.

62. Institute of Medicine. 1978. *Aging and Medical Education*. Washington, D.C.: National Academy of Sciences.

63. Brody, S. J. 1984. Health services: Need and utilization. In *Hospitals and the Aged: The New Old Market*, ed. S. J. Brody and N. A. Persily, 28. Rockville, Md.: Aspen Systems Corp.

64. Collins, G. 1984. Care for far-off elderly: Sources of help. *The New York Times*, Jan. 5.

Fourteen

The Informal System of Health Care

Elaine M. Brody and Stanley J. Brody

The family invented long-term care of the elderly well before that phrase was articulated, making the shift from episodic, short-term care sooner and more flexibly, more willingly, and more effectively than have professionals and the bureaucracy.[1,2] Moreover, the family has always been and continues to be the main provider of long-term health and social support to the aged. The volume of family services dwarfs that provided by the "formal" system of governmental and voluntary agencies and facilities. The family is also the major component of the "informal" or "natural" support system, which includes other unpaid caregivers, such as friends and neighbors.

Reshaping health care for the elderly requires consideration of the main needs of older people, the relationships among those needs, and, therefore, the relationships of the systems that are designed to meet them. The largest areas of need are for income maintenance, medical services, and long-term health and social services. Each of these is interlocked with the others. For example, access to high-quality medical care contributes to the determination of the older person's level of functioning, which in turn dictates the nature and number of supportive services needed. Conversely, a lack of access to supportive services may lead to a neglect of health needs and deterioration in functional capacities, which then necessitate medical care. Similarly, income determines the elderly's ability to obtain supportive health services, prescriptions, proper nutrition, special diets, supportive living arrangements, and the like.

In the last 50 years, public policy has responded unevenly to the needs of the elderly. In the areas of income maintenance and medical services there have been substantial, and for the most part, effective responses, but public policy has faltered in the area of health and social services—that is, in long-term care (LTC).[3] Both the achievements and the failures of public policy have had a direct effect on the family in its role as the provider of economic support for the aged (for day-to-day income and medical care) and as the principal provider of LTC services. As Blenkner pointed out, demographic imperatives have pushed the needs of the elderly beyond the self-solution or the kinship solution to require societal solutions.[4] It follows that the family's capacities dictate the directions public policy should take.

This chapter first summarizes social policy accomplishments (and failures) to date in providing income and medical and mental health care to the elderly. The role of the informal (family) support system is then described. The chapter concludes with a discussion of the respective roles of the formal and informal systems and major issues relating to their integration into a total, balanced LTC system.

Income

During the Depression, more than half of the aged were totally economically dependent on their families, and an additional 13% were similarly dependent on welfare programs.[5] To provide immediate stable relief and to replace the stop-gap Federal Emergency Relief Program, the Social Security Act (SSA) provided an initial income base through Old Age Assistance (OAA), although it varied from state to state. To augment and eventually replace much of the OAA program, social insurance (Old Age Insurance, or OAI) was enacted simultaneously as part of SSA. The avowed purposes of the insurance program were to provide a subsistence base, to encourage older workers to leave the work force to make room for younger entries, and to replace OAA with a more adequate, nationally based program.

All of the goals were achieved. During the 1950s, the number of OAI beneficiaries surpassed the number of those receiving OAA for the first time, providing the beginning of a national subsistence base. The percentage of the aged in poverty dropped from about 75% in 1936 to 35% in 1959 and to 18.6% in 1972.[6] Paralleling this decrease was a virtual elimination of the total economic dependency of the elderly on their adult children, with the rate dropping from 50% in 1936 to 1.5% in 1982. The proportion of those receiving OAA dropped from almost 25% in 1950 to 8% in 1972[5] and to 5% of the successor Supplemental Security Income (SSI) in 1985.[7]

The objectives of the income-maintenance program changed in the late 1960s from minimal subsistence to the replacement of income. In keeping with this agenda, the enactment of the 1972 Amendments to SSA increased OAI by 20%, introduced an annual automatic cost-of-living adjustment (COLA) tied to the consumer price index, and replaced OAA with a national pension program that provided a uniform minimal income floor for the aged.

The effect of the new approach to income maintenance has been to advance substantially the attainment of the goal of the replacement of income for a significant number of retirees. In 1982, the mean income per month of recent retirees was $1956 for couples and $1024 for unmarried individuals. Today's retirees commonly have pension and/or asset income as well.[8]

While the attainment of new goals for income replacement was accelerated by the 1972 SSA Amendments and by the statutory protection of employee pensions (the Employment Retirement Income Security Act, or ERISA), the contemporaneous enactment of Title XVI (SSI), to replace Title I (OAA) as part of these SSA Amendments, provided a new national structure for the assurance of a uniform minimal level of subsistence. SSI created a nationally funded and administered program that replaced the state matching fund requirement and state administrations that served under OAA. As a result, there no longer were wide discrepancies among the states in eligibility requirements and the amount of benefits. The common state restrictions of legally responsible relatives (LRR), liens on beneficiaries' homes, and residency requirements were abolished. The removal of the LRR restrictions was of enormous importance to families, who had often been placed under severe economic stress by the provision in most state OAA programs.[9]

These income-maintenance programs, augmented by public programs like Food Stamps, housing subsidies, and congregate feeding, and by private business, have significantly reduced the economic distress of the elderly. In turn, families have been relieved as well. On the other hand, a significant number of minority elderly women remain in poverty.

The Formal System of Care

Three major components comprise the formal health-care system—medical services, long-term care, and mental health services. Unfortunately, they are marked by a high degree of fragmentation:

> Health services for the aged are multiple, parallel, overlapping, noncontinuous and, at the very least, confusing to the elderly consumer. Rarely do they meet the collective criteria of availability, accessibility, and affordability or offer continuity of care in the holistically organized system. Planning for health services

for the aged is similarly confused. Parallel systems of service have their own planning mechanisms. As a result, the various planning efforts overlap, contradict and are unrelated one to the other.

Virtually all the services are funded by differing public money streams and have varied administrative arrangements, widely ranging eligibility requirements and different benefits for the same or similar services.[10]

The three components of the system are sketched briefly below.

The provision of publicly supported medical services has evolved from the early 1912 reform period, when state legislatures actively considered State Health Insurance, to the 1965 enactment of the age-categorical National Health Insurance program of Medicare (Title XVIII of SSA) and of Medicaid (Title XIX of SSA), enacted for the indigent patient. Through Medicaid and Medicare, the goal of making acute catastrophic medical coverage available was met. This support, when combined with that of the income-maintenance programs, has helped relieve the family of the costs of catastrophic acute medical care.

In 1984, in an effort to control Medicare costs and to protect the viability of the Medicare trust fund, Congress discontinued the practice of paying hospitals on a retrospective charge basis and instituted a prospective payment system through the Health Care Financing Administration (HCFA). In most states this system uses diagnosis-related groups (DRGs) as the basis of payment (see Maddox and Manton, Chapter 4).

Prospective payment has resulted in a sharp drop in lengths of stay as well as admission rates and has had the effect of providing hospitals with incentives to develop step-down services, which have been called short-term long-term care (STLTC)—that is, less-intense levels of service and facilities that are used for a short period of posthospital care.[11] (See Brody and Magel, Chapter 13.) Such services are not consistently available, of course, and there is no information as yet about the effects that earlier discharges have on the elderly patients' families.

Supplementing medical services are various forms of long-term care, which has been defined by the Health Resources Administration as:

> those services designed to provide diagnostic, preventive, therapeutic, rehabilitative, supportive and maintenance services for individuals . . . who have chronic physical and/or mental impairments in a variety of institutional and noninstitutional health care settings, including the home, with the goal of promoting the optimum level of physical, social and psychological functioning.[12]

To date, the major public LTC provision has been for skilled nursing facility (SNF) care under the Medicaid program. Neither Medicare nor Medicaid is permitted to support services other than those that are medically prescribed and administered. Even under Medicaid, few states provide the adult group-care services so critically needed for the respite of family caregivers. The personal health-care services provided are minimal and do not meet the major need for personal maintenance services (i.e., homemaker, shopping, chores, access, etc.). An exception was made (1985) for those elderly who would otherwise be institutionalized. These latter services are provided through Area Agencies on Aging (AAA) under Title III of the Older Americans Act, and in 1981 were funded with less than $1 billion. Also included on the AAA agenda is supporting socially oriented citizen centers. Title XX of SSA (Social Support Services) provides a block grant to states for similar services that also amounts to less than $1 billion for the aged. (A more detailed discussion of LTC services is found in Brody and Magel, Chapter 13.)

The third key element of the formal care system is mental health. (See Cohen and Hastings, Chapter 20, for a more in-depth analysis.) Although the true level of need for mental health care among the elderly has not been fully established,[13,14] evidence that has been accumulating indicates that approximately 25% of older people have significant mental illness symptoms. As with physical disability, persons 75 years old or older are at highest risk.

Unfortunately, the mental health needs of older people are inadequately met, and there is limited access to a full spectrum of appropriate services. For example, the elderly are served at a rate that is less than one-fourth of the rate for the 25- to 44-year-old age group.[15] Moreover, the aged tend to have mental and emotional illness symptoms for longer periods of time, often years, before receiving help.[16] Only 4% of community mental health center patients are elderly, and the elderly comprise only 2% of those served by private practitioners and clinics. Yet many of the mental disorders of the elderly are treatable and reversible.

The barriers to mental health care of the elderly are:

- Inequitable reimbursement structures of federal health-care programs and other financial barriers

- Fragmented, disorganized systems of health and social services available to the elderly

- The low number of mental health professionals who are interested in and trained to provide care to the elderly

- Continued ageism, or negative attitudes toward aging and the aged, on the part of mental health and health professionals

- The limited availability of transportation services and other problems involving accessibility

- "Turf-guarding" by agencies seeking to protect their share of reduced resources.[17]

• Fear of the cost of treating the mentally ill in general

Elderly persons themselves may not seek mental health care because of a lack of awareness of mental health services, distrust and fear based on stigmas created by attitudes toward mental health that were prevalent a generation ago, low levels of self-esteem resulting from loss of meaningful life roles, and beliefs that dementia and other mental conditions are part of normal aging.[18]

The Informal System

Although the formal health-care system has failed to develop a coherent and complete system of health and social services for the aged, families have responded to the vastly increased need. Despite the stubborn and widespread myth that their families do not take care of the elderly, 30 years of research have produced definitive evidence to the contrary and the matter is no longer at scientific issue.

The prevalence of the isolated nuclear family, which was thought to be a consequence of increased industrialization, urbanization, and mobility, has been disproved. The elderly are knitted firmly into the fabric of the family and continue to maintain close contacts and viable relationships with family members.[19] The flow of intergenerational services is primarily downward, from the old to the young, but the flow changes direction when older people become disabled.

It bears repetition that at any given time most older people do not need help, apart from the garden-variety services that family members normally exchange on a day-to-day basis and at times of emergency. It is undeniable, however, that demographic developments have resulted in both an exponential increase in the number and proportion of elderly who depend on their families for help and a dramatic difference in the nature and duration of the help required.

The informal system provides some 80% of the health and social services received by the elderly.[20,21] Data from the national 1982 Long-Term Care Survey show that all formal services together accounted for less than 15% of all "helper days of care" in the community (including home health, homemaker/chore service, adult day care programs, etc.).[22] Families provide the majority of medically related services (such as preparing special diets and giving medications), transportation and shopping, household maintenance, personal care (such as bathing, feeding, dressing, toileting, and supervision), and monitoring, and they often share their homes when the older person can no longer live alone. The family also functions as the real "case manager," linking the older person to available community services and mobilizing or orchestrating the delivery of formal services.

In addition, the family provides many services that do not appear in surveys that examine day-to-day care. Family members provide the expressive support—the affection, emotional support, socialization, and sense of having someone on whom to rely—that is the form of help most desired by the elderly. Families mobilize themselves to meet events that require high-intensity services for the older person: moving from one household to a different living arrangement, acute illnesses and hospitalizations, convalescent and/or rehabilitative care, and, ultimately, terminal care.

In general, the informal support network tends to be structured hierarchically, based primarily on the service provider's relationship to the older person (spouse, near kin, distant kin, and friends), but also on geographic proximity.[23] Spouses, children, and children-in-law play central roles for most of the dependent elderly. Daughters are the most prevalent family helpers for the elderly with disabled spouses and for widowed older people.[24-27] For the most part, friends and neighbors play much smaller roles in the helping network; although they are important resources when children are absent or unavailable, their efforts do not approach those of family members in duration or intensity.[23,28,29] However, friends and neighbors often serve to link the elderly to needed services in the community.[30]

Definitive data on the typical size of the informal networks are limited, since most studies of caregiving focus on the individual who is the "principal caregiver." One review of the literature notes that there have been differing reports on whether the one-caregiver service networks or those service networks comprised of two or more individuals are the most prevalent.[23] The 1982 Long-Term Care Survey found that among older people who need help with ADL, 36.8% have one helper, 30.7% have two, 18.1% have three, and 14.6% have four or more helpers.[31] The most frequently reported informal sources of help, in order of frequency, were spouses (35.6%), daughters (32.6%), sons (32.6%), female relatives (not spouses, daughters, sisters, or daughters-in-law)(14.2%), male relatives (8.1%), daughters-in-law (7.8%), and brothers (1.7%).[31] The proportion who named "other" female or male relatives (22.3%) suggests that grandchildren and possibly nieces and nephews play a significant role.

The size of the informal network may also vary with the characteristics of the dependent person. As might be expected, the amount of help received is directly related to the level of the older person's functional disability.[32,23] In several investigations, the caregiving networks of elderly widows were found to include a greater diversity of providers than the support system of married older people, with more frequent involvement of extended kin, friends, neighbors, and paid sources of help.[28,33] Among the many other relevant variables are family structure, the quality of the relationship between the elderly person and the caregiver, economic resources, other demands on family members' time and energy, the degree of related-ness/blood ties, and urban/rural, socioeconomic, and ethnic factors.

In the main, the distribution of the various kinds of tasks among infor-mal providers is gender-specific and/or based on degree of relatedness. (See Ref. 1 for review.) Personal care and instrumental services are most often provided by spouses (for the married) or by adult daughters (for the wid-owed elderly), while sons tend to help with certain gender-defined services, such as money management. Daughters are three times more likely than sons to share their households with a dependent elderly parent. Within each family network, however, the allocation of the services may be highly diversified, and the number of tasks performed by one family member impressively long.[34]

Caregiving Spouses

As stated above, spouses are the principal providers of care to older people who are married. Due to sex differences in life expectancy and the tendency of men to marry women younger than they are, elderly men are much more likely than elderly women to have a spouse on whom to rely. Most of the 9 million widowed older people are women. At age 65 and over, most older women (52%) are widowed and most older men (77%) are married. Rates of widowhood rise sharply with advancing age, and the imbalance in the proportions of women to men increases. Between the ages of 65 and 74, the ratio of women to men is 131 : 200; between 75 and 84 the ratio is 166 : 100; and at age 85 and over there are 224 women to every 100 men.[35]

Whether they are husbands or wives, older people exert extreme efforts to care for a spouse, but their capacities are limited by their own advanced age, reduced energy and strength, and age-related ailments. Compared with other relatives who provide care, they experience the most stress.[36] Elderly wives who care for disabled husbands, for example, have been found to suffer from low morale, isolation, loneliness, economic hardship, and "role overload" caused by multiple responsibilities.[37] Formal pro-viders, therefore, should pay close attention to such caregivers' need for respite (temporary relief from caregiving activities), concrete helping ser-vices, and emotional support. Since today more couples survive together into advanced old age, such situations are likely to occur with increasing frequency.

Caregiving Adult Children

When an elderly couple has children, they assist the "well" spouse in caring for the disabled parent; when an older person is widowed, the bulk of care is given by adult children.[19,38,39] Accumulated evidence documents the strength of intergenerational ties, the continuity of responsible filial behavior, the frequency of contacts between generations, and the strenuous efforts of adult children to avoid institutional placement of the old.[24]

Most older people realize their preference to live near, but not with, their children,[19] sharing households primarily when reasons of health or economics make it necessary. About 18% of the elderly live with children, about 84% of those with children live less than an hour away from one of them,[19] and 53% have seen their children within the last 24 hours.

Daughters (and to some extent daughters-in-law) have been identified as the principal caregivers to dependent parents and parents-in-law. In addition to providing most of the helping services noted above, daughters predominate among those who share their homes when elderly cannot manage on their own.[24–27,40] Sons also sustain bonds of affection, perform certain gender-defined tasks, and become the "responsible relatives" for the old who have no daughters or none close by.

Parent care is now a normative experience for individuals and families,[1] and responsible filial behavior has persisted despite two broad influential trends that affect the capacity of adult children to provide care.

The first trend is radical demographic developments (see Rice, Chapter 1) that have led to a vast increase in the demands for parent care. Many caregiving adult children are grandparents; the four-generation family has become commonplace, with about 46% of older people with children being at the pinnacle of a four-generation family tree.[41] During the same time span in which the number and proportion of older people in the population increased dramatically, the birth rate fell sharply. People who are now in advanced old age therefore have fewer children to share caregiving responsibilities than used to be the case.

In addition, since parents and children age together, the adult children of the greatly increased number and proportion of people in advanced old age most often are in middle age, and some are in their sixties or seventies. To illustrate: between 1900 and 1976, the number of people who experienced the death of a parent before the age of 15 dropped from one in four to one in twenty, while the number of middle-aged couples with two or more living parents increased from 10% to 47%.[42] In the early 1960s, about 25% of people over the age of 45 had a surviving parent, but only a decade later, 25% of people in their late fifties had a surviving parent.[43] By 1980, about 40% of people in their late fifties had a surviving parent (some had both parents), as did about 20% of those in their early sixties, 10% of those in their late sixties, and 3% of those in their seventies.[44] Ten percent of all people now 65 years old or older have a child over the age of 65! Another clue to the ages at which adult children may be called on to provide parent care are data showing that the median age of the children of an 85-year-old woman (in 1985) is 59.[45] The need to provide parent care, then, occurs at a time of life when the adult children themselves may be experiencing age-related interpersonal losses, the onset of chronic ailments, and lower energy levels, and may be retired or approaching retirement. Their responsibilities often extend both upward to the old and downward to the younger generations.

The second broad trend has been the rapid entry of middle-aged women into the work force. Sixty percent of women between the ages of 45 and 54 work, as do 42% of women between the ages of 55 and 64.[46] Some work because of career commitment, but most because the money is needed. Millions of women, therefore, find themselves confronted with multiple roles that often compete: the traditional roles of wife, homemaker, and mother, and the role of paid worker as well as that of helper to an elderly parent.

For many women the need to care for the old arises (whether or not they do paid work) at a time when most people expect to have "empty nests"; instead, they find that those empty nests are refilled (literally, or in terms of increased responsibility) by impaired older people in need of care.[24] As women advance from 40 years of age to their early sixties, for example, those who have a surviving parent become more likely to have that parent be dependent on them, to spend more time caring for the parent, to do more difficult caregiving tasks, and to have the parent in their own household.[47] Middle-aged women, then, not only may be experiencing their own age-related problems but also may be facing their peak responsibilities, rather than diminishing cares, at this stage in their lives.

Caregiving to elderly parents is not limited to the middle-aged, of course. As many as one-third of caregiving daughters may be either under 40 or over 60. Younger caregivers may still have their own children at home. Older women may have age-related declines and chronic ailments that limit their caregiving capacities.

Effects of Family Caregiving

The caregiving efforts of families have been found to have social as well as economic costs. Evaluation of the service needs of the elderly therefore requires a perspective that includes the situations and problems of the families concerned: the unique family constellation, the family's capacities, and family members' anxieties and symptoms of stress.

Recently, research on the effects of caregiving has been accelerating. To put the matter in perspective: in the main, having an elderly parent is gratifying and helpful. Older people are a resource to their children, providing many forms of assistance. Most people help their parents willingly when need be and derive satisfaction from doing so. Some adult children negotiate this stage of life without undue strain. However, there can be severe strain when there is an increase in reliance on children to meet a parent's needs.

While some caregivers experience financial hardship and some experience declines in their physical health, study after study has identified the most pervasive and most severe consequences as emotional strain. Mental illness symptoms, such as depression, anxiety, frustration, feelings of helplessness, sleeplessness, lowered morale, and emotional exhaustion, are related to restrictions on time and freedom, isolation, conflict from the competing demands of various responsibilities, difficulties in setting priorities, and interference with lifestyle and social and recreational activities.[25,48–55] Moreover, such findings are not unique to the United States. Similar information is emerging from other countries.[56,57] Caregiving daughters appear to be more vulnerable to such effects than sons. When sons do become principal caregivers, they do less, are helped by their wives, and experience less strain.[58]

The women who are the principal caregivers and who often are under considerable stress from their multiple competing responsibilities have been characterized as "women in the middle."[59] The pressures they experience place them at high risk of mental and physical illness symptoms. Their other family members are affected as well. Among the family strains that have been identified are relationship problems, lack of privacy, changed routines and patterns of social activities, and postponement of vacations and future plans.

Very recently, attention has been called to another kind of cost to the family that is a consequence of caregiving. Some caregiving spouses and children are deterred from participation in the labor force.[60] Others leave their jobs or cut back on working hours because of the care needs of elderly husbands and parents, resulting in sharp reductions in family income.[1] National data indicate that among caregivers to older people, 13.5% of wives, 11.6% of daughters, 11.4% of husbands, and 5% of sons quit their jobs to care for elderly relatives; many more reduce their working hours, rearrange their work schedules, or take time off without pay.[61]

Information about the effects of parent care on women's work force participation is just beginning to emerge. Scattered findings indicate that working women continue to meet their responsibilities to their families, their elderly parents, and their jobs, but give up their own free time and opportunities for socialization.[49,62,47] One recent study found that disabled parents of working women and nonworking women received the same amount of care from all sources of services together.[63] Both employed and nonworking daughters provided equal amounts of emotional support, service arrangement, financial management, shopping, and transportation. When the daughters worked, however, the family purchased more help for personal care, but there was no increase in the utilization of services subsidized by government/agencies.

The Elderly Without Close Family

Elderly individuals without family or whose family members are not close at hand and whose illness or disability is severe or likely to be prolonged are at high risk. They therefore require special attention from formal system providers.

A significant minority of older people do not have a close family member on whom to rely, and the proportion who are deprived in that respect rises with advancing age. At age 74 and over, for example, 68% of women and 24% of men are widowed, in addition to the 9% of women and 7% of men who are divorced or who have never married. About 20% of people who are now 65 and over have never had a child, and an undetermined number are childless because they have outlived their children.[35] Although the vast majority of those with children see them frequently, 11% (almost 2 million old people) do not see a child as often as once a month.[27] For most, geographic distance precludes the availability of a child for day-to-day supportive health care; for a minority, little or no help can be expected due to long-standing alienation. Over all, more than 1 in 20 (5.3%) of all people 65 and over are entirely kinless—that is, without spouse, children, or siblings.

Family Relationships of the Institutionalized Aged

Despite the widespread notion that old people are "dumped" into nursing homes by hard-hearted, uncaring families, research has established definitively that such placement is made only after families have made prolonged and strenuous efforts to avoid it.

The 5% of those 65 and over who are in institutions at any one time are outnumbered two to one by equally disabled noninstitutionalized old people who are cared for by their families,[64,65] a proportion that did not change between 1962 and 1975.[27] The role of social support in the form of family is highlighted by the fact that, in contrast to those who live in the community, the vast majority (88%) of the institutionalized aged are not married (being widowed, divorced, or never married), more of them (about half) are childless, and those who have children have fewer children than the noninstitutionalized.[59]

Although most research on the family relationships of older people has focused on noninstitutionalized older people, existing information refutes the notion that family ties are severed when institutionalization takes place. Families continue to be interested and concerned, to visit their elderly relatives regularly, and to experience many emotional strains.[2,66]

The Role of the Formal System Vis-à-vis the Role of the Informal System

A major social policy issue concerns the relationship of the formal system to that of the family. In recent years, as part of an effort to shrink the formal system to save public dollars, there has been an insistent call for the family to increase its efforts to care for the disabled elderly. To summarize the information that bears on that issue:

- Research findings indicate that today the family provides more care and more difficult care to more elderly people over longer periods of time than ever before in history.[1,2]

- Community care for severely disabled older people is not cheaper than institutional care,[67,65,68] nor does it reduce their rates of institutionalization.[69]

- Nursing home beds are deficient in both number and quality. It is primarily the Medicaid-eligible older person or the one who requires "heavy care" who has access problems.[21] Such people are likely to be those who suffer from Alzheimer's disease or a related disorder.[70]

- When formal services are provided they are add-ons, not substitutes for existing services.[69] Such add-on services supplement family services and strengthen the family's caregiving capacities.[25,71–73]

After a careful review of cost-comparison studies, Weissert[69] concluded: "The challenge . . . must be to find ways to finance this new mode of care for this new class of patients, not to continue to try fruitlessly to justify community care as something it is not—a substitute for nursing home care or a way to save money."

Despite the accumulated knowledge about the role of the family and the strains it experiences as a result of caregiving, social policy has made virtually no response to the needs of families. For example, respite care and day care are scarce and not universally or adequately available. There is limited regular public or private funding for their consistent support; the programs that do exist are episodic and discontinuous, and vary greatly among the states.[74] Economic supplements to caregiving families (e.g., attendance allowances, Social Security credits for caregivers remaining at home) are much more prevalent in other industrialized nations.[75] Community health and social services are limited and disproportionately underfinanced when compared to acute-care services for the aged.[10] Enormous inequities exist among the various states in their expenditures for Medicaid services, both for nursing home care and community-based services.[21]

The "alternatives" issue that characterized the 1970s—that is, the notion that community services are cheaper, better, and could substitute for institutional services—proved to be spurious. Both types of services are needed to serve a heterogeneous population whose needs change over time. The goal, then, is to develop a viable partnership between the formal and informal support systems—for the formal system to supplement and support the efforts of the informal network and to substitute for those efforts when the family becomes overburdened and when the disabled elderly lack or lose informal supports.

In responding to the implications of an aging society, policy should monitor changes that affect the family's caregiving capacities. For example, it is not known how the current high rates of divorce and remarriage will affect filial care in the future when adult children have multiple loyalties. Other trends to be monitored include the rise in the number of single-parent families, one-child and childless couples, and the later ages at which women have a first child.

Problems of organizational and individual case management have been recognized as major issues in service delivery. Although many of the elements of the array of services needed are in place in most communities, they are often uneven regionally, are in short supply, are underdeveloped, lack consistent funding, and are unavailable to many people who need them. The goal is to rationalize these varied planning and service-delivery agencies so that they constitute a system in each community and can make a coordinated response to each individual and family in need.

The problem at the level of organizational systems inevitably is reflected at the level of the individual and family, for whom it is a baffling problem to mobilize and coordinate the needed services. The existence of an array of services is not equivalent to their actual utilization. Among the barriers to obtaining services is the lack of administrative linkages. Other barriers are the client's lack of knowledge about the service, inability to connect with it, unpalatable eligibility criteria or humiliating assessment procedures, the tendency of service agencies to perceive need only in terms of the services they offer, the complexities of entitlements, and bewildering regulations. Interventions designed to deal with these issues are variously called information and referral service, service management, outreach, case management, matrix management, channeling, and other names.

More subtle issues also impede service utilization and highlight the need for counseling. There are psychological barriers to using needed services. There are differences in the acceptability of services to different socioeconomic and ethnic groups of older people and families with different personalities and expectations. Therefore, whatever the label given to the process that is now most commonly referred to as case management, it must include the enabling process called counseling or case work. Case management should not be artificially divided into the mechanical manipulation or arrangement of services on the one hand and the offering of help with psychological issues on the other hand.

Finally, society's responsibility to support the efforts of caregiving families goes beyond ethical or humanistic considerations. All available information indicates that the well-being of the generations is interlocked collectively as well as on the level of the individual family. Because of the linkages among the generations (economically, socially, and psychologically), the situations of the elderly person and family members affect each other reciprocally. It is therefore a practical necessity to integrate the efforts of the formal and informal systems, so that their combined efforts constitute what Lebowitz has called a "balanced service system."[76]

References

1. Brody, E. M. 1985. Parent care as a normative family stress. *Gerontologist* 25:19–29.
2. Brody, E. M. 1985. The role of the family in nursing homes: Implications for research and public policy. In *Mental Illness in Nursing Homes: Agenda for Research*, ed. M. S. Harper and B. Lebowitz. Washington, D.C.: Government Printing Office.
3. Brody, E. M., Brody, S. J. 1987. Aged: Services. *Encyclopedia of Social Work, 18th Edition*. Silver Spring, Md.: National Association of Social Workers.
4. Blenkner, M. 1965. Social work and family relationships in later life with some thoughts on filial maturity. In *Social Structure and the Family: Generational Relations*, ed. E. Shanas and G. F. Streib. Englewood Cliffs, N.J.: Prentice Hall.
5. Upp, M. 1982. A look at the economic status of the aged then and now. *Soc Secur Bull* 45:16–22.
6. United States Department of Health and Human Services. 1982. *Social Security Bulletin. Annual Statistical Supplement, 1982*. 64. Washington, D.C.: Government Printing Office.
7. United States Department of Health and Human Services. 1985. Social Security in review: Program operations. *Soc Secur Bull* 48(8):49.
8. Maxfield, L., Reno, V. 1985. Distribution of income resources of recent retirees: Findings from the beneficiary survey. *Soc Secur Bull* 48(1):7–13.
9. Schorr, A. L. 1960. *Filial Responsibility in the Modern American Family*. Washington, D.C.: Government Printing Office.
10. Brody, S. J. 1979. The thirty-to-one-paradox: Health needs and medical solutions. *Natl J* 11(44):1869–1873.
11. Brody, S. J., Magel, J. S. 1984. DRG: The second revolution in health care for the elderly. *J. Am Geriatr Soc* 32(9):676–679.

LIBRARY ST. MARY'S COLLEGE

12. United States Health Resources Administration, Division of Long-Term Care. 1977. *The Future of Long-Term Care in the United States—The Report of the Task Force.* Washington, D.C.: Government Printing Office.
13. Butler, R. N., Lewis, M. 1973. *Aging and Mental Health: Positive Psychosocial Approaches.* St. Louis, Mo.: C. V. Mosby.
14. Schuckit, M. A. 1974. Unrecognized psychiatric illness in elderly medical-surgical patients. Paper presented at 27th Annual Meeting of the Gerontological Society of America, Portland, Oreg.
15. President's Commission on Mental Health. 1978. *Report to the President,* Vol. 1. Washington, D.C.: Government Printing Office.
16. Eisdorfer, C., Lawton, M. P. (eds.) 1973. *The Psychology of Adult Development and Aging.* Washington, D.C.: American Psychological Association.
17. United States Senate, Special Committee on Aging. 1982. *Developments in Aging: 1981,* Vol. 1. Washington, D.C.: Government Printing Office.
18. Hagebok, J. E., Hagebok, B. R. 1983. Meeting the mental health needs of the elderly: Issues and action steps. *Aging* 335-6:26–31.
19. Shanas, E. 1979. Social myth as hypothesis: The case of the family relations of old people. *Gerontologist* 19:3–9.
20. United States General Accounting Office. 1982. The elderly should benefit from expanded home health care but increasing these services will not insure cost reductions. *Report to the Congress by the Comptroller General.* IPE-83-1. Washington, D.C.: Government Printing Office.
21. United States General Accounting Office. 1983. Medicaid and nursing home care: Cost increases and the need for services are creating problems for the states and the elderly. *Report to the Congress by the Comptroller General.* Washington, D.C.: Government Printing Office.
22. Doty, P., Liu, K., Wiener, J. 1985. An overview of long-term care. *Health Care Financing Rev* 6(3):69–78.
23. Spivak, S., Haskins, B., Capitman, J. 1984. A review of research on informal support systems. Appendix F of *Evaluation of Coordinated, Community-Oriented Long-Term Care Demonstration Projects: Final Report,* DHHS, Contract No. 500-80-0073. Berkeley, Calif.: Berkeley Planning Associates.
24. Brody, E. M. 1978. The aging of the family. *Ann Am Acad Political Soc Sci* 438:13–27.
25. Horowitz, A. 1982. *The Role of Families in Providing Long-term Care to the Frail and Chronically Ill Elderly Living in the Community.* Final Report submitted to the Health Care Financing Administration. New York: Hunter College, Brookdale Center on Aging.
26. Myllyuoma, J., Soldo, B. J. 1980. Family caregivers to the elderly: Who are they? Paper presented at the 33rd Annual Meeting of the Gerontological Society of America, San Diego, Calif.
27. Shanas, E. 1979. The family as a social support system in old age. *Gerontologist* 19:169–174.
28. Cantor, M. H. 1979. Neighbors and friends: An overlooked resource in the informal support system. *Res Aging* 1:434–463.
29. Stoller, E., Earl, L. 1983. Help with activities of everyday life: Sources of support for the noninstitutionalized elderly. *Gerontologist* 23(1):64–70.

LIBRARY ST. MARY'S COLLEGE

30. Koser, G. 1981. *Enhancing and Sustaining Informal Support Networks.* Albany, N.Y.: State Health Planning Commission, Health Advisory Council.
31. Macken, C. L. Undated. *1982 Long-Term Care Survey: National Estimates of the Number and Degree of Functional Impairments and Sources of Support Among Elderly Medicare Beneficiaries Living in the Community.* Washington, D.C.: Health Care Financing Administration.
32. Caro, F. G., Blank, A. E. 1984. Burden experienced by informal providers of home care for the elderly. Paper presented at 37th Annual Meeting of the Gerontological Society of America, San Antonio, Tex.
33. O'Brien, J., Wagner, D. 1980. Help-seeking by the frail elderly: Problems in network analysis. *Gerontologist* 20:78–83.
34. Frankfather, D. L., Smith, M. J., Capers, O. 1979. Family maintenance of the disabled elderly. Paper presented at meeting of the American Orthopsychiatric Association, Washington, D.C.
35. Allan, C., Brotman, H. 1981. *Chartbook on Aging in America.* Washington, D.C.: The White House Conference on Aging.
36. Horowitz, A., Shindelman, L. W. 1981. Reciprocity and affection: Past influences on current caregiving. Paper presented at 34th Annual Meeting of the Gerontological Society of America, Toronto, Canada.
37. Fengler, A. P., Goodrich, N. 1979. Wives of elderly disabled men: The hidden patients. *Gerontologist* 19:175–183.
38. Sussman, M. B. 1965. Relationships of adult children with their parents in the United States. In *Social Structure and the Family: Generational Relations,* ed. E. Shanas and G. F. Streib, 62–92. Englewood Cliffs, N.J.: Prentice Hall.
39. Tobin, S. S., Kulys, R. 1980. The family and services. In *Annual Review of Gerontology and Geriatrics,* Vol. 1, ed. C. Eisdorfer, 370–399. New York: Springer-Verlag.
40. Troll, L. E. 1971. The family of later life: A decade review. *J Marriage Fam* 33:263–290.
41. Shanas, E. 1980. Older people and their families: The new pioneers. *J Marriage Fam* 42:9–15.
42. Uhlenberg, P. 1980. Death and the family. *Fam Hist* 5:313–320.
43. Murray, J. 1973. Family structure in the preretirement years. *Soc Secur Bull* 36:25–45.
44. National Retired Teachers Association and the American Association of Retired Persons. 1981. National Survey of Older Americans. (Unpublished data.) Washington, D.C.: National Retired Teachers Association and the American Association of Retired Persons.
45. Torrey, B. B. 1985. Sharing increasing costs on declining income: The visible dilemma of the invisible aged. *Milbank Memorial Fund Q* 63:377–394.
46. United States Bureau of Labor Statistics. 1981. Labor force by sex, age and race. *Earnings and Employment* 28:167.
47. Lang, A., Brody, E. M. 1983. Characteristics of middle-aged daughters and help to their elderly mothers. *J Marriage Fam* 45:193–202.
48. Archbold, P. 1978. Impact of caring for an ill elderly parent of the middle-aged or elderly offspring caregiver. Paper presented at the 31st Annual Meeting of the Gerontological Society of America, Dallas, Tex.

49. Cantor, M. H. 1983. Strain among caregivers: A study of experience in the United States. *Gerontologist* 23:597–604.
50. Danis, B. G. 1978. Stress in individuals caring for ill elderly relatives. Paper presented at the 31st Annual Meeting of the Gerontological Society of America, Dallas, Tex.
51. Frankfather, D. L., Smith, M. J., Caro, F. G. 1981. *Family Care of the Elderly: Public Initiatives and Private Obligations.* Lexington, Mass.: Lexington Books.
52. Gurland, B., Dean, L., Gurland, R., Cook, D. 1978. Personal time dependency in the elderly of New City: Findings from the U.S.–U.K. cross-national geriatric community study. In *Dependency in the Elderly of New York City,* 9–45. New York: Community Council of Greater New York.
53. Hoenig, J., Hamilton, M. 1966. Elderly patients and the burden on the household. *Psychiatr Neurol* 152:281–293.
54. Robinson, B., Thurnher, M. 1979. Taking care of aged parents: A family cycle transition. *Gerontologist* 19:586–593.
55. Sainsbury, P., Grad de Alercon, J. 1970. The effects of community care in the family of the geriatric patient. *Geriatr Psychiatry* 4:23–41.
56. Gibson, M. J. 1982. An international update on family care of the ill elderly. *Ageing Int* 9:11–14.
57. Horl, J., Rosemary, L. 1982. Assistance to the elderly as a common task of the family and social service organizations. *Arch Gerontol Geriatr* 1:75–95.
58. Horowitz, A. 1981. Sons and daughters as caregivers to older parents: Differences in role performance and consequences. Paper presented at 34th Annual Meeting of the Gerontological Society of America, Toronto, Canada.
59. Brody, E. M. 1981. "Women in the middle" and family help to older people. *Gerontologist* 21:471–480.
60. Soldo, B. J. 1980. Family caregivers to the elderly: Who are they? Paper presented at the 33rd Annual Meeting of the Gerontological Society of America, San Diego, Calif.
61. Stone, R., Cafferata, G. L., Sangl, J. 1987. Caregivers of the frail elderly: A national profile. *Gerontologist.* 27:616–626.
62. Horowitz, A., Sherman, R. H., Durmaskin, S. C. 1983. Employment and daughter caregivers: A working partnership for older people? Paper presented at 36th Annual Meeting of the Gerontological Society of America, San Francisco, Calif.
63. Brody, E. M., Schoonover, C. 1986. Patterns of care for the dependent elderly when daughters work and when they do not. *Gerontologist* 26(4):372–381.
64. Brody, S. J., Poulshock, S. W., Masciocchi, C. F. 1978. The family caring unit: A major consideration in the long-term support system. *Gerontologist* 18(6):556–561.
65. Comptroller General of the United States. 1977. *The Need for a National Policy to Better Provide for the Elderly.* HRD-78-19. Washington, D.C.: General Accounting Office.
66. George, L. K. 1984. *The Dynamics of Caregiver Burden.* Final Report submitted to the American Association of Retired Persons' Andrus Foundation. Durham, N.C.: Duke University.

67. Fox, P. D., Clauser, S. B. 1980. Trends in nursing home expenditures: Implications for aging policy. *Health Care Financing Rev.* 1(2):65–70.
68. Palmer, H. C. 1983. The alternatives question. *Long-Term Care: Perspectives from Research and Demonstrations*, ed. R. J. Vogel and H. C. Palmer, 255–305. Washington, D.C.: Government Printing Office.
69. Weissert, W. G. 1985. Seven reasons why it is so difficult to make community-based long-term care cost effective. *Health Serv Res* 20(4):424–433.
70. Brody, E. M., Lawton, M. P., Liebowitz, B. 1984. Senile dementia: Public policy and adequate institutional care. *Am J Public Health* 74:1381–1383.
71. Sherwood, S., Morris, S., Morris, J. N. 1984. Relationships between formal and informal service provision to frail elders. Paper presented at 37th Annual Meeting of the Gerontological Society of America, San Antonio, Tex.
72. Zawadski, R. T. 1983. Research in the demonstrations: Findings and issues. *Home Health Care Serv Q* 4:209–228.
73. Zimmer, A. H., Sainer, J. S. 1978. Strengthening the family as an informal support for their aged: Implications for social policy and planning. Paper presented at the 31st Annual Meeting of the Gerontological Society of America, Dallas, Tex.
74. Meltzer, J. W. 1982. *Respite Care: An Emerging Family Support Service.* Washington, D.C.: Center for the Study of Social Policy.
75. Gibson, M. J. 1984. Women and aging. Paper presented at International Symposium on Aging, Georgian Court College, Lakewood, N.J.
76. Lebowitz, B. D. 1978. Old age and family functioning. *J Gerontological Soc Work* 1:111–118.

Fifteen

Health-Care Cooperatives

James P. Firman

Most proposals for improving health-care arrangements for older Americans advocate more direct economic regulation, greater reliance on market forces, or the development of new provider organizations. However, the potential of each of these strategies is limited unless older persons are able to become better informed and more rational consumers. During the past 20 years, senior citizens have been exercising greater political power. During the next several decades, organized groups of older Americans will begin flexing their economic muscles in an attempt to become a more effective "third force" in the health-care marketplace.

The Limitations of Current Proposals for Reforming the Health-Care Marketplace

Each of the current proposals for ensuring that older persons can get high-quality and affordable health care has shortcomings and is likely to be of limited success.

Proponents of marketplace strategies claim that increased competition among health-care providers is the best way to achieve efficiency and cost containment, but critics argue that market strategies do not address adequately the issues of access, equity, and control of public spending. Furthermore, because of the complexity of the health-care marketplace, it is

278

claimed that consumers cannot and "should not" be expected to act as rational decision makers.[1] If market strategies will not work, the logic goes, more direct governmental intervention is the only reasonable alternative.

Proponents of greater reliance on regulation argue that more governmental intervention is needed to control costs, to weed out inefficient providers, and to ensure access to health care for disenfranchised groups. But critics of more direct economic regulation argue that it leads to uneconomic behaviors, including reduction of innovation, subsidy of inefficient operations, and inappropriate reimbursement systems, all of which result in excessive costs.[2]

Another shortcoming of regulatory approaches in the United States is the fact that government and consumer concerns are often different. For example, whereas the government wants to contain Medicare and Medicaid expenditures, consumers are primarily concerned about out-of-pocket costs. The case has been made that, whereas market strategies lead to distributional inequities based on income and wealth, regulatory strategies lead to inequitable distributions of influence and power. In this view, regulatory strategies have contributed to a shift in the balance of influence and power from consumers to government and providers.[3] Unfortunately, regulatory agencies may not be very effective representatives of consumer interests, since regulators may be more influenced by the sharp and concentrated interests of producers than by the broad and diverse interests of consumers.[4]

Others believe that physicians, or provider organizations controlled by physicians, should be given greater responsibility for protecting the interests of individual consumers. The conventional wisdom is that physicians should function as decision-makers and controllers of consumer demand because only they can recognize the health needs of individual patients and understand the value of alternative therapies. However, this conventional wisdom is becoming increasingly difficult to accept, as evidence mounts that physicians may be creating unnecessary demand. At least one study has strongly supported the hypothesis that geographical variations in surgical rates are largely explained by the ratio of physicians (particularly specialists) to the general population.[5] Many believe that differences in the ways physicians are taught to use technologies account for these discrepancies. Because of an expected oversupply of specialists and subspecialists, most of whom believe strongly in the value of the therapies that they are trained to provide and in their right to function as entrepreneurs, the prospect of unchecked physician control of health-care expenditures is troubling. If physicians are able to control effective demand for services and if the oversupply continues, as it is likely to for at least the next three or four decades, health-care costs will continue to spiral upward.

A number of new contractual arrangements and prepaid provider organizations, including health maintenance organizations (HMOs) and social health maintenance organizations (SHMOs), are designed to improve the efficiency and effectiveness of health care for the elderly. It is hypothesized that these organizations can reduce unnecessary utilization of hospitals and specialists and lead to a greater emphasis on health promotion and disease prevention. Although these proposals are theoretically attractive, experience with HMOs for both the aged and nonaged suggests that their ability to "skim" healthy patients exceeds the ability of regulatory mechanisms to compensate through quotas or differential reimbursement rates. It still remains to be demonstrated that regulatory strategies can ensure harmony between corporate financial objectives and public policy concerns.

Empowering Medicare Beneficiaries through a Consumer Cooperative

Given the vagaries of regulatory and marketplace strategies, older consumers may need to intervene directly and collectively to make health-care systems more accessible, effective, and affordable. Proponents of both market and regulatory strategies are likely to agree on the value of a more informed and educated group of citizens/consumers. Consumers capable of deciding intelligently among alternatives and making judgments on quality and price are essential to an effective market strategy. Better organized and informed consumers could also improve the effectiveness of regulations to control abuse and promote compliance with industry or governmental standards.

One approach for empowering older consumers of health care is a Medicare consumers' cooperative. The cooperative organization would help older persons bargain for, choose, and pay for needed medical and social care. The prototype organization would be independent and consumer financed, providing its members a variety of cooperative purchasing, consumer information, and financial services.

Group Bargaining and Cooperative Purchasing Services

Unlike adults in the labor force, most retired individuals negotiate with providers as individuals, rather than as groups. Whereas unions and employers organize and represent workers in the purchase of health insurance, usually at substantial discounts, older persons negotiate individually, with little economic leverage. This situation is particularly ironic considering that the elderly comprise the largest single health-care consumer group, as evidenced by membership in Medicare.

A Medicare consumers' cooperative could gain for individuals the group benefits of substantial discounts and/or expanded service benefits. This group-bargaining and cooperative purchasing approach may apply to every sector of the health-care economy, including hospitals, physicians, nursing homes, and home health agencies, as well as to prescription drugs, hearing aids, and eyeglasses.

Group purchasing generates significant benefits not only for group members, but also for cooperating providers, who have the opportunity to increase their service volumes and reduce their marketing costs. For example, in the industry of HMOs for the elderly, marketing costs are projected to run as high as 40% of gross revenues. Group purchasing arrangements may encourage providers to shift resources from advertising to expanded services and benefits.

The Metropolitan Senior Federation of Minneapolis/St. Paul (70,000 members) is currently the leading example of a local organization of older persons that has been able to produce substantial benefits to members through group bargaining and cooperative purchasing arrangements. Since 1971, the Metropolitan Senior Federation has negotiated significant price discounts from a variety of health-care providers, including dentists, doctors, pharmacies, hearing aid dealerships, and HMOs. These discounts are available to older persons for a modest annual membership fee ($7 in 1984). The organization has also demonstrated its ability to work with providers to make available new services and products, including the nation's first catastrophic insurance plan.[4]

Consumer Health Information Services

As the health-care industry becomes increasingly complex, many older individuals find it difficult to understand and assess the range of health-care options available to them. Information on providers, including their credentials, the services offered, fee structures, and hours of service, is usually difficult if not impossible to obtain. Consequently, the choice of providers, often made under stressful circumstances, is too often haphazard or serendipitous. Uninformed decision making often leads to inadequate choices and hardly promotes effective competition among providers. A Medicare consumers' cooperative can provide essential information to older persons on the availability and characteristics of the full spectrum of health services.

In addition to objective information, consumers might derive substantial benefit from subjective consumer ratings on many aspects of care that are legitimately in their domain. For example, ratings of physicians might indicate how well the physician explains diagnoses and treatment plans to the patient, how concerned the physician seems to be with the patient's total well-being, how much time the physician spends with the patient, how accessible the physician is to telephone queries outside of office hours, and how considerate the physician's staff and office arrangements are of the needs of older patients.

Older consumers also need better information on health promotion and disease prevention, in terms they can understand. The nature of their disabilities should be explained in ways that support sound decision making about the types of providers they should see and the kinds of medical and social services they should have. Also not generally accessible and understood are second-opinion services and major surgery and long-term care placement, both of which could help individuals feel more confident in making major decisions involving significant costs to themselves, their families, and society. All of these information services, designed to help consumers make better choices, could be provided through a consumer cooperative.

Financial Services

Consumer cooperatives can play an important role in alleviating several of the financial concerns that face older persons. One mundane but serious concern of most older consumers is the unintelligible Medicare bill. Most older individuals are unable to understand their bills, and if they detect an apparent discrepancy, they are often unable to negotiate effectively with their third-party fiscal intermediary. Financial planning services designed specifically for the elderly can also be of great value. Currently most financial planning models emphasize asset accumulation, but the actual financial planning needs of most older persons are for asset preservation or for gradual decumulation. Designing and delivering these tailored financial counseling services, perhaps through peer counselors, is another logical and needed service of a Medicare consumers' cooperative.

Another common problem among older persons is lack of access to credit markets. Millions of older individuals are house-rich but cash-poor and are unable to meet medical or social care expenses. Retired homeowners, despite their wealth, are usually unable to borrow money from banks, which look at income as the primary investment criterion. Enabling older homeowners to borrow money without having to sell their homes could provide needed help to millions, particularly those with health impairments. A recent study estimates that if home-equity conversion plans were available, two-thirds of all elderly homeowners could afford an adequate long-term care insurance policy and more than three-fifths of the "high-risk" single elderly could afford comprehensive home care for the rest of their lives.[6]

A consumer cooperative could play an instrumental role in enabling members to gain access to needed credit in a manner that would guarantee members lifetime tenancy in their homes. A variety of consumer and investor concerns remain to be overcome before home-equity conversion plans are more widely available, but none appears to be insurmountable.[7] Increasing the ability of members to pay for needed services would also enhance the ability of individuals and the collective membership to bargain and to pay for needed care.

Cooperative Work Programs

Consumer cooperatives may also prove to be excellent vehicles for promoting exchanges of labor among older persons. Many retirees have the time and the inclination to be of service, but they have a difficult time finding paid employment and are reluctant to work without any compensation. Through a cooperative, older persons may be able to provide services to others (e.g., peer counseling, chores, friendly visiting, home-delivered meals) and in return earn credits that they can redeem for similar or other services in the future. A major barrier to the development of cooperative work programs has been the lack of an ongoing source of funding for the administrative costs of such a program. In a consumers' cooperative, a portion of membership revenues could be allocated for this purpose.

Benefits to Providers and Government

A Medicare consumers' cooperative could benefit older individuals, providers, and government. For provider groups, the opportunity to offer services to and through an organization of informed and interested consumers can be a means of increasing volume and reducing marketing costs. This could lead to both improved benefits and/or reduced prices for consumers as well as significant savings for providers. A consumer cooperative with an effective marketing research arm could also help providers to design and implement services that respond directly to the needs and preferences of elderly consumers. Finally, the development of consumer credit and other financing services could enable more consumers to pay for services, thereby reducing bad debts and accounts receivable.

Consumer cooperatives could also aid government in controlling health-care costs and improving the quality of services. Group purchasing arrangements established by consumer cooperatives can lead directly to reduced costs. Information services are likely to lead to more appropriate use of available resources and technologies. Consumer credit services enhance the ability of older individuals to pay for their own care or insurance, and an active consumer organization could strengthen the enforcement of regulatory procedures. The demonstrated benefits to Medicare of consumer cooperatives may eventually be sufficiently compelling to justify expansion of current coverage to include modest membership fees.

Financial and Market Feasibility

Although the feasibility of a Medicare consumers' cooperative has not yet been demonstrated, preliminary financial and market analyses suggest its potential for success. A membership of 30,000 or more in an urban area would provide group-bargaining and consumer health-information services at an estimated cost of $25 per person per year. This fee is considerably less than 1% of the average older person's expenditures in 1986. A recently conducted marketing study indicates that 45% of the elderly in one area would be interested in paying a modest fee to join this type of organization.

In 1986, a real market test of a Medicare consumers' cooperative began in the greater Washington, D.C. area. The United Seniors Health Cooperative (USHC) is now offering many of the services described herein to local senior citizens. Membership was 10,000 as of December 1988 and USHC's leadership projects enrollments of 15,000 in 1989 and 20,000 in 1990.

Perspectives on Consumer Cooperatives

Cooperatives hold an unusual place in American political and economic thought: they appeal to conservatives and capitalists as well as liberals and socialists. As Paul Starr notes: "Although cooperatives express some of the fundamental concerns of socialism for equality and collective actions they make no direct challenge to the capitalists' order."[8]

Despite their broad philosophical appeal, the development of cooperatives in the U.S. health-care marketplace has been limited. The leading examples of medical cooperatives in the United States have been consumer-owned provider organizations (the Ross-Loos Clinic, was founded in 1921 in Elk City, Oklahoma, and The Group Health Association in Washington, D.C., started by federal employees in 1937), which were formed to provide services not otherwise available to their members. In virtually all cases, these cooperatives provide primary and acute medical services on a prepaid basis. In 1980, there were only 20 known health-care cooperatives in the United States. They had an estimated membership of 740,000 and an annual volume of about $750 million.[9]

One reason for the scarcity of consumer cooperatives has been organized opposition by local medical societies afraid of competing provider groups. Another barrier has been the substantial amount of capital necessary to establish a prepaid provider organization and the difficulties of raising such sums from individuals.[10] Because it would not be a direct provider of health services, the prototypical organization proposed here would require only a fraction of the capital needed to purchase or build hospital and clinic facilities.

Consumer cooperatives are somewhat more abundant in the financial services industry, where they have not been hindered by the same kinds of organized opposition and onerous capital requirements. More than 21 million Americans belonged to credit unions in 1981, although their total assets represent only 2% of the assets of all thrift institutions.[11] The impetus for the formation of credit unions (i.e., the need for members to gain better access to credit markets) is the same problem faced today by millions of retired homeowners.

Congress has recognized the broad-based political appeal of consumer cooperatives and the difficulty these organizations face in gaining access to capital markets. The National Consumer Cooperative Bank was formed under federal charter in 1978, and authorized:

> to provide for consumers a further means of minimizing the impact of inflation and economic depression by narrowing the price spread between costs to the producer and the consumer of needed good services, facilities, and commodities through the development and funding of specialized credit sources for, and technical assistance to self-help, not-for-profit cooperatives and for other purposes.[10]

The Bank, dedicated to promoting the development of cooperatives, particularly those that serve low-income or elderly persons, may be an important source of financing for such organizations in the United States.

International Models

Health-care consumer cooperatives have fared well in the mixed economies of other nations. In Sweden, for example, a consumer cooperative was formed in 1905 to provide fire insurance for members. The resulting organization, Folksam, started to grow rapidly after World War II and soon developed into one of the largest Swedish insurance companies. By 1977, Folksam was responsible for 21% of the nation's personal sickness and accident policies and 41% of all group sickness and accident policies. Overall, almost half of all Swedes are members of at least one consumer cooperative.[12] To a lesser extent, consumer cooperatives are also active in Israel, Denmark, and Norway. The economies of these countries are dominated by privately owned businesses, with a relatively high degree of government intervention but a relatively low degree of government ownership. As the American economy, and particularly the health-care marketplace for the elderly, begins to resemble the mixed economies of other nations, the need to adopt consumer approaches that thrive elsewhere becomes more apparent.

Conclusions

Is consumerism dead, or is there a place for consumer initiatives in health care and other marketplaces of the future? Paul Bloom and Steven Greyser studied consumerism as a "product" subject to a standard "product life cycle." They concluded that, far from being dead, consumerism may be entering an important new stage:

> We foresee a quieter but still active consumer movement during the 1980's. We think the public will shift from its past role as largely cheering spectators to one of active participants. We envision participative consumerism as a major characteristic of this marketplace.[13]

Older persons, individually and collectively, must choose the role they will play in shaping the health-care marketplace of the future. From a traditional perspective, their choices are to continue to rely almost exclusively on political strategies aimed at reforming Medicare and/or Medicaid, in the hope of making coverage more comprehensive and reducing out-of-pocket expenses, or to rely on providers and an increasingly competitive environment to protect their interests. The strategy proposed here—participatory consumerism—stands in contrast to these traditional choices and deserves greater attention. The concept of a Medicare consumers' cooperative, designed to help the elderly and disabled bargain for, choose, and pay for health care, appears to be feasible, has promise of being cost-effective, and can complement both regulatory and competitive strategies for health-care reform.

During the past 20 years, older Americans have begun to exercise increased political power. Ideally, during the next 20 years, older citizens/consumers will begin to flex their economic muscles and become a more effective "third force" in the health-care marketplace.

References

1. Vladeck, B. 1981. The market vs. regulation: The case for regulation. *Milbank Memorial Fund Q* 59(2):88–106.
2. McClure, W. 1981. Structure and incentive problems in economic regulation of medical care. *Milbank Memorial Fund Q* 59(2):107–144.
3. Wolf, C., Jr. 1979. A theory of non-market failures. *Public Interest* 4(3):114–133.
4. Metropolitan Senior Federation. 1983. *A Decade of Action: The Metropolitan Senior Federation.* St. Paul, Minn.: Metropolitan Senior Federation.
5. Wennberg, J., Barnes, B., Zubkoff, M. 1982. Professional uncertainty and the

problem of supplier-induced demand. *Soc Sci Med* 9(3):811–824.
6. Jacobs, B., Weissert, W. 1984. Home equity financing of long-term care for the elderly. In *Long-Term Care Financing and Delivery Systems: Exploring Some Alternatives*. Conference Proceedings, January 24. Washington, D.C.: Government Printing Office.
7. Firman, J. 1983. Reforming community care for the elderly and disabled. *Health Aff* (2):67–82.
8. Starr, P. 1983. *The Social Transformation of American Medicine*. New York: Basic Books.
9. Cooperative League of the U.S.A. 1980. *Facts about Cooperatives*. Washington, D.C.: Cooperative League of the U.S.A.
10. National Consumer Cooperative Bank Act, PL 95-351 12 U.S.C. 3001 et seq.
11. United States League of Savings Associations. 1980. *Savings and Loan Factbook, 1980*. Chicago Ill.: League of Savings Associations.
12. Swedish Information Service. 1983. The cooperative movement in Sweden. In *Fact Sheets on Sweden*. Stockholm: Swedish Information Service.
13. Bloom, P., Greyser, S. 1981. The maturing of consumerism. *Harvard Business Rev* (November–December), 130–139.

Part Four

Special Problems of Geriatric Health Care

Planners seeking broad strokes with which to revise health policy for the elderly usually review financing techniques, legislative reform, and sources of care. Ironically, the particular health problems of an aging population, the strides made in improving its medical care, and the challenges that practitioners and researchers still face are often neglected. This section, which is unified by its clinical orientation, redresses these oversights by focusing on specific elements of geriatric illness and medical treatment.

Two related articles carry a plea for a medical specialty devoted exclusively to geriatrics. The elderly commonly suffer from multiple conditions, take multiple medications that increase the risk of adverse interactions, and suffer the damaging stresses of fear and loss. Furthermore, while the young generally expect to recover fully from illness, the elderly often can hope only to minimize their discomfort or to learn to cope with chronic pain. The result, argue both James Williamson and Lambert N. King, is that older people are best served by health professionals trained to understand their distinct set of needs.

James Williamson draws upon the British experience, where general practitioners commonly provide primary care to the elderly and refer their patients to geriatric specialists for secondary care needs. The author identifies three systems of geriatric care: the selective referral model, in which an expert geriatric assessment team steers a patient to an appropriate general

289

practitioner, internist, orthopedist, psychiatrist, etc.; the age-related model, in which all hospital patients over a certain age receive care from a geriatric unit; and the integrated model, in which geriatric experts work within a hospital's internal medicine department.

In the United States the proposal to develop geriatric medicine as a practice specialty is of very recent vintage and remains highly controversial. Lambert N. King argues persuasively that geriatric medicine is a discipline broad and distinct enough to include academic research, teaching, and clinical subspecialty practice. Board-certified geriatricians need not compete with internists, to play a useful role coordinating care in both acute and long-term settings, asserts King.

Helen L. Smits, Lisa F. Berkman, and Mary C. Kapp select two common surgical procedures—intraocular lens implant and prosthetic hip replacement—and two clinical problems—hypertension and diabetes—to illustrate the strengths and weaknesses of current medical practices. Judiciously applied treatment can enhance life or extend it, affirm the authors; less certain is how satisfied patients are with the care they receive and how they respond to medical admonishments to change their behavior.

The skeleton of alcoholism rattles in many closets, but until recently problem drinking among the elderly has been overlooked or ignored. Philip W. Brickner and Linda K. Scharer reveal how the physiological, emotional, and social characteristics that distinguish older drinkers from younger ones also cloud the diagnostic picture. They identify clues to alcoholism in the over-65 population, describe the hazards of the disease that are peculiar to the elderly, look at model treatment programs, and propose techniques for financing rehabilitation.

Like alcoholism, mental health care for the elderly has often been a stepchild neglected by pressures to treat more obvious illness and disability. But as evidence mounts that psychological and physical well-being are inextricably linked, a sensitivity to mental disorders has simply become part of the practice of responsible medicine. Within that context, Donna Cohen and Margaret M. Hastings take a comprehensive look at past, present, and future mental health policies for the elderly, describing the need, analyzing social attitudes, and calling for a better-coordinated, more cohesive system of care.

An ounce of prevention is worth a pound of cure, goes the adage, which is nowhere more true than in combatting illness among the elderly. William R. Hazzard analyzes the health system's bias toward diagnostics and treatment of disease at the expense of primary prevention and recommends a shift in emphasis. The weight of his proposals could alter patterns of physician education, clinical practice, cost containment, and hospital use.

Sixteen

The Need for a Geriatrics Specialty: Lessons from the United Kingdom

James Williamson

Many people assume that differences in health care between the United States and the United Kingdom are due to the latter's National Health Service, often described by Americans as socialized medicine. However, the differences are more profound and stem from contrasting ideas about the actual role of medical care in society that date back several centuries. In the United Kingdom, physicians derived prestige and status from established institutions, such as Royal Colleges and Corporations. In the United States, on the other hand, the medical profession had no such establishments and hence physicians adopted a much more entrepreneurial approach within a free and highly competitive market. When scientific and technological advances became available, American doctors seized them and offered them to patients. This practice has led to a very rapid and indeed extreme specialization within American medicine.[1]

One important result in the United States has been the decline in the standing of general practice, which has seriously affected health care for the elderly. While a similar trend occurred in the United Kingdom in the 1950s, very deliberate efforts were made to resuscitate general practice in the 1960s; now it is a popular calling that attracts many of the best medical graduates. The persistence of a "personal doctor" for each citizen, unimpeded by financial barriers, has indirectly contributed to the development of a comprehensive system of care for the elderly. In this system, primary care of the elderly is provided by general practitioners, who make referrals to secondary tiers of care as they judge is appropriate. The resurgence of interest in family medicine in the United States, although it started later than in the United Kingdom, also surely offers a good prospect for fruitful collaboration with any developing geriatric teams.

Demographic and Health-Care Data

In 1980 the aging of the U.K. population was at about the same stage as that projected for the United States at the end of this century (see Table 16.1). Projections into the next century indicate that the oldest groups will undergo the greatest increases; females age 85 and over will increase from about 450,000 in 1981 to almost 900,000 in 2021. Many old people live alone, especially aged females. Almost half the over-75 female population live in single-person households, and this proportion is steadily increasing.

Middle-aged married women have been shown to play key roles in support of the elderly in industrial societies, but in many countries these women are now much more likely to have paid employment outside the home. In the United Kingdom the percentage of employed married women age 55–59 rose from 26.4% in 1961 to 51.9% in 1981; for those age 45–54, the figures were 31.1% in 1961 and 66.8% in 1981.[2] The percentage of employed married women age 45–54 in the United Kingdom in 1981 was higher than the 62% reported by Brody for the United States.[3] Thus, the available "middle-aged woman time" per aged person in the United Kingdom has declined sharply, both relatively and absolutely.

Unfortunately, accurate and up-to-date statistics on the living arrangements of elderly persons of different ages are not available for the United Kingdom. However, Table 16.2 shows where persons of pensionable age were in 1981.

About 96.7% of pensionable persons live in private houses, and for all persons aged 65 and over, the figure is about 95%, which is very similar to that for the United States. Only a very small proportion (1.2%) are in hospitals, and only a few more (1.9%) are in residential homes. It is important to stress that hospital care in the United Kingdom is entirely free. It is not possible to estimate the extent to which free hospital care in the United States would result in increased demand.

Some information is available on relative costs of health care in the two countries. In 1982, the expenditure on health care was 5.3% of the GNP in the United Kingdom and 9.9% in the United States. The cost of health care per person was $4831 in the United Kingdom and $8291 in the United States.[4] Since there is no evidence that health care is any more effective in the United States than in the United Kingdom, as judged by the usual criteria of mortality and morbidity rates, it seems that the British taxpayer

Table 16.1.   Percentages of Elderly, by Age Group, in the
Population of Great Britain, 1981

Age Group	Male	Female	Total
65+	12.2%	17.8%	15.1%
75+	3.9%	7.6%	5.8%
85+	0.5%	1.6%	1.1%

Source: Extracted from 1981 Census, Office of Population Censuses
and Surveys, HMSO, London.

Table 16.2.   Living Situations of Persons of Pensionable Age in Great Britain, 1981

Living Arrangement	Males (65+)	Females (60+)	Total
Private House	97.5%	96.3%	96.7%
Hotel/Boarding House	0.15%	0.06%	0.1%
Hospital/Homes (psychiatric)	0.5%	0.06%	0.6%
Hospital/Homes (other)	0.5%	0.7%	0.6%
Homes for Old and Disabled	1.4%	2.2%	1.9%
Other	0.2%	0.14%	0.2%

Source: Extracted from 1981 Census. Office of Population Censuses and Surveys, HMSO,
London.

receives a bargain from the National Health Service. Those of us who work
in the geriatric service like to think that we have contributed significantly
to this value for money.

In all developed countries, the elderly are heavy and increasing consumers of health and social services. In the United Kingdom in 1981–
1982, the per capita health cost for the 75 and over group was £750,
compared to £320 for the 65–74 group and only £80 for the 16–64 group.
Rates for annual consultation with general practitioners increase with age,
the 75 and over group averaging about six consultations, compared to four
for the 45–64 age group.[4]

The elderly are also high users of hospital and institutional services.
Table 16.3 shows the very high usage of bed-days by the 65 and over group.
Especially striking is the fact that half of the female bed-days used were
taken by the 75 and over group, although this group comprised only 7.6%
of the total female population (see Table 16.1).

Contrasting Health Services for the Elderly in the United Kingdom and the United States

The National Health Service (NHS), financed by general taxation, provides the most notable contrast between the health-care systems of the
United Kingdom and the United States. The NHS provides mostly free

Table 16.3. Usage of Hospital Bed-Days (Excluding Psychiatric Beds),
Expressed as Percentage of Age and Sex Groups (Scotland, 1981)

	Age Group		
Sex	65–74	65+	75+
Male	24.6%	52.1%	27.5%
Female	20.0%	70.1%	50.0%
Total	21.7%	63.3%	41.6%

Source: Extracted from Scottish Hospital Inpatient Statistics 1981, Information Services Division, Scottish Health Service, Common Services
Agency.

health care for all citizens at the time of contact. The NHS is by no means
perfect, and it is often derided by outsiders, but there is no doubt that it has
greatly helped the development of a comprehensive system of geriatric
care. It is also, along with the monarchy, one of the most popular institutions in Britain, according to numerous opinion polls. In 1986 and 1987
the public reaffirmed its high opinion of the NHS in the form of an outcry
against alleged cuts in funding by the Tory government. It is notable that
this reaction came from all political quarters.

A most important difference between the United Kingdom and the
United States is the United Kingdom's strong and thriving system of primary medical care based upon general practitioners (GPs). Virtually all
citizens are registered with GPs, who are then responsible for each individual's health needs. The GPs may deal with these needs themselves or
they may work as part of a primary care team with representatives from a
range of agencies, such as community nursing services (also free under the
NHS) and social services, which includes a very well-organized homemaker service. Certain social services are also provided by the social work
departments of local authorities, so there is sometimes an administrative
barrier between health and social services, which can appropriately be
overcome with the skilled intervention of a geriatrician. It should be
emphasized that a person may register with any GP and may elect to
transfer from one to another. All specialists, including geriatricians, are
secondary services, that is, almost all patients are referred to them by GPs.
This contrasts with American practice, in which patients may refer themselves to specialists; both systems have certain advantages and disadvantages.

A most important difference is the method of remuneration of doctors in
the United Kingdom. General practitioners are paid an annual capitation
fee (which is higher for patients aged 65 and over) plus a series of induce-
ment payments to encourage good standards of care and practice. A limited
list of services are paid for by item of service (for example, house calls by

GPs done "out of hours"). Hospital specialists are paid by salary, the level being set annually by an independent review body that tries to keep doctors' earnings in line with those in comparable professions. Hospital specialists receive very limited income from item-of-service payment, although their house calls are remunerated at a fairly generous level. Some geriatricians may have their basic salary increased by as much as 25% through house-call remuneration. For many years British physicians were relatively poorly paid by international standards, but most doctors no longer think this is the case.

Patterns of remuneration of doctors are vitally important in health care, but it is almost impossible to devise a comprehensive geriatrics service based upon item-of-service payment. Much important work with the elderly and their families cannot be evaluated in terms of time and cost in a reasonably rational fashion. For example, often the geriatrician's most important contribution is a conversation with the elderly patient's worried daughter that explains the patient's condition and indicates sources of support in the coming months or years. How would this service be priced by the auditors of Medicare/Medicaid?

Another important difference between the United Kingdom and the United States is the existence of geriatric medicine as a fully accepted practice specialty in Britain. Every Health District now has a Geriatric Medicine Department staffed by consultants who have elected to pursue a career in care of the elderly. They are supported by junior medical staff, who either are training for a career in geriatric medicine or are rotating through it as part of their training for another specialty. By contrast, the need to accredit geriatrics as a practice specialty is hotly contested in the United States, as King discusses in Chapter 17.

Finally, it may be postulated that the NHS, with all its shortcomings, does offer the chance to plan and deliver health care in response to the true needs of individuals and communities. This is much more difficult to achieve within the American system, based as it is largely upon response to market forces.

Historical Development of Geriatric Medicine in the United Kingdom

Contrary to widely held belief, geriatric medicine existed in the United Kingdom as a separate entity prior to the inception of the NHS.

The first steps were taken by Dr. Marjory Warren in the late thirties. Working as a physician in a London teaching hospital, she made several fundamental observations that are still valid. She noticed that elderly patients in the "chronic wards" of her hospital had often not received full diagnostic investigation but had instead been admitted directly to what was, in effect, a medical backwater. She found that some responded to treatment, with resultant improvement and the possibility for return home. She showed that elderly patients with irrecoverable conditions (such as stroke or arthropathy) could often be successfully rehabilitated and returned to the community. She showed that many elderly patients fared badly in an acute medical ward, where staff were often less than fully interested in their special needs and where they were in competition with other groups of patients with more acute and more "interesting" and "re-warding" conditions. She emphasized the need for health workers to be much more knowledgeable about medical care of the elderly. She stated, "The medical profession, having succeeded in prolonging the life of men and women, must no longer fail in its responsibility to the elderly when they fall sick or become infirm."[5]

She then acted upon these observations by taking two practical steps: 1) She required that no elderly patient be admitted to any chronic-care facility without first receiving full geriatric assessment and attempts at treatment and rehabilitation, and 2) she established a special assessment ward into which elderly patients were admitted in order to have their needs accurately and fully identified.

This was the dawn of geriatric medicine in Britain. It is interesting that at about this time Warren wrote, "It is noteworthy that geriatrics has received more attention in America than in this country and much of the literature on the subject has emanated from American writers."[6] What happened to the "more attention" shown by Americans, and why did their interest seem to wane? A major factor must have been the burgeoning of medical technology, which has proved to be such a dominant influence in medical education and practice in the United States. The fact that British medicine never became so obsessed with technology is partly due to the historical differences in professional attitudes already discussed, but an-other factor must be the advent of the National Health Service. The NHS had one indisputable effect: providers of health care could not possibly fail to be aware of pressures and needs within the community, since everyone, including the old, the poor, and other "unattractive" patient groups, was equally entitled to medical care under the NHS.

The infant specialty of geriatric medicine was alive and thriving by the mid-forties, but it faced many hazards and hindrances, including apathy and hostility from within the medical profession. Other pioneers joined Warren's band, and assessment units were set up in several centers. At first these units were largely hospital oriented, but movement into the commu-nity soon started. This was encouraged by the practice of preadmission home visiting, which in these early days was mainly done for the purpose of assessing priority and determining which patient on the waiting list would qualify for the next vacancy.[7] Some observers then noticed that home visiting by geriatricians often brought significant extra benefits, and in many cases the patients did not require hospitalization at all but could be appropriately dealt with in some other way.[8] An inevitable result of the practice of home visiting was a demand for better community and domiciliary support, mostly nursing and homemaker services.

The next development came with the realization that many patients were coming to the attention of geriatric services at a very late stage in their condition, when it was often impossible to achieve significant improvement. Surveys showed a large amount of unreported disability among the elderly at home.[9] This finding heralded the era of preventive geriatrics, in which GPs, community nurses, and members of the public with elderly relatives were encouraged to think in terms of earlier detection, for example, by case finding.[10,11]

During the fifties to the mid-seventies, geriatrics grew much faster than any other specialty in the United Kingdom. It eventually awakened academic interest, and medical schools began to establish chairs and departments of geriatric medicine, but it remained difficult to attract British graduates, nurses, and therapists to the programs, and many senior medical posts went to overseas graduates. It is not difficult to understand this situation: most students had had no exposure to geriatric medicine and had generally regarded older patients as uninteresting, often referring to them as "bed blockers." Gale and Livesley[12] showed that while preclinical medical students possessed a reasonably open mind toward geriatrics, senior students and interns often had highly negative attitudes. The main reason for recruitment problems, however, was the remarkable expansion in the specialty. Between 1967 and 1976, consultant posts in geriatric medicine increased by 111%; the next greatest increase was in anesthesiology, where the expansion was a mere 41%, and yet there were also recruitment problems in this specialty.

In recent years the picture has altered completely, and now formal geriatric medicine courses are offered in all but one British medical school.[13] Thus student doctors have usually received some introduction to modern care of the elderly, and many have done clinical clerkships in geriatric units. This education, combined with reduced career prospects in traditional specialties, has resulted in considerable numbers of British graduates deciding to specialize in geriatric medicine. Even more now seek geriatric internships and residency training as a means of equipping them for a career in some other broadly based specialty, since they appreciate that they will inevitably be increasingly involved with aged patients.

The Present and Future of Geriatric Medicine

The recent history of geriatric care in the United Kingdom may well represent the immediate future of geriatric care in the United States. Ideally,

America will benefit from British experience by adopting the measures that have proven successful and by avoiding its mistakes.

It is a common American error to imagine that the British socialized health system has only a single model of geriatric care. In fact, our varied approaches have resulted in responses that range from custodial institutional care to acute-care units that purport to cope with every medical emergency in old age.

Dr. William Barker, of the University of Rochester, found that British medicine has three main models of geriatric care: a system of selective referrals, an age-related pattern (as in pediatrics), and care that is fully integrated with internal medicine.[14,15] The relative merits and effectiveness of each model are hotly debated. It is worth considering each in detail before deciding what elements, if any, are transplantable to the United States and other countries.

Selective Referral

Selective referral is, in most respects, directly related to the original model of the pioneers of geriatrics. The current emphasis is upon close collaboration with other specialties, so that the skill, expertise, and methods of the geriatric team may be used to the maximum advantage of all patients. The principal specialties, general practice, internal medicine, orthopedic surgery, and psychiatry, are all increasingly involved in medical care of older patients. Early referral is sought in order to reverse or to arrest disability and to ensure that caregivers receive support at a stage when they can most effectively assist a patient. Located in a general hospital, the geriatric unit has access to full diagnostic and therapeutic resources, with emphasis upon rehabilitation. In my own department, this model has coped with the demands of a total defined population of about 20,000 old persons (65 and over) without delays or waiting lists for admission; referred patients are seen within 24 hours. About one-third of patients require admission to our wards, and in over 90% of cases they are admitted in less than 24 hours. We pay regular visits to internal medicine wards and to the acute orthopedic unit, where all geriatric patients are seen automatically, without referral for consultation. Our contribution within the acute medical wards succeeded in reducing the mean length of stay of elderly patients and increased the proportion who went home. Among the most aged group (85 and over), the mean stay of females in acute medical wards was reduced from 49 to 22 days.[16]

We are often asked whether we are not, in effect, usurping the function of GPs. We do not believe so, and we have always seen our service as complementing that of the GPs. This impression has been confirmed by a survey of GPs that used an anonymous questionnaire. The results of this investigation showed that 98% of GPs shared our view of geriatric practice.[17]

A continuing challenge, of course, is to ensure that GPs (and others who refer patients) are well enough informed to make suitable selection for referral. Twenty-five years ago, many patients were referred at a late stage,[9] but now late referral is the exception and usually happens if the patient is difficult and resists assistance, or if the referring GP has failed to appreciate the benefits of the referral model.

Age-Related Model

The age-related model requires that the geriatric unit accept responsibility for all patients over a certain age, generally 75, who need hospital care (and therefore once again the service requires the full resources of a general hospital). One advantage claimed for this service is that it ensures that all patients who need geriatric expertise will receive it from the time of admission to hospital. It is also claimed that the full range of acute work offered enhances the job satisfaction of geriatricians and their junior colleagues. The converse implicit in this claim is less vehemently stated: the rest of the work with the elderly may be dull and unrewarding. Objections to this model are varied:

- It concentrates too much upon hospital care. Since 98% of the elderly are not in the hospital, it gives a lopsided view of health care of the elderly.

- If adopted on a wide scale, it would require a massive transfer of resources from the acute sector, which has been increasingly involved with the elderly. There is a danger of developing two standards, one for the young and middle-aged and another for the old. No one need doubt which would be the more privileged service.

- It could lead to duplication of expensive equipment.

- It means that internists would be denied the chance to work with the aged, a situation that would not be in anyone's long-term interest. It would also perpetuate the professional isolation of the geriatrician.

- It diverts attention from the other equally important aspects of modern geriatrics, such as prevention and community support for caregivers.

- Most importantly, it aims to please physicians rather than best meeting patients' needs.

This model has attracted much greater interest in England than in Scotland. Furthermore, the claim that it attracts more graduates to geriatrics is belied by the fact that, in 1978, the proportion of consultant posts in geriatric medicine held by British graduates was only 57% in England and Wales, while in Scotland it was no less than 95%.[18,19]

The Integrated Model

In the integrated model the geriatric service is fully integrated into the general hospital's internal medicine department, which is staffed by internists with subspecialty interests, such as gastroenterology, respiratory medicine, and cardiology. The geriatrician thus becomes an internist with a special interest in geriatrics and is involved in the acute care of all adult age groups but assumes special responsibility for the elderly and those requiring rehabilitation and long-term care.[20] One objection to this model is, again, an overconcentration upon hospital care. This model also tends to presuppose that the clinical medicine of old age equates with geriatric medicine, although geriatric medicine is actually concerned with the much wider considerations of community care, prevention, and long-term care. Geriatric medicine also demands considerable management skills and leadership to use scarce resources effectively and to ensure good teamwork. Many doubt whether it is feasible for a single physician to be fully competent in the whole field of adult internal medicine and also have a sufficient knowledge of geriatric medicine.

Variants of these models exist throughout the United Kingdom. Frequently the particular model developed in an area evolved because of local circumstances, and it might not be acceptable or appropriate elsewhere. Still, debate continues about the merits of each model—and this debate can only benefit us all.

Principles and Practice of Geriatric Care

The Nature of Need in Old Age

Many of the problems in coping with the medical care of an aging population stem from an inaccurate and incomplete understanding of need in old age. In traditional medicine, need is established by the process of medical diagnosis, that is, the localization of a lesion and the identification of its pathological nature, but medicine has only belatedly come to accept that in old age multiple pathology is commonplace, and often this has meant involvement of several subspecialists, each intent upon scrutiny of a particular organ or system or upon performance of a special procedure.

For younger persons and the younger old, the traditional model of health care may be successful; indeed, it may yield dramatic benefits to individual patients. However, for the old-old, the traditional model is increasingly unsatisfactory, because at this stage in the life span, the changes that come with age become increasingly important. For example, from early adulthood on, about 1%–1.5% of renal function is lost per year.[21] By age 85, individuals may have lost 60%–80% of kidney function from age changes alone. A male patient who has had significant prostatism or a female with recurrent urinary tract infection may experience even greater loss, so that by age 85 renal reserves may be close to zero. Similar age- and disease-related decreases may occur in cardiac, pulmonary, skeletal, and liver function, so that the aged individual leads an existence of extreme precariousness. Any stress may provoke organ or system failure, which can in turn initiate multiple failure, characterized by an increasing difficulty in maintaining homeostasis. Therefore, since the old-old are the most rapidly growing group in the population, medical care must take into account age-change features.

Not only do age changes become increasingly important, but so do the effects of environmental stress. Some effects are easy to comprehend, such as hypothermia brought about by the stress of low ambient temperature. Frequently, however, the stress may be much more subtle and difficult to detect, let alone to quantify. For example, the psychological and emotional stresses that are common in old age can arise from widowhood and loneliness, loss of role satisfaction, inadequate income, and, perhaps most important, the stress of trying to cope with disabling illness. In recent decades an increasingly common stress for urban elderly has been relocation to new and often impersonal housing developments. For someone who has spent a lifetime in the close-knit community of a downtown area, relocation may be a severe strain.

While stress of this sort may manifest itself with overt signs of anxiety, it is also commonly translated into somatic symptoms, which may lead the unwary physician to initiate extensive or hazardous investigations or to prescribe medication. The patient is thus exposed to the hazards of treatments while the underlying stress remains undetected. At best this represents a "papering over," and at worst the patient may suffer an adverse drug reaction without any prospect of benefit. Frequently, adverse reaction to drugs or treatment leads to further investigation and the prescribing of yet another drug. Thus a vicious circle may be set up in which the patient becomes more and more afflicted and dependent.

The precariousness and vulnerability of aged persons thus must be understood as resulting from a combination of age changes, disease changes, and the stress of environmental factors. For some patients, traditional approaches offer cure, rehabilitation, and return to previous levels of function. A substantial proportion, however, survives, but in a much more dependent state. Aged patients, with their complex needs, often do not fit into the traditional models of acute and chronic health care. The particular kind of care they need has given rise to the specialty of geriatric medicine.

Family Support for the Elderly

All studies confirm the immense importance of satisfactory family support to the welfare of the elderly. The myth that modern families do not care about their elderly has been debunked. The elderly are in frequent contact with their offspring, and in the United Kingdom about two-thirds of elderly persons have seen a younger relative "today or yesterday" and close to 90% "within a week." Even in the highly mobile American society, these contact figures are only slightly lower. [22]

Therefore, patient assessment must include the strengths and weaknesses of family aid, and the family must receive suitable support so that they may continue to help the elderly for as long as possible.

Finally, functional assessment, including determination of mental function, mobility, continence, ability in activities of daily living, and the retention of social skills, extends the requirements of geriatric assessment far beyond the limits of traditional medical diagnosis.

Practical Requirements for Geriatric Assessment and Service Delivery

Assessment

A detailed and comprehensive assessment of an elderly person, which involves medical diagnosis, functional assessment, and identification of sources of stress in the patient and caregivers, necessitates a multidisciplinary team approach. Assessment cannot be achieved by professionals working in isolation, nor can it be achieved by professionals sending reports, however detailed, to a committee or panel that then makes the assessment, a method favored in some parts of North America.

Furthermore, because of the precariousness of function in old age and the importance of keeping family stress within tolerable limits, this age group is always urgent.

Using a house call to make an initial assessment has several important advantages:

- It enables the service to respond at once. Two-thirds of patients referred to our service are seen within three hours, and 90% are seen on the day of referral.

- It is the aged person's ability to function in the home environment that is crucial. Functions observed in an outpatient department, a hospital ward, or, worst of all, in an emergency room may give a very misleading impression.

- An adequate clinical assessment can be made in almost all home visits. Blood and urine can be collected for analysis and an ECG may readily be performed.

- Much nonclinical and paraclinical information is obtained in the home, including detection of hazards in the home, stress or exhaustion in caregivers, and medication in the house not mentioned by the referring physician. [17]

Full geriatric assessment will be completed when the nurse, the physiotherapist, the occupational therapist, and the social worker have obtained a complete picture of medical, psychological, social, and family need.

Resources

The next requirement is ready access to a wide range of resources in balanced supply so that the appropriate service may be selected to meet each identified need. This essential requirement is termed the *continuum of care.* (Few countries provide this balanced continuum. In the United States, inadequate community resources and overprovision of institutions have inevitably led to unnecessary institutional care.)

The resources ranged along the continuum include good primary medical care (GP and community nurses), recreational opportunities, adequate income, adequate housing (including radio alarm systems for the specially vulnerable who live alone), day care (ranging from lunch and social clubs to highly staffed day hospitals), residential homes, geriatric assessment wards, acute-care facilities, and inpatient care for those who need long-term nursing and medical care. An overarching, important requirement is good coordination of all these resources and a swift, flexible response to the often rapidly changing needs of the elderly and their caregivers. For example, an increasingly valuable service that the United Kingdom provides is planned respite care, which may simply allow the family to take a vacation or offer them a guaranteed break at regular intervals.

How Does the British Experience Relate to the United States?

How can the British experience be useful in improving the care of the elderly in the United States? What elements of the British system could and should be transplanted to the United States, and what are the problems involved?

A few items are of special importance:

- A modern society cannot meet the very complex needs of its elderly without enthusiastic and dedicated teams of workers who have elected to specialize in the health care of the elderly. The so-called Beeson Report[23] did not recommend the establishment of a formal practice specialty in geriatrics, and this is readily understandable in the prevailing climate of opinion against further medical subspecialization. However, geriatric medicine is not just another subspecialty. It is a different way of practicing medicine, combining new knowledge, ideas, attitudes, and concepts with a rediscovery of some older and previously valued forms of practice, such as the house call.

- The importance of the team approach must be recognized, especially by physicians, who must acknowledge that clinical diagnosis is only part of the geriatric assessment and that the nurse's, therapist's, and social worker's contributions are generally just as important as the physician's.

- The whole range of services must be available at the time of need, and services must be provided in a balanced fashion with efficient coordination and close collaboration between the providers of each individual service. Good relations must exist between service providers at every level, from those in contact with patients and families to administrators and managers, and, where relevant, even to politicians at the local and national levels. Health and social services must work closely and harmoniously, which requires some changes in standard practices.

   It is just as important to ensure that an elderly patient being discharged from the hospital will receive adequate homemaker support at home as it is to see that the proper drugs are prescribed to control the patient's congestive cardiac failure. Since these basic services are as fundamentally important as purely medical services, they must be available to all patients who need them. No patient should be denied any services because of inability to pay. The result of denial will certainly be a longer hospital stay or inappropriate, unnecessary, and expensive institutional care. The present limitations of Medicare and Medicaid funding for domiciliary services (see Harrington, Chapter 2, for further details) are totally illogical.

- Services aimed at helping families to continue their support should be provided as part of the continuum of care. Although this may be contrary to the American ethic of self-sufficiency, experience suggests that if families are offered prompt and continuing support, they will generally continue to care for their elders within their capability and bounds of tolerance. Once caregivers have been stretched beyond their limits, however, the breakdown of support is too often permanent and irreversible.[24]

- In many respects the most frustrating area is the remuneration of doctors. Calculating remuneration on the basis of items of service is impossible for many fundamental components of geriatrics. A salaried service may be required, and while this may be contrary to the entrepreneurial instincts of the American medical profession, it is by no means impossible.

- Americans must look critically at each of the current British models of geriatric service and decide which could most appropriately be adapted to their needs. Selected referral, with its very strong emphasis upon close collaboration with general practice, internal medicine, orthopedic surgery, and emergency room service, is, in my opinion, the most favored model for modern geriatric medicine and could most readily be transplanted, wholly or partially, into North America.

Summary

The experience of the growth of geriatric medicine in the United Kingdom provides an interesting episode in recent medical history. Its successes and failures are worth detailed study by those in other countries who are seeking to adapt to the needs of their aging populations. It is easy to find defects and failures in British geriatric medicine, but, as pointed out by Campion,[25] "It is not that British geriatrics has won all the battles in long-term care, but at least someone has been showing up for the fight."

The great energy and inventiveness of American medicine, freed of the shackles of inappropriate models of health care, will undoubtedly rise to the challenges of geriatric care. Time is short, however, and the need for fundamental changes in some professional attitudes is extremely urgent.

References

1. Stevens, R. 1976. The evolution of the health care systems in the United States and the United Kingdom: Similarities and differences. HEW Pub. No. (NIH) 77-1288. Washington, D.C.: Government Printing Office.
2. Central Statistical Office. 1984. *Social Trends*. London: Her Majesty's Stationery Office.
3. Brody, E. M., Campbell, R., Johnson, P. T. 1983. Women's changing roles and help to the elderly: Attitudes of women in the U.S. and Japan. Paper presented at the 37th Annual Meeting of the Gerontological Society of America, San Francisco, Calif., November 1983.
4. Office of Health Economics. 1984. *Compendium of Health Statistics*, 5th ed. London: Office of Health Economics.
5. Warren, M. W. 1946. Care of the chronic aged sick. *Lancet* 1:841–842.
6. Warren, M. W. 1943. Care of the chronic sick. A case for treating chronic sick in blocks in a general hospital. *Br Med J* 2:822–823.
7. Brooke, E. B. 1948. The place of the outpatient department in caring for old people. *Med Press* 219:400–402.
8. Amulree, Lord, Exton-Smith, A. N., Crocket, G. S. 1951. Proper use of the hospital in treatment of the aged sick. *Lancet* 1:123–126.
9. Williamson, J., Stokoe, I. H., Gray, S., Fisher, M., Smith, A., McGhee, A., Stephenson, E. 1964. Old people at home: Their unreported needs. *Lancet* 1:1117–1120.

10. Lowther, C. P., McLeod, R. D. M., Williamson, J. 1970. An evaluation of early diagnostic services. *Br Med J* 3:275–277.
11. Anderson, W. F., Cowan, N. 1955. A consultative centre for older people. *Lancet* 2:239.
12. Gale, J., Livesley, B. 1974. Attitudes towards geriatrics: A report of the King's survey. *Age Ageing* 3:49–53.
13. Smith, R. G., Williams, B. O. 1983. A survey of undergraduate teaching of geriatric medicine in British medical schools. *Age Ageing* 12(Suppl.):2–6.
14. Barker, W. H. 1983. Hospital based geriatric services in Great Britain: Implications for the U.S. Report on a World Health Organisation Travel Study Project. Rochester, N.Y.: University of Rochester Medical Center.
15. Barker, W. H. 1987. *Adding Life to Years: Organized Geriatric Services in Great Britain and Implications for the United States.* Baltimore, Md.: Johns Hopkins University Press.
16. Burley, L. E., Currie, C. T., Smith, R. G., Williamson, J. 1979. Contribution from geriatric medicine within acute medical wards. *Br Med J* 2:90–92.
17. Arcand, M., Williamson, J. 1981. An evaluation of home visiting by physicians in geriatric medicine. *Br Med J* 283:718–720.
18. O'Brien, T. D., Joshi, D. M., Warren, E. W. 1973. No apology for geriatrics. *Br Med J* 2:277–280.
19. Bagnall, W. E., Datta, S. R., Knox, J., Horrocks, P. 1977. Geriatric medicine at Hull: A comprehensive service. *Br Med J* 2:102–104.
20. Evans, J. G. 1983. Integration of geriatric with general medical services in Newcastle. *Lancet* 1:1430–1433.
21. Shock, N. W. 1952. Age changes in renal function. In *Cowdry's Problems of Ageing*, ed. A. I. Lansing. Baltimore, Md.: Williams & Wilkins.
22. Shanas, E., Townsend, P., Friis, H., Milhoj, P., Stenhouwer, J. 1968. *Old People in Three Industrial Societies.* New York: Atherton Press.
23. Institute of Medicine. 1978. *Aging and Medical Education.* Washington, D.C.: National Academy of Sciences.
24. MacMillan, D. 1960. Preventive geriatrics. *Lancet* 2:1439–1441.
25. Campion, E. W. 1980. Personal view. *Br Med J* 281:1002.

Seventeen

The Need for a Geriatrics Specialty: Reality in the United States

Lambert N. King

Racing against demographic imperatives, the geriatric medicine movement in the United States has stimulated interest in the health and health
care of older persons. However, despite this growing interest there has been
little support for the creation of a new practice specialty of geriatrics.[1-5] In
fact, since 1978, many of the nation's powerful organizations representing
physicians' interests have issued reports opposing the establishment of
geriatrics as a clinical specialty. Organizations that have taken official
positions include the Institute of Medicine, the Association of American
Medical Colleges, the Federated Council for Internal Medicine, the American College of Physicians, and the American Geriatrics Society. These
diverse organizations reached an unusual consensus asserting that a new
practice specialty of geriatrics is both unnecessary and undesirable, but that
accelerated development of geriatrics as an academic discipline within
existing specialties, particularly internal medicine, is essential. The consensus position advocates enhanced teaching of gerontology and geriatrics
within the undergraduate medical curriculum and in residency training
programs in family practice and internal medicine. In 1984, only sixteen
university-affiliated internal medicine residencies sponsored mandatory ro-
tations in geriatric medicine.[6] Yet the American College of Physicians has
stated that internists are increasingly trained in the formal basic aspects of

geriatrics and that certification in internal medicine reflects expertise in geriatric medicine.[7]

Opposition to the emergence of geriatric medicine as a practice specialty is based upon at least four major contentions. First, there is the belief that a new specialty of geriatric medicine would deplete already limited academic resources needed to educate primary care physicians in the principles and content of geriatrics. Second, there is concern that a geriatric practice specialty will reinforce medical–institutional models, rather than social and community models, to meet the needs of the elderly. Third, the emergence of geriatric medicine may inhibit growth of the numbers of nonphysician providers—nurse practitioners, physician assistants, social workers—and the multidisciplinary teams best equipped to affordably serve elderly patients. Finally, there is the view that for geriatrics to succeed academically, it must first establish more comprehensive research programs to form the basis for fellowship training.[8]

In the United States, discussion of geriatric medicine as a practice specialty is a recent event. In contrast, the medical practice of geriatrics developed in the United Kingdom before the inception of the National Health Service in 1948. While controversy regarding its future continues, the specialty of geriatrics in Great Britain has become firmly established by virtue of its responsibility for caring for well-defined patient populations. Williamson, in Chapter 16, acknowledges that the operation of geriatric services in the United Kingdom cannot easily be transplanted to the United States, but argues that only an integrated system of geriatric care can adequately meet the needs of the elderly in the United States. Another commentator, after a comparative analysis of geriatric medicine in the United States and Great Britain, has questioned whether the present form of health-care delivery in the United States can systematically meet the challenge posed by future numbers of disabled elderly patients, and asked whether specific economic interests are served by a health-care delivery system that opposes a comprehensive practice specialty of geriatric medicine.[9]

Another critical dissent from the official consensus opposing geriatric medicine as a practice specialty has come from Kane et al., who in 1980 projected that geriatric medicine in the United States will require between 7000 and 10,300 geriatricians by the year 1990.[10] Along with these projections, the authors identified the following factors as favoring formal geriatric practice beyond the academic center.

- The medical care of the elderly requires a body of knowledge and skills distinct from those offered by other physicians.

- Geriatricians are the logical choice to provide care to a substantial portion of the elderly with dementia and depression.

- Improving the currently unsatisfactory quality of medical care of the elderly requires leadership and participation of geriatricians in the community, not just in the teaching hospital.

- Geriatricians will undoubtedly be needed to assume primary care responsibilities for many patients over age 75 whose previous primary care physician no longer can best deal with the patient's geriatric problems.

- Geriatricians will be needed in larger skilled nursing facilities, residential complexes, and agencies for home-based long-term care.

- There will be significant public demand for geriatric services.

The growth and adaptation of geriatric medicine to meet the health-care needs of older persons, especially the most aged, are by no means assured. Dr. Robert Butler described geriatrics as being at a beginning, primitive stage and noted: "We're still a long way from creating what we need—mainly, trained people to teach primary caregivers how to do geriatrics." Butler observed continuing resistance in the medical community to geriatrics, both as a perspective and an academic discipline, and expressed concern that geriatrics may not be able to survive under a reimbursement system that favors medical procedures over diagnosis and prevention.[11]

Official positions that have been taken by medical organizations concerned with the future of geriatrics need to be examined. Is the present consensus well founded? Will it lead to practices that meet the needs of frail elderly persons? Are there alternative strategies better suited to achieve the objectives of the geriatrics movement in reforming undergraduate and graduate medical education and in developing the programs and service networks required to serve elderly patients in the future? To answer these questions, the reasons used to justify opposition to geriatric medicine as a new practice specialty have to be considered. Then geriatric medicine, as it exists today, must be examined in light of its scientific and technical content, its efficacy in solving health-care problems, and the social determinants affecting health-care systems and institutions.

Why Not a Geriatrics Practice Specialty?

In a review of the findings in an Institute of Medicine committee's report on aging and medical education, Dans and Kerr discussed the conclusion that the care of the aged should continue to be the responsibility of well-trained primary-care physicians, rather than board-certified specialists in geriatrics.[12] Among the reasons were:

First, although there is a developing body of knowledge about aging and care of the aged that should be a part of medical education, much of this knowledge is not easily separable from its parent disciplines. Therefore, increased training and research resources in gerontology and geriatrics will enhance the development of existing fields and allow for better dissemination of knowledge to students, house staff, and practicing physicians.

Second, development of a specialty of geriatrics could draw attention, energy, and resources away from needed improvements in the numbers and training of the nurses, nurse practitioners, and allied health personnel who provide the bulk of the day-to-day care of the aged. It was noted that most problems of the elderly do not require the services of geriatricians, but rather a multidisciplinary team approach that includes patients, their families, and community groups.

Finally, geriatrics should be an academic discipline without a specialty board, in order to de-emphasize the negative features of subspecialization while retaining its benefits.

These arguments against a separate geriatrics practice specialty will be further considered after an examination of the factors affecting professional specialization and the contemporary position of geriatric medicine.

Factors Affecting Medical Specialization

Twentieth-century medicine has been fertile ground for those seeking to promote new clinical practice specialties or biomedical disciplines. In an effort to make external controls unnecessary, physicians wishing to be identified as specialists instituted their own certifying boards, which in turn impose standards for individuals wishing to be recognized as specialists in the field concerned. The first such specialty was ophthalmology, established in 1916, followed by otolaryngology in 1924, obstetrics and gynecology in 1930, dermatology and syphilology in 1932, pediatrics in 1933, orthopedic surgery, psychiatry, neurology, and radiology in 1934, urology in 1935, pathology and internal medicine in 1936, and surgery in 1937.[13] Since 1936, internal medicine subspecialties have grown to include allergy and immunology, cardiology, endocrinology, gastroenterology, hematology, infectious diseases, nephrology, pulmonary medicine, and rheumatology. More recently, residency programs and certification in the new practice specialties of family practice and emergency medicine have been initiated. Whatever else may have resulted from this increasing trend toward specialization, there is no doubt about the effectiveness of these actions in increasing the professional standing of physicians certified in these fields, both among professional colleagues and among patients. There can also be little doubt about the success of specialty and subspecialty boards in garnering support for medical education and research in their respective areas.

Along with the proliferation of new practice specialties, there has been rapid development of other biomedical disciplines, such as neurophar-macology, behavioral immunology, molecular biology, medical genetics, and clinical pharmacology. The 1978 Institute of Medicine Study on Aging and Medical Education emphasized similarities between geriatrics and the disciplines of clinical pharmacology and genetics, which have emerged as areas of concentration for a small number of faculty members, rather than as new practice specialties requiring formal board certification. This rela-tively narrow categorization of geriatrics as an essentially academic disci-pline would limit geriatricians mostly to large teaching hospitals and a small number of affiliated teaching nursing homes.

It is regarded as axiomatic that the growth of scientific and technical knowledge has been an important factor in the development of the highly differentiated occupational structure of medical care. Financial and pres-tige incentives, however, have been concomitant factors. Indeed, most of today's practice specialities emerged well in advance of the remarkable growth in medical knowledge that has occurred since the end of World War II. More recently, the specialty of family practice developed in the United States not so much in reaction to a new body of knowledge, but in an effort to integrate existing knowledge in the context of a biopsychosocial model of the patient and family. Furthermore, emphasis upon technological inno-vation as the explanation for specialty differentiation does not explain how geriatric medicine achieved successful specialty status in Great Britain, but not in the United States.[14] Nonetheless, the size and content of the body of knowledge of contemporary geriatric medicine are important factors to be considered in relation to the question of a new practice specialty.

Does the Base of Knowledge Justify Geriatrics as a Practice Specialty?

Geriatric medicine today consists of an increasing body of scientific knowl-edge concerning health and disease in relationship to aging. The success of geriatric medicine is measured by its success in restoring and maintaining functional capacity and preventing iatrogenic illness. Finally, geriatrics integrates medical care with a concern for the entire range of social, family, financial, and psychological resources and support available to the elderly patient. Is the knowledge base of geriatric medicine large and unique enough to justify acceptance as a new practice specialty?

Currently, to be accepted, a new practice specialty or subspecialty must provide a foundation of scientific knowledge and skills not easily assimi-lated or provided by existing physician specialty groups. This body of knowledge must justify additional clinical training and experience and must be objective enough to provide meaningful content for a certification exam. Furthermore, the core knowledge of a new specialty must promote the growth of new knowledge, methods, and techniques, and must provide

previously unavailable or more effective consultative services to other disciplines. Finally, the emerging specialty must be effective in communicating its value to other physicians, although the viability of an emerging
specialty may be a classic "cart–horse" phenomenon. The decision to
organize a specialty or subspecialty board, to institute specific training
requirements, and to provide for certification by examination tends to
promote credibility. Conversely, a reluctance to assert that a special body of
clinically applicable knowledge exists may imply that the emerging discipline is not likely to occupy an important consultative or practice role.
Therefore, those who advocate that geriatric medicine should be defined
primarily as an important academic, teaching, and research endeavor and
not as a certified practice specialty may be consigning the field to an
unnecessarily narrow role.

There has been only limited discussion in the medical literature about
whether geriatric medicine represents a body of knowledge and skills sufficient to justify a new practice specialty. However, several sources provide a
starting point from which to examine this question. The Executive Council of the Association of American Medical Colleges (AAMC) recently
published a report titled *Preparation in Undergraduate Medical Education for
Improved Geriatric Care—A Guideline for Curriculum Assessment.*[15] The
report presented a detailed description of the attitudes, basic knowledge,
and clinical skills in geriatrics that should be conveyed in undergraduate
medical education. The guidelines emphasize the personal attitudes as well
as the socioeconomic and psychosocial knowledge necessary for compassionate and effective geriatric care. Theories of aging, both biological and
psychosocial, are stressed. The report also contains an important section
on clinical skills, including the special aspects of medical interviewing and
of recording the medical history and physical examination of the elderly.
Judicious approaches to laboratory studies, medical interventions, and
drug therapy are specifically encouraged based upon detailed empirical
information. Finally, the importance of patient and family education in
promoting optimal independence and function are discussed. If all physicians in training were to master this material by the end of even their
graduate medical education, elderly patients would greatly benefit in their
interactions with physicians and hospitals. Equally relevant, however, is
the fact that these guidelines are a distillation of a larger base of knowledge
and skills that constitute contemporary geriatric medicine. This distillation is the result of significant basic research in the mechanisms of aging,
systematic investigations in the social sciences, and substantial clinical
investigation, including hypothesis-based studies and controlled trials.
The quality and scope of the knowledge base reflected in the AAMC
guidelines compare favorably with the published literature underlying the

relatively new specialties of family practice and emergency medicine.

A second rough measure of the knowledge base of geriatric medicine can be obtained through a retrospective look at the growth of published literature. A survey of the literature shows that publications on gerontology and geriatrics have burgeoned within the last ten years. The number of articles identified by a Medline search as having implications for clinical practice increased from 1055 during 1977–81 to 1756 during 1982–6. This trend, still accelerating, demonstrates the capacity for geriatric medicine to increase its knowledge base.

Published articles in geriatrics are drawn from nearly every branch of medical activity, including most of the recognized subspecialties as well as an even more diverse group of disciplines, including psychology, sociology, medical social work, medical economics, nursing, religion, physiotherapy, podiatry, pharmacy practice, demography, education, ethics, law, and health-care administration. The effective practice of geriatric medicine, in contrast to many other medical subspecialties, requires mastery of a very broad set of multidisciplinary information and skills.

Another source documenting the knowledge base of contemporary geriatric medicine is the geriatrics bibliography compiled by Rosenthal in the *Journal of the American Geriatrics Society.*[16] The bibliography is strongly oriented toward clinical medicine and reflects a dynamic and productive knowledge base. Most of the references are less than five years old, and two-thirds of the references cited in the second edition of the bibliography were replaced by more current or more detailed articles. A total of 692 publications are cited, the majority of which are refereed. Approximately 75% of the citations in the bibliography are from journals not specifically dedicated to gerontology, geriatrics, or aging research and clinical practice. This high percentage of geriatrics articles published in other specialties' publications reflects contributions from virtually all of the medical and surgical subspecialties. The involvement of these varied medical and surgical subspecialties with the health problems of elderly patients is relevant to the question of geriatric medicine as a practice specialty. The geriatrician's special role in supervision and integration of care for frail elderly patients with complicated acute and chronic multisystem disease arises partly from mastery of this diverse body of knowledge.

In both acute and long-term care, geriatric medicine presents special challenges. Eliciting the medical history and performing the physical examination of elderly patients require more time, energy, and skill than are required for younger patients. Multisystem disease is more prevalent, and a single explanation for the patient's illness is less likely. Nonspecific and unusual disease presentations are common, and a complicated interplay with biopsychosocial factors is the rule rather than the exception. Geriatric medicine also requires maturity, wisdom, and experience. Primary-care physicians with the requisite skills in geriatric medicine are rare and are likely to remain so.

The Efficacy of Geriatric Medicine

There is limited but growing evidence in the geriatric medicine literature of a capacity to benefit elderly patients in both acute and long-term care settings. The most convincing demonstration of the efficacy of geriatric medicine has occurred in the area of comprehensive assessment. Comprehensive assessment emphasizes quantification of all relevant medical, functional, and psychosocial attributes and deficits in order to achieve a rational basis for therapy and resource planning in the care of elderly patients. Although comprehensive assessment should be assumed to be a health-care goal for patients of any age, younger patients do not present multisystem medical and psychosocial problems as often as the frail elderly do. The purposes of geriatric assessment include: screening for treatable disease, accurate diagnosis, rational therapeutic planning, ensuring appropriate use of services and avoiding inappropriate use of services, determining optimal placement, and documenting change over time. Published reports on geriatric assessment units or programs suggest associations between these programs and improvements in the outcome of care, including improved diagnostic accuracy, improved placement location, enhanced functional status, and more appropriate use of medications.[17]

More recently, Rubenstein and colleagues reported the results of a randomized controlled study conducted in a Veterans Administration hospital that compared patients cared for on a special geriatric evaluation unit (GEU) with patients given standard care and discharge planning.[18] The typical patient in the study was 78 years old, male, white, married, and living at home before admission. The patients had an average of four medical conditions, requiring substantial nursing care and four prescribed medications. After 1 year of follow-up, the mortality in patients treated in the GEU was 24%, in contrast to 48% mortality in the control group. Seventy-three percent of the GEU patients were discharged to home or a boarding facility, compared to 53% of the control patients. Only 13% of the patients treated in the GEU were discharged to nursing homes, in comparison to 30% of the control patients. There was a lower rehospitalization rate in the GEU patients and greater improvement in functional and mental status scores. Costs for the follow-up year were adjusted to reflect differences in survival and showed that the mean institutional care cost per year survived was substantially lower for the patients treated in the GEU. Although the patients studied have special selection characteristics (an entirely male group in a VA hospital), these findings demonstrate a capacity to improve the quality of care for frail elderly patients in a cost-effective manner.

Other efforts to evaluate the utility of geriatric medicine have yielded less conclusive results. Campion et al. studied the effects of comprehensive assessment by a Geriatric Consultation Team (GCT) on acute-care hospital patients.[19] The study patients had multiple illnesses and received an average of at least three medications. Functional assessment showed that 59% of the patients frequently depended upon others for ambulation, 52% were cognitively impaired, and 11% were clinically depressed. Over 10.5 months of follow-up, the GCT and non-GCT patients had similar hospital readmission rates (43%). The authors did note an increase in the number of patients placed in rehabilitation and specialty hospital settings, and they emphasize a range of qualitative benefits of a GCT in a teaching hospital. Given the high hospital readmission rate of the frail elderly patients in this study, the critical role of a GCT in promoting continuity of care and in minimizing excessive diagnostic interventions merits further evaluation.

Another factor to be considered is the publicly perceived efficacy of a new specialty or discipline in meeting the needs of patient populations. Remarkable changes in medical care have occurred as a result of public perceptions of specialized initiatives to meet widespread medical care needs. For example, major resources have been devoted to the development of coronary care units at hospitals throughout the United States, which were advocated by cardiologists and widely accepted by hospitals long before there was any rigorous demonstration of their effectiveness.[20] Furthermore, expansion of the concept of coronary care further stimulated the growth and acceptance of the specialty of cardiology. Another example is family medicine, the growth of which was predicated mainly upon the potential of this specialty to meet special geographic and demographic needs for competently trained primary-care practitioners. Therefore, public perception of the capacity of geriatric medicine to meet the future health-care needs of growing numbers of elderly patients may influence support not only for geriatric medical education but also for the multidisciplinary programs and facilities required for comprehensive long-term care systems.

To some degree, public opinions of geriatric medicine will depend upon how geriatric physicians define and project their discipline. At the same time, other external forces will also have effects, sometimes unpredictable, on the evolution of geriatric medicine. For example, Medicare's prospective payment system (see Maddox and Manton, Chapter 4), together with federal and state efforts to limit nursing home and home-care costs, may result in major underprovision of care for elderly patients and exclusion of clinical geriatric medicine from the medical care system. The possible extension of prospective payment systems to physician reimbursement would have decisive effects upon division of income among medical specialties. Indeed, Dr. Knight Steel has cautioned that naive unconcern about fiscal matters may be the downfall of many geriatric medicine programs in the next decade.[21]

Geriatric medicine remains in the early stages of demonstrating its social and medical utility. Research in geriatric medicine presents special challenges, including the difficulty of measuring treatment outcomes for patients with multiple chronic illnesses. The measurement of restoration or maintenance of functional capacities is more complicated than more narrowly defined outcomes of cure or improvement in pathophysiological parameters. The influence of the role of the geriatrician may often not be demonstrably separable from the effect of the multidisciplinary team or unit. Nonetheless, through its growing research efforts and the initiation of validated clinical programs, geriatric medicine offers the promise of significant improvements in the quality and economy of health-care services.

The Need for a Geriatrics Practice Specialty

The developing knowledge base of geriatric medicine today necessarily results from a large range of other disciplines and specialties. Yet there is little evidence to date that most primary-care internists are effectively assimilating and using the knowledge base of geriatrics. As the number of complicated frail elderly patients accelerates, how will thousands of practicing physicians with substantial experience and skills in geriatric medicine be trained?

Initiation of an accredited practice specialty of geriatrics might draw some attention, energy, and resources away from certain educational efforts directed at students in general, physicians in graduate internal medicine and family practice training programs, practicing physicians, and a range of other health practitioners required for multidisciplinary long-term care programs. On the other hand, hospitals already have shown considerable interest in training nonphysician staff to provide multidisciplinary long-term care and case-management services. It is also reasonable to predict that creation of a nationally recognized specialty or subspecialty of geriatrics would stimulate greater interest among medical students and primary-care residents in the future of geriatric medicine. Physicians whose practice patterns have included considerable experience in geriatrics, and who might be eligible for a certification exam, may enhance their knowledge in preparation for the exam, as well as become role models in conveying the principles and philosophy of geriatric medicine to other physicians. Finally, a board-certified specialty of geriatrics is more likely to effectively mobilize resources and support for new programs and facilities to meet the needs of elderly patients than is a loosely organized network of teaching-hospital academic units.

Would a geriatrics practice specialty increase or alleviate the fragmentation of care that frail elderly patients encounter in acute-care hospitals? It is incorrect, I believe, to view the emergence of geriatric medicine as just another example of reductionism or medicalization of the elderly. If the philosophical base of contemporary geriatrics is respected and enhanced, geriatricians practicing in acute-care hospitals could be instrumental in protecting and serving the interests of the most vulnerable patients, who may require multiple subspecialty services but who also need knowledgeable clinicians to supervise and integrate their care. Board-certified geriatricians may well be successful in minimizing use of subspecialty services for patients and in setting an influential example for general internists and family practitioners, who will continue to care for the majority of older patients.

In its effort to reshape medical education and health-care services to the benefit of increasing numbers of elderly patients, the geriatrics movement should not lose sight of two harsh facts. First, resources to support services that incorporate the principles of geriatric medicine will have to be extracted largely from existing total health-care expenditures. Second, geriatrics will inevitably have to compete with other interest groups such as hospitals, proprietary home-care programs, and existing specialties, all of which have more clearly defined agendas and targeted strategies. The question remaining is: How effectively will geriatric medicine—with its philosophy of minimizing unnecessary diagnostic and therapeutic interventions—interact with existing subspecialties which are likely to continue to be more procedurally and less holistically oriented to the needs of the elderly?

Writing in *The Journal of the American Geriatrics Society*, David Greer questioned whether geriatrics should attempt to establish a significant position in clinical medicine:

> Geriatric medicine is still amorphous: its place within the medical profession and its social role remain to be defined. To prosper, geriatric medicine must meet two principal criteria. It must establish a unique and credible role within the profession; what professional void will it fill? It must demonstrate its social utility; what perceived need in society will it fulfill? In times of economic restraint, a third factor could be critical to the development of geriatric medicine: will it have a salutory effect on health care costs?[22]

Greer noted that the aged and their families are frustrated with traditional medicine, and that the profession has so far remained unresponsive. He criticized the traditional disease orientation and mechanistic approach to illness and the continued emphasis on providing medical services in institutional settings that are toxic to the elderly. Greer argued that attempts to establish a foothold for geriatrics in clinical medicine will involve geriatricians in territorial battles with academic medical centers and general hospitals. Instead of such an approach, he advocated that geriatricians expand their roles to address broad deficiencies in education, research, and service, which would favor integrated community systems rather than medical centers, team practice rather than a medical model, quality-of-life objectives rather than diagnostic medicine, and milieu therapy rather than polypharmacy.

In an editorial comment, David Rogers found Greer's thesis appealing and agreed that physicians have overmedicalized many of the natural or inevitable events of human life. He questioned whether physicians are the persons best equipped to develop the integrated mix of social, technical, and health services for older people. While not advocating that geriatricians compete with traditional specialists in the care of certain specific but complex medical problems of the elderly, Rogers remained uncertain about where geriatrics fits as a practice specialty. Noting that demographic statistics suggest that all physicians must become more skilled in caring for the aged, Rogers suggested that specialty geriatricians can serve two specific functions: using their special expertise to assist in the care of other physicians' patients, and using their special skills and perspectives in assessment, which is a critical process in the delivery of multidisciplinary chronic care.[23]

Rogers suggested that in the first role, the geriatrician can be seen as serving a function analogous to that of an infectious-disease consultant. But if this role is valid, why should the geriatrician, a skilled clinician with experience and knowledge in the assessment and care of complicated frail elderly patients, be less recognized and probably less influential than a board-certified subspecialist in infectious disease? The development of a subspecialty board and certification in infectious diseases has in no way inhibited the growth of academically oriented divisions of infectious disease in teaching hospitals. On the contrary, it is far more likely that the academic role of all medical subspecialties in teaching hospitals has been enhanced by board certification. In its zeal to convey the principles of geriatric medicine to all primary-care physicians, is it wise for geriatric medicine to cast aside well-deserved legitimacy as a practice specialty?

Summary

The geriatric medicine movement in the United States has worked to stimulate the interest of both medical practitioners and medical organizations in the health and health care of older persons. While the proponents of geriatrics in the United States constitute a highly decentralized network, they have forged a consensus concerning the priorities for physicians and organizations interested in the future of geriatrics. Emphasis has been placed upon increasing instruction in the principles of geriatric medicine for both undergraduate and graduate students of medicine, upgrading the quality of long-term care for disabled and chronically ill elderly, and increasing the quality and quantity of basic and clinical research in aging and geriatric care. Gradually, academic geriatrics units with associated fellowship programs have emerged in more than fifty medical schools, and the number continues to grow.

In 1987, two historic actions were taken that are likely to enhance greatly the growth of geriatrics as a practice specialty in the United States. After years of consideration, the American Board of Family Practice and American Board of Internal Medicine jointly announced certification and examination requirements for geriatric medicine.[24] In addition, a single set of proposed guidelines for fellowship training programs in geriatric medicine was jointly completed and submitted to the residency review committees for internal medicine and family practice.[25] These actions provide for recognition of competence in geriatric medicine on the basis of formal training and passing of a written examination prepared by members of both boards. Successful candidates will be awarded a Certificate of Added Qualifications and will be designated as Diplomates in Geriatric Medicine. Diplomates will be responsible for revalidating the certificate within 7 years by a recertification process to be developed. One provision is of special relevance to the growth of geriatrics as a practice specialty. Four years after they have been certified in family practice or internal medicine, physicians whose practices have included substantial experience in caring for the elderly will be admitted to examination in geriatric medicine. (This provision is applicable for a period of 5 years after the first examination in geriatric medicine in 1988.)

The long-delayed initiation of a certification process in geriatric medicine, especially a process encompassing both internists and family practitioners, provides a foundation for marked expansion of geriatric research, teaching, and clinical practice. Recruitment is likely to be enhanced by growing awareness of certification in geriatric medicine and the equivalency established with other officially recognized specialties. These developments also increase the potential for third-party reimbursement for geriatric medicine services, generating funds that might be partially redistributed within academic geriatric programs to support multidisciplinary geriatric teams and units.

The balance of evidence now available indicates that geriatric medicine is becoming a major research, teaching, and clinical specialty, but some barriers still remain to block its emergence. Everyone sharing commitment to geriatric medicine needs to remember the advice of Samuel Johnson, who noted, "Nothing will ever be attempted if all possible objections must first be overcome."

References

1. Institute of Medicine. 1978. *Aging and Medical Education.* Washington, D.C.: National Academy of Sciences.
2. Butler, R. 1979. Geriatrics and internal medicine. *Ann Intern Med* 91:903–908.
3. Swanson, A. 1979. The role of geriatrics in medical education. *J Med Education* 54:59–61.
4. Reichel, W. 1981. Geriatric medical education: Developments since the American Geriatrics Society conferences on geriatric education, 1976–1977. *J Am Geriatr Soc* 29:1–9.
5. Federated Council for Internal Medicine. 1981. Geriatric medicine: A statement from the Federated Council for Internal Medicine. *Ann Intern Med* 95:372–376.
6. Calkins, E. 1984. Clinical experience: House staff and subinterns. Paper presented at the New York Academy of Medicine conference on the Geriatric Medical Education Imperative, New York, October 11.
7. American College of Physicians, Health and Public Policy Committee. 1984. Long-term care of the elderly. *Ann Intern Med* 100:760–763.
8. Beck, J. C. 1985. Development of pediatrics and family practice from a historical perspective: Lessons for geriatrics. *J Am Geriatr Soc* 33:727–729.
9. Carboni, D. 1983. *Geriatric Medicine in the United States and Great Britain.* Westport, Conn.: Greenwood Press, 127.
10. Kane, R., Solomon, D., Beck, J., Keeler, E., Kane, R. 1980. The future need for geriatric medicine manpower in the United States. *N Engl J Med* 302:1327–1332.
11. Geriatric Medicine Slow to Spread in U.S. *Grey Panther Network,* Winter 1985, p. 2.
12. Dans, P., Kerr, M. 1979. Gerontology and geriatrics in medical education. *N Engl J Med* 300:228.
13. Stern, B. F. 1941. *Society and Medical Progress.* Princeton, N.J.: Princeton University Press, 96.
14. See Ref. 9, p. 9.
15. Association of American Medical Colleges. 1983. Preparation in undergraduate medical education for improved geriatric care: A guideline for curriculum assessment. *J Med Ed* 58:503–526.
16. Rosenthal, M. 1986. Geriatrics: An updated bibliography. *J Am Geriatr Soc* 34:148–171.
17. Rubenstein, L. 1983. The clinical effectiveness of multidimensional geriatric assessment. *J Am Geriatr Soc* 31:758–762.

18. Rubenstein, L., Josephson, K., Wieland, G., English, P. Sayre, N., Kane, R. 1987. Effectiveness of a geriatric evaluation unit: A randomized clinical trial. *N Engl J Med* 311:1664–1670.
19. Campion, E., Jette, A., Berkman, B. 1983. An interdisciplinary geriatric consultation service: A controlled trial. *J Am Geriatr Soc* 31:792.
20. Waitzkin, H. 1983. *The Second Sickness.* New York: Free Press, 90–110.
21. Steel, K. 1984. Geriatric medicine is coming of age. *Gerontologist* 24:370.
22. Greer, D. 1983. Hospice: Lessons for geriatricians. *J Am Geriatr Soc* 31:67–70.
23. Rogers, D. 1983. Where does the geriatrician fit? *J Am Geriatr Soc* 31:124–125.
24. American Board of Family Practice and American Board of Internal Medicine. 1987. Joint announcement on certification for advanced training in geriatrics. *J Am Geriatr Soc* 35:700–701.
25. Ad Hoc Committee of the American Geriatrics Society. 1987. Guidelines for fellowship training programs in geriatric medicine. *J Am Geriatr Soc* 35:792–795.

Eighteen

The Value of Medical Care: Four Case Studies

Helen L. Smits, Lisa F. Berkman, and Mary C. Kapp

The effects of the existing health-care system on the elderly are uneven. Certainly, many failures can be documented, but so can many successes, and a redesign of medical and social services for the elderly requires a careful study of both. This chapter focuses on some successes within the practice of modern medicine to elucidate the policies that best support and enhance good-quality health care for the elderly.

The Selection of the Areas Studied

Four commonly occurring conditions have been chosen to illustrate the positive effects of modern medicine on the health of the elderly: two surgical procedures, the use of the intraocular lens and prosthetic replacement of the hip, and two clinical problems, hypertension and diabetes. The surgical procedures are typical of the life-enhancing techniques that have been used with increasing frequency on elderly patients. Lens implantation has been controversial, while prosthetic hip replacement has been accepted with considerably less debate. The treatment of the two chronic clinical conditions has been hypothesized to be life extending. Treating hypertension clearly prolongs life, but treating diabetes has less clear-cut benefits. Because the four conditions selected for study avoid areas where relatively little can be done, as in the treatment of stroke, our observations may overstate the benefits of medical management.

Intraocular Lens Implant

Surgery to remove a lens or lenses opacified by cataract is the most common operation in patients over 65[1] and has been claimed to be the most frequent major surgical procedure in the world.[2] The demand for vision-restoring surgery has long been high among those affected with cataracts; the surgical removal of cataracts antedates the use of anesthesia by over 100 years. The first series of cataract extractions was reported in 1756 by Daviel, who operated on a total of 434 cases, with only 50 failures.[2] Reports of large series of extractions and debate about the best approach to cataract removal can be found in the surgical literature throughout the nineteenth and twentieth centuries.

Precise statistics on the prevalence of senile cataract are difficult to obtain. In one large sample of the noninstitutionalized population in the United States, lens opacities were found in approximately 60% of those age 65–74, with half of the affected individuals displaying decreased vision.[3] The Framingham Study, which used a somewhat different definition of opacity, found cataracts in 18% of persons age 65–74, and in 46% of those 75–84.[4] Because cataract extraction is frequently performed on outpatients while the best nationwide data on surgical procedures are obtained from hospital discharges, it is also hard to know how often lens removal takes place. Probably the best information is available from the Food and Drug Administration (FDA) through its surveillance of intraocular lenses. The FDA reports 409,000 lens implants in persons of all ages between August 1981 and August 1982 and estimates that approximately 525,000 cataract procedures were performed over the same period.[5] The total number of lens extractions performed annually has risen rapidly since the passage of Medicare, a phenomenon that is viewed by at least one author as evidence of "acute remunerative surgery,"[6] but is seen by others as proof of improved access to care, coupled with increased demand for surgical repair of decreased vision.[7]

A patient who simply has an opacified lens removed has little more vision than before surgery, unless additional corrective measures are taken. There are three approaches to the treatment of loss of lens (aphakia): 1) corrective spectacle lenses, 2) corrective contact lenses, and 3) implantation of an artificial intraocular lens (IOL). Of the three, spectacle lenses are at once the safest and the least satisfying to patients who use them. Spectacles carry no risk beyond the risk of the surgery itself. Unfortunately, however, vision with spectacles is relatively poor. Common serious problems found even in properly fitted lenses include false orientation and distortion, "swim," and aberrations and restrictions in the peripheral visual fields.[1] The weight of thick lenses and the need to keep track of glasses can present additional problems for the elderly. Contact lenses, by contrast, provide better vision, but 50% of the elderly cannot cope with lenses, which must be removed daily. Extended-wear contact lenses may improve on this figure, but even they are often unsuccessful in the elderly because of dry eyes or chronic eyelid infections.[8]

An implanted lens, by contrast, produces vision far superior to either of the other corrective measures. Magnification is only 1% to 3%, as contrasted with 30% for spectacles and 5% to 10% with ordinary contact lenses. In addition, none of the problems with spatial disorientation or abnormal peripheral vision that are associated with spectacles occurs.[8] However, intraocular lenses carry a risk of complications that is greater than the risk associated with cataract surgery alone. A recent FDA review showed that persistent, vision-threatening complications were present in from 1.6% to over 6% of all eyes with IOLs one year after surgery, with the rate depending on the type of lens implanted. The posterior chamber lens, which is associated with the lowest complication rate, is now the lens most frequently implanted in the United States. The FDA did not estimate how much excess risk IOL implantation represents over cataract surgery alone, but the return for any excess risk is a high success rate; over 85% of all IOL cases achieve vision of 20/40 or better.[5]

The FDA study shows a marked rise in the number of IOLs implanted since the beginning of 1980; the majority of ophthalmologists and patients have obviously accepted the procedure as being effective and having a reasonable level of risk. Improvements in the lenses themselves and in surgical technique have apparently convinced many previously skeptical surgeons that the procedure is worthwhile. To the critical reviewer, however, the available work on IOLs leaves a good deal to be desired. Although the FDA has carefully defined and monitored the risks of surgery, it has been less successful in defining and monitoring either its benefits or the indications for surgery. A high degree of patient satisfaction with successful procedures is described anecdotally but does not appear to have been measured empirically. Objective tests of important aspects of visual function, such as measures of peripheral vision, are also lacking. As Jaffee notes, a measure such as 20/40 vision does not indicate how well the patient actually sees, since the test measures only central vision.[8] Peripheral vision, depth perception, and night vision are not assessed. More analysis is also needed concerning the 10%–15% of patients who have neither a vision-threatening complication nor a "successful" outcome. How well they see, and how well they might have seen had an alternative corrective measure been used, are very important elements in decisions about the risks and benefits of surgery.

Finally, the literature on IOLs, like that on cataracts in general, does not deal in sufficient detail with appropriate indications for surgery. The conservative approach of 20 years ago, in which cataracts were allowed to "ripen" until the patient was close to functionally blind, is clearly unsuitable for a healthy and active elderly population. Modern surgical techniques, coupled with excellent visual results from IOLs, appear to justify earlier surgery, but new indications should be based on careful visual testing before surgery and on evaluation of the patient's need and desire to improve vision. Cataract surgery is unique among common procedures in that examination of the pathologic specimen is useless, so that tissue committees do not provide an adequate safeguard against unnecessary surgery. In the absence of careful pre- and postoperative visual testing, Taylor's question remains both disturbing and unanswered: Are we doing cataract surgery before patients need it?[6]

Total Hip Replacement

Replacement of a hip with an orthopedic prosthesis is also a relatively common procedure, performed annually on approximately 45,000 persons over age 65.[9] The surgery is aimed primarily at relieving pain, with restoration of function an important secondary benefit. Actually, the two outcomes are closely linked, since in arthritics, who comprise the bulk of patients, pain is frequently the primary cause of loss of function. No randomized controlled trial has been conducted to evaluate hip replacement, but its acceptance is widespread. Most reported case series focus on uncontrolled results from the use of a particular prosthetic design or surgical protocol, with infection rates or mortality as the outcome indicator. Despite the fact that pain is the primary reason for hip replacement, ratings of pain and functional status are frequently not included in the published reports. One problem with the evaluation of hip replacement arises because complications or failures may occur years after surgery, so a satisfactory short-term result may be a poor indicator of the benefits of the procedure.

One study of 300 patients 4 to 7 years after operation included follow-up data on 251 of the initial group. Of these individuals, 94.3% reported no pain or mild pain 2 years after surgery; 97% still reported no pain or mild pain 5 years after surgery. By contrast, 96.4% were in moderate to severe pain in the preoperative period. Overall hip evaluation, including pain, function, motion, and the absence of deformity, was measured on a 100-point scale using the Harris hip evaluation scoring system. At 5 years the average score was 92; preoperative average scores were 45. Although this study is comprehensive and deals with the outcome issues of most importance to patients, its impact is reduced by the wide ranges in the ages of patients (39–84) and the wide variety of underlying conditions.[10]

In 1982, a consensus panel of the Swedish Medical Research Council noted that there was no randomized controlled trial of hip replacement but concluded that "The operation has meant a revolutionary change in the lives of many . . . . a change from a sedentary and painful life to a painless and mobile life."[11] A National Institutes of Health (NIH) panel reached similar conclusions at approximately the same time. Precise identification of the risks of surgery is difficult. Operative mortality is less than 1%; the worst complication is deep infection, which occurs in approximately 1% of patients. Because of the difficulty inherent in treating infection with a foreign body in place, this complication is catastrophic, requiring removal of the prosthesis and holding out little possibility of future replacement. Dislocation occurs in 0.8% to 2.4% of all patients, with the better results occurring at centers that perform the procedure more frequently. Heterotropic bone formation (abnormal growth of new bone) is frequently seen on x-rays but limits function in less than 2% of cases. Despite a general tone of enthusiasm and optimism, the NIH consensus panel concluded there is need to establish multi-institutional studies of different types of patients, prosthetic designs, materials, methods of insertion, and postoperative protocols.[9]

Those who study hip replacement have made a serious effort to quantify the degree of pain, limitation of motion, and nature of gait. A variety of "hip rating scales" have been developed and compared, but all have the disadvantage of attempting to lump together pain and function, which may obscure important clinical distinctions in some groups.[12] None of the studies of hip replacement seems to have considered the possibility of measuring patient satisfaction, reported activity levels, or the ability to perform the instrumental activities of daily living as a way of quantifying the "revolutionary" effects of this procedure.

Diabetes

Diabetes mellitus is divided into two main types. The first, which was formerly known as juvenile type, is now appropriately described as insulin-dependent, ketosis-prone diabetes. This condition is associated with changes in the frequency of certain histocompatibility antigens (HLA) on chromosome 6 and islet-cell antibodies. It occurs most commonly in children but may have its onset at any age. The second type of diabetes, formerly known as adult-onset diabetes, is now properly described as non–insulin-dependent, non–ketosis-prone diabetes; it commonly occurs after age 40 but may occasionally be found in younger individuals. Non–insulin dependent diabetes is further subdivided according to whether obesity is present. Other, much smaller, subclasses of diabetes include diabetes secondary to other illnesses and gestational diabetes. The discussion here is confined to non–insulin-dependent, non–ketosis-prone diabetes (NIDD), the only class with any substantial effect on the health of the elderly.

The first problem in dealing with NIDD is deciding who has it. With the exception of some American Indian and Micronesian populations, among whom diabetes is exceedingly prevalent, the distribution of plasma glucose levels among populations studied (with diagnosed diabetics excluded) is unimodal.[13] As a result, epidemiology does not provide clues to the most appropriate distinction between the diabetic and nondiabetic population. The problem is further compounded by a rise in average plasma glucose and increased impairment in glucose tolerance with increasing age. The inevitable result has been both debate and confusion regarding the appropriate criteria to be used for the diagnosis of diabetes. In one study, twenty well-qualified American and European diabetologists showed no consensus on either the lowest 2-hour glucose considered "clearly abnormal" or the highest value considered "clearly normal." The study notes that "interindividual differences in criteria up to 70 or 80 mcg per 100 ml were occasionally observed and differences of 20 mcg per 100 ml were quite common."[14] A more recent effort by the National Diabetes Data Group (NDDG) to define blood levels for fasting patients and for 1 hour and 2 hours after an oral glucose tolerance test should help to reduce the disagreement among experts.[15] The World Health Organization subsequently endorsed the criteria for diabetes mellitus developed by the NDDG,[16] but the extent of the use of NDDG criteria in practice is still unclear. Davidson[17] cautions that the diagnosis of diabetes should be reserved for individuals with fasting hyperglycemia, in order to avoid the social, employment, and insurance side-effects of overdiagnosis.

Disputes about the exact definition of abnormal blood glucose levels, coupled with the practical difficulties involved in obtaining blood samples from large populations, make estimates of the true prevalence of the disease uncertain. Because of the large number of undiagnosed and asymptomatic cases, self-reporting is not a very satisfactory substitute for direct measurement. Using pre-NDDG criteria and data from the 1960–1962 National Center for Health Statistics survey, Knowles estimated a 2.6% prevalence of known diabetes in the United States, a 0.6% prevalence of unknown diabetes, and a 2.8% lifetime risk of developing diabetes.[18] Melton reevaluated data collected between 1945 and 1969 using the NDDG criteria and noted that these criteria reduce the incidence of diabetes by about 20%, by eliminating a number of NIDD cases.[19]

Despite the difficulty of distinguishing non–insulin-dependent diabetics from the normal population, there is no question that NIDD is a serious health risk. Diabetes occurring after the age of 60 is associated with a life expectancy of only 10 years, and this figure has not increased since 1950.[17] Excess mortality associated with diabetes can be observed as late as the eighth decade, with most of the increase explained by cardiovascular disease.[20] Even after adjusting for other major risk factors, the relative risk of cardiovascular disease was twice as great for diabetics in the 45–74-year-old Framingham cohort.[21]

Short-term treatment of elevated blood glucose levels may be needed to avoid or eliminate life-threatening hyperglycemia, whether ketotic or nonketotic, to facilitate the treatment of secondary conditions (such as infections), or to enable the patient to withstand major surgery. Treatment for these reasons is accepted as good practice, and no population-based figures are available on incidence or outcome. The merits of long-term treatment are much more uncertain. Although there is a general consensus among experts that blood-sugar levels should be kept as normal as possible, debate continues about the effect of diabetic control on complications and about the merits of "good" as opposed to "poor" control, over the long run. This debate is as old as the discovery of insulin; several generations of diabetologists have now followed their mentors into either the "rigid" or the "loose" school of diabetic therapy. In 1976 and 1977 the editorial pages of the *New England Journal of Medicine* presented both sides as well as the editor-in-chief's summary and conclusion.[22–24] Little has occurred since that time to resolve the debate as it applies to the elderly.

The complications of diabetes include atherosclerosis, neuropathy, microvascular changes, renal disease, and a variety of ocular lesions, including retinopathy, maculopathy, neovascularization, and cataracts. Blindness may be a long-term result of the ocular lesions; azotemia may arise from the renal disease. All complications increase markedly as the disease progresses. The most important complication of diabetes in the elderly group is atherosclerosis, particularly cardiovascular disease; acceleration of cataract formation may be presumed to occur as well. Some authors have hypothesized that elderly diabetics do not live long enough after diagnosis to experience neuropathy or microvascular disease; others argue that at least some complications may in fact be part of the underlying pathology of insulin-dependent diabetes rather than the result of prolonged hyperglycemia. There is, however, good laboratory evidence to show that neuropathy, nephropathy, and retinopathy can be induced in animals as a result of hyperglycemia alone, evidence that supports the position of the first group. Although a physiological explanation for the association between diabetes and atherosclerosis has been proposed, the evidence from animal experimentation indicating that elevated blood glucose directly affects atherosclerotic lesions is not convincing.[25]

The overall goal of treatment of diabetes is to achieve as close a return to a normal metabolic state as is possible without enhancing risk. Behavior modification, particularly diet and exercise to reduce weight, should be the first approach to treatment of the non–insulin-dependent diabetic. This approach should be supplemented with insulin or oral hypoglycemic therapy only if control is not satisfactory. While behavior modifications are difficult to achieve at any age, decreased physical mobility and a reluctance to change long-standing eating habits make this modification even more difficult in the elderly. The traditional drug treatment of NIDD has been oral hypoglycemic agents, an approach that has been widely questioned following the long-term prospective clinical trial conducted by the University Group Diabetes Project.[26] This study showed little difference between insulin therapy and diet alone in stable adult-onset diabetes. The conclusions were based on mortality rates, nonfatal vascular complications, and serious microvascular complications. This same study showed increased risk associated with oral hypoglycemic agents; whether these conclusions are valid is still being debated.

Despite convincing laboratory evidence of the association between microvascular complications and elevated blood-glucose levels, firm clinical evidence that good control reduces these effects is hard to find. One reason may well be that in most studies control has been measured in terms of a blood-sugar measurement taken, at most, once a month. Such levels may have little to do with the average blood-sugar level over time and may well have been most influenced by the strength of the individual patient's desire to appear to be under good control when visiting the doctor, a desire that can lead to careful management of diet and drugs for the last few days before the test. The question of the relationship between good control and complications should be answered with some precision in the next few years. The most recent advance in the treatment of diabetes is the development of mechanical insulin pumps that administer insulin throughout the day. At their most sophisticated, these devices sample blood glucose and adjust insulin administration accordingly. While the devices themselves do not appear to offer potential benefits to the elderly non–insulin-dependent diabetic, the information collected from their use in a group of younger diabetics can greatly enhance understanding of the association between treatment and complications.

The debate about the need for good control of diabetes arises largely because treatment can carry significant risk. Ideally, management of the elderly diabetic should be a delicate balancing act. Hypoglycemic episodes, which may occur with either insulin or oral agents, may be particularly serious in the frail elderly because of interaction with other risk factors. Falls associated with hypoglycemia, for example, can produce fractures in the presence of osteoporosis; unconsciousness secondary to hypoglycemia may go unnoticed and untreated in the isolated individual for so long that permanent brain damage occurs. At the same time, serious hyperglycemia can be difficult to manage in the elderly patient whose impaired renal and cardiovascular function enhances the risks of dehydration and complicates fluid replacement. A final element in the balancing act is the difficult choice of treatment agents. Behavior changes are believed to be difficult for the old to achieve and physicians are skeptical of their utility; oral hypo-glycemics raise the question of enhanced risk; and, at best, insulin is unattractive to elderly patients, while at worst it is impossible to administer accurately.

Review of the evidence in this field reveals another interesting and disturbing fact. Although much is known about the diagnosis of diabetes and about the merits and demerits of the various forms of treatment, very little is known about actual patterns of treatment. If the surgical literature can be faulted for inadequate attention to outcomes that are difficult to measure, the medical literature has to be faulted for its failure to report the outcomes of average practice. Only two firm conclusions can be drawn from a review of the literature on diabetes: 1) overtreatment appears to pose as serious a threat to the elderly as undertreatment, and 2) properly managed medical care of the diabetic has potential benefit in terms of the reduction of short-term ill effects of hyperglycemia.

Hypertension

Hypertension, like diabetes, is an extremely common condition in the elderly, with well-identified disease risks. Hypertension, usually defined as a systolic blood pressure of 160 mm Hg or greater and/or a diastolic blood pressure of 95 mm Hg or greater, is present in up to 50% of older men and women in the United States. The prevalence is greater in blacks than whites and greater in women than men.[27] In the elderly, as in younger people, hypertension is a major risk factor for cardiovascular and cere-brovascular morbidity and mortality.[28-32] The concept that old people tolerate hypertension well appears to be largely mythical. It may stem from the idea that high blood pressure or large increases in blood pressure are a part of the normal aging process—another myth, since in some popula-tions blood pressure does not seem to increase with age. Many people in developed countries, including at least 50% of the elderly in the United States, do *not* have hypertension, and most studies have shown hyperten-sion to be associated with serious pathologic changes. The evidence that hypertension is associated with congestive heart failure, angina pectoris, myocardial infarction, transient cerebral ischemic attacks, and strokes in the elderly has been reviewed in several recent papers,[27,33,34] but the focus here is on the efficacy of medical management of hypertension.

There are three main areas of concern in management of hypertension.

First, are there treatment regimens that successfully lower blood pressure in the elderly to normal ranges? Does lowering blood pressure lead to a reduction in morbidity and mortality risks? For many reasons, lowering blood pressure does not necessarily lower an individual's risk of poor health outcomes. Especially in older people, current hypertension may represent an *accumulation* of decades of exposure to high blood pressure. It may also be that hypertension is not causally linked to cardiovascular complications but represents a similar endpoint, and both are caused by some underlying pathologic process. Second, are the treatment methods available acceptable to elderly people? Does the management of hypertension have other serious side-effects, making the risks of management outweigh the benefits? Since elderly people frequently do not tolerate pharmacologic agents as well as younger people, and since drug therapy is the most common approach to hypertension, this is a serious issue. Third, can optimal management approaches be successfully implemented on a national scale across diverse populations of elderly and of medical practitioners?

Does Treatment Lower Blood Pressure and Reduce Complications?

Several investigators have addressed the issue of whether pharmocologic treatment of hypertension is effective in the elderly. The most recent and convincing of these studies is the Hypertension Detection and Follow-Up Program (HDFP), conducted on 2376 men and women age 60–69 at entry. The evidence from this study indicates that elderly people who received aggressive and systematic treatment in stepped care (SC), rather than referred care (RC), experienced a 16.4% reduction in 5-year mortality after entry into the study.[35] The 5-year incidence of fatal and nonfatal stroke was reduced by 45.5% (5.5/100 vs. 3.0/100) in this group.[36] The difference in diastolic blood pressure for the SC group versus the RC group ranged from 5.1 to 7.7 mm Hg. Thus, this study shows that blood pressure can be substantially lowered in an older age group, with resultant drops in overall and stroke mortality. As HDFP investigators have pointed out, the reduction in risk in the SC group is remarkable considering the fact that the HDFP was not a classical clinical trial of active drug therapy versus placebo. Instead, the trial compared the morbidity and mortality outcomes in a population treated with blood-pressure medication prescribed in a timed, stepwise protocol (SC) to a similar population treated by a variety of community care resources (RC). The investigators also note that many of the community resources were effective, although about 20% more of the older people in SC achieved the HDFP goal diastolic blood pressure as compared to the RC group.

Other small and less well-controlled trials also support the contention that lowering blood pressure in hypertensive elderly people has beneficial effects in terms of reducing cardiovascular disease, particularly congestive heart failure, and cerebrovascular disease, although the evidence is mixed with regard to changes in the rate of myocardial infarction.[37,38] Radin and Black's helpful and balanced review of this literature[33] shows that while the weight of the evidence clearly falls on the side of treatment, there are ambiguous areas where further research is needed and in some cases is currently underway: First, there are currently no reports of completed clinical trials indicating the efficacy of therapy in isolated systolic hypertension but there is a large multicenter trial, Systolic Hypertension Project in the Elderly, in progress. Such studies are essential since most findings indicate that isolated systolic hypertension in the elderly is as important a risk factor for all-cause mortality as other types of hypertension.[30,39–42] Second, the effect of antihypertensive therapy in patients with a prior stroke is less certain than the benefit for those without a prior stroke.

Are There Serious Side-Effects to Pharmacologic Therapy?

Many investigators and clinicians have expressed concern that treating hypertension in elderly persons with existing cerebrovascular disease may precipitate cerebral infarctions; others are similarly concerned that the benefits of treatment may be outweighed by less life-threatening, yet still considerable, side-effects. Many side-effects, such as changes in affect and cognitive function, have been poorly defined. Because elderly people are generally more vulnerable to the toxic effects of drugs than younger people are, and since elderly people may be taking other medications regularly, it is logical to approach the pharmacologic management of elderly hypertensives cautiously. Although antihypertensives vary widely in their effects, generally they should be used to reduce pressure slowly, since rapid and severe reductions in blood pressure bring about many adverse effects.[33] Interactions of antihypertensives with other drugs, in some cases not prescribed by the same physician, must be monitored.

Problems associated with the use of drugs suggest that attempts to control and to reduce blood pressure through nonpharmacologic approaches may be useful and acceptable to patients. Nonpharmacologic measures include diet modification, decreased salt intake, weight control, physical exercise, and stress reduction.[43] Although behavior modification is rarely attempted among the elderly and there are few data demonstrating subsequent reductions in morbidity and mortality, the time may be right to assess the effectiveness of this intervention in this population group.[44] There is as of yet little information on the acceptability of such therapies to the elderly.

Shapiro and Jacob[43] cogently argue that "the asymptomatic nature of hypertension, its relative mildness in the majority of patients, the slowness of the development of target organ damage, the reluctance of patients and providers to take or give potentially harmful, or at least inconvenient, medications, and the multifaceted nature of the ailment that requires simultaneous or consecutive treatment of different types, all constitute adequate reasons for studying and using nonpharmacologic therapies." The nonpharmacologic methods might be used as adjuncts to other methods or as first steps in the treatment process that can delay the use of drugs if goals are achieved. While most clinicians agree that a carefully monitored SC drug therapy protocol should be beneficial for the elderly hypertensives, it is not without its risk in terms of troublesome side-effects, such as weakness, depression, postural hypotension, and the risk of serious disease, especially precipitation of congestive heart failure and angina. Behavior-oriented approaches have the advantage of being safe, free of side-effects, and probably cheaper than drug therapy, although they may require a significant amount of the health-care team's time for implementation.

Can Optimal Management Approaches Be Implemented on a National Scale?

Pharmacologic and nonpharmacologic treatments are available for optimal management of elderly hypertensives. All the evidence indicates that these treatments have a very beneficial effect on patients and that the benefits outweigh the associated risks. In this sense, the medical community has been successful in treating a very common disorder. On the other hand, the HDFP experience indicates that there is room for improvement in the community, since the HDFP SC group achieved significantly better results than the RC group. Several factors may stand in the way of the general practitioner's successful treatment of the elderly person with hypertension: 1) a belief that older people tolerate hypertension well and that it may even be beneficial for them to have somewhat higher levels than younger people; 2) lack of knowledge concerning the most appropriate ways to achieve blood pressure control or reluctance to undertake complete programs requiring the use of several drugs and the close monitoring of their effects; 3) a general tendency to avoid methods of control in treating most patients, coupled with a belief that such methods are especially inappropriate for older adults. Since behavior modification is often difficult to achieve and requires special training of the provider, it is again not surprising that such treatments tax the art of the primary care physician.

It is possible that these three impediments to successful treatment can be remedied by educating the medical community in the most up-to-date pharmacologic treatment and its effects. Allocation of resources within medical institutions for training both physicians and other health-care providers in nonpharmacologic methods of treatment would also enhance average practice patterns. Although optimal methods of treating elderly hypertensives will continue to change, particularly in those with isolated systolic hypertension, great progress can be made through the widespread implementation of the best methods already available.

Observations and Conclusions

The elderly can derive measurable benefits from traditional medical care. Even for the old-old, life extension (e.g., treatment of hypertension), and life enhancement (lens implant and hip prostheses) are possible. However, there are limitations to existing knowledge about medical care and to traditional approaches to treatment.

Benefits of Care

Technological advances have had a striking effect on the care of the elderly. Neither lens implantation nor prosthetic hip replacement was commonly performed a decade ago; both procedures are now widely used, and both offer marked improvements over earlier treatment methods. Both methods also offer promise of further development in related areas, such as the use of prostheses to replace joints other than the hip. Each of these procedures enhances independence and reduces disability; a prosthetic hip may not eliminate a patient's need for social and supportive services, but it will often reduce the nature and intensity of that need.

Projections for the future suggest that the contributions of technological development to the care of the elderly will continue and accelerate. Affordable mechanical devices that read printed text to the blind or display the spoken word to the deaf are only two examples of the kinds of technology that will continue to make independent living more feasible for the disabled. What is needed, then, is neither an uncritical acceptance of all technological advances nor a complaisant dependence on human helpers, but instead a careful balancing of the most advanced medical care with appropriate supportive services. In particular, critics of medical care must learn to distinguish between high technology with little or no return, such as the overuse of life support in the dying patient, and high technology that offers, as these two procedures do, increased independence and improved function.

Limitations of Knowledge

There are some basic problems in the medical literature. Within the field of surgery, the morbidity and mortality of commonly performed procedures are much better known than their benefits. "Soft" results, such as improvements in function, tend to be described anecdotally rather than measured with precision. Patient satisfaction, which is really the ultimate test of any life-enhancing procedure, is rarely measured. Satisfaction was not measured in any of the ophthalmologic studies reviewed, despite the fact that enhanced satisfaction is the only reason to accept the excess risk associated with lens implant. The need to better evaluate the outcomes of common procedures has been argued for some years by authors interested in the patterns of surgical practice.[45] However, the outcomes measured need to be the right ones.

Despite its limitations, the surgical literature does often record the gross outcomes of common practice. A variety of large data sets are now available that include standardized information from all hospital-discharge abstracts for a specific area or a specific set of patients. Since the hospital-discharge data set includes major surgical procedures, associated diagnoses (including diagnoses attributable to complications), length of stay, and whether a given patient was discharged alive, calculations of average mortality as well as calculations of some morbidity measures are possible. The resulting reports provide a reasonable estimate of the expected mortality and length of stay for a procedure performed by a surgeon of average competence at an average hospital. This information provides a standard against which a local hospital's or physician's practice can be judged.

The medical literature, in contrast, tells much about the results of "ideal" practice and very little about the results of common practice. A careful literature review provides a good estimate of how both diabetes and hypertension ought to be treated, but, with the exception of the HDFP, which used community practice as a control, there are no hints about how a patient would fare in the office of an internist or family practitioner of average competence. Without this information, clinicians have no real standard against which to judge themselves or their colleagues. Without information on common treatment methods, complications, or treatment failures, they cannot even decide whether patients are receiving appropriate care.

A corollary to this lack of office practice information is the lack of population-based information about whether patients with conditions like those described here are receiving any effective treatment at all. The growing evidence of benefits derived from the treatment of hypertension, even in very old patients, contradicts the old clinical precept that the elderly tolerate hypertension well and should not be treated for mild elevations. In their review articles and the advice given to general practitioners, experts in hypertension clearly articulate their belief that the condition is frequently undertreated, particularly in the very old. However, no firm data exist on the size of the problem or on recent trends in practice patterns, so little can be deduced about how serious the problem is and how much physician re-education is warranted. Population-based studies of the care that the average patient receives in the average office are a badly needed element in any attempt to improve office care or the links between patient and office.

Limitations of Treatment Methods

The literature on the two nonsurgical conditions reviewed here illustrate another serious problem in current patterns of practice. Both diabetes and hypertension are "lifestyle" diseases in which genetic factors interact with controllable aspects of daily life, such as eating habits, smoking, exercise patterns, and stress. Physicians have never been enthusiastic about prescribing a change in behavior before they prescribe a medication. Judging from the literature, they are even less willing to do so in the care of the elderly, who are perceived as rigid or inflexible (i.e., "set in their ways"). The few modest trials of stress reduction in hypertension, for example, have focused largely on younger patients.

However, because the elderly are so vulnerable to the complications of drug treatment, physicians *should* focus on changing the behavior of their elderly patients. In fact, retirement, with the associated increase in leisure and the resulting freedom from job-site influences, may make behavior change easier for the elderly than the majority of professionals believe.

A case in point is the successful low-salt, low-cholesterol cookbook recently published by Craig Claiborne, a leading food writer.[46] In his preface, the author, in his sixties at the time, recounts the advice he received from a physician regarding the need to eliminate salt and cholesterol from his diet. He then describes both his old and new eating habits in some detail before proceeding to present a series of varied and attractive recipes that suit the diet. Mr. Claiborne recounts the initial consultation with his physician. The doctor offered little in the way of specific suggestions other than noting that the patient might indulge himself (within reason) "on occasion," and might be permitted alcohol in moderation. Weight loss and increased exercise were also prescribed, although, even secondhand, one has the sense that the physician was not overly optimistic about the ability of an obese food writer whose income was dependent on dining out and testing recipes to change his eating patterns.

The patient in this case took the challenge seriously, and he set about learning how to change his habits without abandoning his interest in food. The book is filled with the kind of detail essential to a successful alteration in diet: the flavors that make sodium reduction less noticeable, the change in taste sensation that results when overall salt is markedly reduced, the benefits of using fresh produce. The conclusions to be drawn are that older patients can change and that they can do so even when there are compelling reasons to make change unlikely. The lesson to professionals is that change must be individual and must reflect the patient's own needs and interest. If Craig Claiborne can lose 20 pounds, lower his blood pressure, and still make money on cookbooks by developing low-salt chili con carne, then perhaps a more sympathetic and responsive approach from professionals can help others to achieve the same health goals. A research focus on effective methods of behavior change could do much to provide elderly patients with treatments that carry the lowest possible risk.

The Conclusions for Practice

In the last analysis, the most important conclusion to be drawn is simple: the care of the elderly is mainstream medicine. The elderly benefit from techniques employed by a variety of specialists, orthopedists, and ophthalmologists, as well as internists and family practitioners. The benefits to be derived from care depend on technological advances and will continue to do so in the future. Evidence presented elsewhere in this volume also shows that the elderly visit doctors frequently and avail themselves of new techniques like those described in this chapter. System "reform," therefore, should focus on improvements in identified weak areas in practice, rather than on developing entirely new ways to deliver medical care. Needed improvements include better attention to personal outcomes, especially satisfaction; more research on behavior modification and, in particular, more efforts in understanding how, and in what circumstances, the elderly can modify their behavior; and more research on actual practice patterns, especially in nonsurgical areas. Modern medicine has many benefits to offer the elderly patient, benefits that are sometimes overlooked when medicine's very real limitations are too strongly emphasized.

References

1. Dabezies, O. H., Jr. 1979. Defects of vision through aphakic spectacle lenses. *Ophthalmology* 86:352–379.
2. Henkind, P. 1983. No pun intended, intraocular lenses are in. Editorial. *Ophthalmology* 90:27A–28A.
3. Leske, C. M., Sperduto, R. D. 1983. The epidemiology of senile cataracts: A review. *Am J Epidemiol* 118:152–165.
4. Kini, M. M., Leibowitz, H. M., Colton, T., Nickerson, R. J., Ganley, J., Dawber, T. R. 1978. Prevalence of senile cataract, diabetic retinopathy, senile macular degradation, and open-angle glaucoma in the Framingham eye study. *Am J Ophthalmol* 85:28–34.

5. Stark, W. J., Worthen, D. M., Holladay, J. T., Bath, P. E., Jacobs, M. E.,
    Murray, G. C., McGhee, E. T., Talbott, M. W., Shipp, M. D., Thomas, N. E.,
    Barnes, R. W., Brown, D. W. C., Buxton, J. N., Reinecke, R. D., Lao, C-S.,
    Fisher, S. 1983. The FDA report on intraocular lenses. *Ophthalmology* 90:311–
    317.
6. Taylor, J. M. 1981. Medicare payments and changes in the rate of cataract
    extraction. *Ophthalmology* 88:41A–46A.
7. Jaffee, N. S. 1983. The way things were and are: Changing indications for
    intraocular lens implantation. *Ophthalmology* 90:318–320.
8. Jaffee, N. S. 1981. The current status of intraocular lens implant surgery. *Mt
    Sinai J Med* 48:539–542.
9. Total hip-joint replacement in the United States. *JAMA* 248:1817–1821.
10. Beckenbaugh, R. D., Ilstrup, D. M. 1978. Total hip arthroplasty. *J Bone Joint
    Surg* 60-A:306–313.
11. Total hip-joint replacement in Sweden. *JAMA* 248:1822–1824.
12. Langan, P., Weiss, C. A. 1981. Hip rating scales: A clinical analysis. *Int Surg*
    66:331–333.
13. Williams, F. T. 1981. Diabetes mellitus. *Clin Endocrinol Metab* 10:179–194.
14. West, K. M. 1975. Substantial differences in the diagnostic criteria used by
    diabetes experts. *Diabetes* 24:641–644.
15. National Diabetes Data Group. 1979. Classification and diagnosis of diabetes
    mellitus and other categories of glucose intolerance. *Diabetes* 28:1039–1057.
16. World Health Organization. 1980. *WHO Expert Committee on Diabetes
    Mellitus. Second Report.* Technical Report Series 646. Geneva, Switzerland:
    World Health Organization.
17. Davidson, M. B. 1981. The continually changing 'natural history' of diabetes
    mellitus. *J Chronic Dis* 34:5–10.
18. Knowles, H. C., Meinert, C. L., Prout, T. E. 1976. Diabetes mellitus: The
    overall problem and its impact on the public. In *Diabetes Mellitus*, ed. S. S.
    Fajans, 11–32. HEW Pub. No. (NIH) 76–854. Washington, D.C.: Govern-
    ment Printing Office.
19. Melton, L. J., Palumbo, P. J., Dwyer, M. S., Chu, C-P. 1983. Impact of recent
    changes in diagnostic criteria on the apparent natural history of diabetes
    mellitus. *Am J Epidemiol* 117:559–565.
20. Agner, E., Thorsteinsson, B., Eriksen, M. 1982. Impaired glucose tolerance
    and diabetes mellitus in elderly subjects. *Diabetes Care* 5:600–604.
21. Kannel, W. B., McGee, D. L. 1979. Diabetes and cardiovascular disease. The
    Framingham study. *JAMA* 241:2035–2038.
22. Cahill, G. F., Etzwiler, D. D., Freinkel, N. 1976. 'Control' and diabetes. *N
    Engl J Med* 294:1004.
23. Siperstein, M. D., Foster, D. W., Knowles, H. C., Jr., Levine, R., Madison,
    L. L., Roth, J. 1977. Control of blood glucose and diabetic vascular disease. *N
    Engl J Med* 296:1060–1063.
24. Ingelfinger, F. J. 1977. Debate on diabetes. Editorial. *N Engl J Med* 296:1228–
    1229.
25. Brownlee, M., Cerami, A. 1981. The biochemistry of the complications of
    diabetes mellitus. *Annu Rev Biochem* 50:385–432.

26. University Group Diabetes Program. 1982. Effects of hypoglycemic agents on vascular complications in patients with adult-onset diabetes. VIII. Evaluation of insulin therapy: Final report. *Diabetes* 31(Suppl. 5):1–81.
27. Ostfeld, A. M. 1978. Elderly hypertensive patient: Epidemiologic review. *NY State J Med* 78:1125–1129.
28. Kannel, W. B., Gordon, T. 1978. Evaluation of cardiovascular risk in the elderly: The Framingham study. *Bull NY Acad Med* 54:573–591.
29. Ostfeld, A. M., Shekelle, R. B., Tufo, H. M., Wieland, A. M., Kilbridge, J. A., Drori, J., Klawans, H. 1971. Cardiovascular and cerebrovascular disease in an elderly poor urban population. *Am J Public Health* 61:19–29.
30. Colandrea, M. A., Friedman, G. D., Nichaman, M. Z., Lynd, C. N. 1970. Systolic hypertension in the elderly: An epidemiologic assessment. *Circulation* 41:239–245.
31. Kannel, W. B., Wolf, P. A., Verter, J., McNamara, P. M. 1970. Epidemiologic assessment of the role of blood pressure in stroke: The Framingham study. *JAMA* 214:301–310.
32. Shekelle, R. B., Ostfeld, A. M., Klawans, H. L. 1974. Hypertension and risk of stroke in an elderly population. *Stroke* 5:71–75.
33. Radin, A. M., Black, H. R. 1981. Hypertension in the elderly: The time has come to treat. *J Am Geriatr Soc* 29:193–200.
34. Radin, A. M. 1983. Hypertension in the elderly. *Primary Care* 10:135–139.
35. Hypertension Detection and Follow-Up Program Cooperative Group. 1979. Five-year findings of the hypertension detection and follow-up program. II. Mortality by race, sex and age. *JAMA* 242:2572–2577.
36. Hypertension Detection and Follow-Up Program Cooperative Group. 1982. Five-year findings of the hypertension detection and follow-up program. III. Reduction in stroke incidence among persons with high blood pressure. *JAMA* 247:633–638.
37. Veterans' Administration Cooperative Study Group on Antihypertensive Agents. 1972. Effects of treatment on morbidity in hypertension. III. Influence of age, diastolic pressure, and prior cardiovascular disease: Further analysis of side effects. *Circulation* 45:991–1004.
38. Hypertension-Stroke Cooperative Study Group. 1974. Effect of antihypertensive treatment on stroke recurrence. *JAMA* 229:409–418.
39. Garland, C., Barrett-Connor, E., Suarez, L., Criqui, M. H. 1983. Isolated systolic hypertension and mortality after age 60 years: A prospective population-based study. *Am J Epidemiol* 118:365–376.
40. Kannel, W. B. 1981. Implications of the Framingham study data for treatment of hypertension: Impact of other risk factors. In *Frontiers in Hypertension Research*, ed. J. H. Laragh, F. R. Buhler and D. W. Seldin, 17–21. New York: Springer-Verlag.
41. Ostfeld, A. M., Shekelle, R. B., Klawans, H., Tufo, H. M. 1974. Epidemiology of stroke in an elderly welfare population. *Am J Public Health* 64:450–458.
42. *Blood Pressure Study 1979*. 1980. Chicago, Ill.: Society of Actuaries and Association of Life Insurance Medical Directors of America.
43. Shapiro, A. P., Jacob, R. G. 1983. Nonpharmacologic approaches to the treatment of hypertension. *Annu Rev Public Health* 4:285–310.

44. Black, H. R. 1979. Nonpharmacologic therapy of hypertension. *Am J Med* 66:837–842.
45. Wennberg, J. E. 1984. Dealing with medical practice variations: A proposal for action. *Health Aff* 3:6–32.
46. Claiborne, C., Franey, P. 1980. *Craig Claiborne's Gourmet Diet.* New York: Times Books.

Nineteen

Alcoholism among the Elderly

Philip W. Brickner and Linda K. Scharer

The problem of alcoholism among the elderly requires special consideration. It is a poorly understood, pernicious, unappreciated—and treatable—disorder.

The Extent of the Problem

The prevalence of alcoholism in elderly people is not known. Our best
evidence indicates that problems with alcohol affect about 1.6 million
people among the 20 million individuals aged 65 and older living in the
United States.[1] A frequently cited figure for the prevalence of alcoholism
among older people is 2–10%, information based on a community survey,
circa 1965, limited to males in New York City.[2] Although this information
is more than 25 years old, it appears to remain valid and is supported by
more recent analyses.[3]

Efforts to understand the background of the problem tend to increase the
uncertainty about its prevalence. For instance, broad studies have indicated that, starting at about age 50, people begin to drink less.[4] The
explanations[5] for this finding may include the following:

1. Faulty sampling. Older people surveyed may understate their drinking, as a result of deliberate or unconscious denial, or there may be a
   bias in research technique.

2. Alcoholism may be a self-limiting disease. People who drink heavily early in life tend to die early. Estimates[6] indicate that drinkers lose 10–15 years of life expectancy compared to nondrinkers. Studies of Skid Row men reveal that those who began drinking relatively late in life are few. Bahr[7] interviewed 94 Bowery men and found that a mere 7% began heavy drinking after age 45. However, one study[4] suggests with irony that after heavy drinkers, abstainers are statistically the next to die, and that moderate drinkers live longer.

3. People may, in fact, actually drink less as they get older. One explanation may lie in the "wisdom of the body." With the same alcohol intake, older persons develop higher blood alcohol levels than do younger people,[8–11] as a result of age changes in body composition. Older people may therefore sense that less is enough. Furthermore, difficulties in speech, locomotion, and equilibrium may be more disturbing to older people, and the effects of alcohol, such as feeling high, euphoria, and uninhibited behavior, may be less attractive than when they were younger. Concerns about the consequences may result in a deliberate attempt to decrease alcohol intake. Also, the social atmosphere that previously encouraged drinking may no longer be available. Drinking could be a consequence of stress, which, according to Kenneth Weiss,[12] is based on drives for territory, mates, and competition within the species, concerns that decrease with age in humans.

4. Women are the majority among older people[13] and are less likely than men to be heavy drinkers.

5. Death certificates may inaccurately state the cause of death to save the surviving family members from social stigma.[13]

Three groups can be identified among elderly heavy drinkers: 1) The few survivors of many years of heavy drinking, often people who have alienated their family and friends, have medical problems as a result of drinking, and are likely to be identified through community surveys rather than through their own efforts to seek help. 2) Intermittent heavy drinkers, individuals who have consistently lapsed throughout adult life in response to stress. 3) Reactive problem drinkers, who managed to cope earlier in life but start drinking under the pressures of advancing age. Accounting for this group leads to certain contradictions. If, for instance, retirement can be considered a cause of drinking, it also appears to be a cause of abstinence. Since heavy drinking decreases markedly at about age 65,[4] equal numbers of people probably stop drinking because of job loss as start drinking.

Causes of Drinking in Older People

Why do people drink? This question remains unresolved in alcoholism research. One view holds that alcoholism is a disease that results from the chemical nature of alcohol, combined perhaps with a genetic predisposition and the individual's nature or personality.[5] Others stress the social and cultural background of the drinker, placing emphasis on life circumstances.

Why do *old* people drink? Many older people must bear loneliness, isolation, alienation, and lack of self-esteem.

Certain subgroups of the elderly are estimated to have high rates of alcoholism.[14–17] These include individuals in trouble with the police, widowers, people with medical problems, the brain-damaged, those who are hospitalized, and residents of long-term care institutions. Other than for the latter group, prevalence rates are not known.

People in nursing homes, in general, fulfill the criteria for alcoholism at a rate of about 20%.[14] It is particularly noteworthy that studies of nursing homes in the Midwest[15] show that the proportion of residents with alcohol problems is in the range of 40–60%.

For people faced with life in an institution, Robert Butler's phrase "houses of death," describing nursing homes,[18] perhaps makes the point. For some of the elderly, drinking may be seen as one of life's few remaining joys, an act that makes life bearable when all personal control is removed. A heavy-drinking patient in a project for the homebound aged, the Chelsea-Village Program in New York City, responded to remonstration by saying: "I'm trying to think of something else I can do which will give me any pleasure in life."

Establishing the Diagnosis in the Elderly

It is a general truth that older people do not exhibit the classical features of addictive alcoholism because of their decreased ability to metabolize the drug.[19] As a result, their presenting behaviors differ from those of younger drinkers. Older people are more likely to demonstrate a problem through a combination of physical, mental, and social symptoms: self-neglect,[20] falls leading to fractures, confusion, and behavior that leads to family quarrels.[21]

The major criteria for diagnosis of alcoholism established by the National Council on Alcoholism[22] are often poorly applicable to older people. They include:

- Drinking a fifth of whiskey per day, or its equivalent in wine/beer, for a 180-pound person
- Alcoholic "blackouts"

- Withdrawal syndromes: gross tremors, hallucinosis, convulsions, delirium tremens (DTs)
- Blood alcohol level >150 mg/100 ml without the appearance of intoxication
- Continued drinking despite medical advice
- Family and/or job problems caused by drinking.

Psychiatric terminology, as used in DSM-III,[23] is equally inapplicable to older people. For alcohol dependence (alcoholism) to be established as a diagnosis, DSM-III requires the presence of both a pattern of pathological alcohol use or alcohol-related impairment in social or occupational functioning, and signs of either tolerance or withdrawal. However, most older alcoholics have no opportunity for occupational malfunction because they are no longer employed; many are not evident social misfits because they are isolated; and many older people who start drinking late in life cannot ingest enough to develop tolerance.

Perhaps the most useful approach to defining problem drinking in older people requires discrimination between the expected consequences of normal aging and the problems that arise from excessive drinking in later years.[15,24] A sensible definition of alcoholism among the elderly should be pragmatic and take into account physical and psychological addiction, societal norms, genetic and racial factors, and social problems.[6]

Barriers to Diagnosis

Problems in diagnosis constitute perhaps the greatest barrier to effective treatment of older alcoholics. Older drinkers do not fit the alcoholic stereotype and thus may escape recognition.

The diagnostic effort is complicated further because many older people avoid contact with agencies that care for alcoholics, break off relations with caregivers before the diagnosis is established, or receive treatment for other conditions while their problem with alcoholism remains undetected.[25]

The issue is sometimes clarified when patients are hospitalized and their alcohol intake suddenly drops. The ensuing withdrawal symptoms can provide the basis for diagnosis.[26] Among other clues for the recognition of alcoholism among the elderly, beyond the obvious discovery of empty bottles under the bed, are unexplained depression, a change in sexual performance or interest (impotence), confused states, staggering, falling, injuries, loss of appetite or decreased interest in food, an attack of gout, or agitation, anxiety, and insomnia.

Mixed Etiologies

The tendency to neglect alcoholism as part of a differential diagnosis is compounded by the fact that behavior that would identify alcoholism in younger people may be passed off in the elderly as eccentricity. Problems caused by alcohol abuse blend into pathological states that arise from the sociological or physical consequences of aging. The interconnections between alcohol and depression, the use of multiple medications, and the stresses of late life cloud diagnostic efforts.

As people age, nutritional demands for maintenance of optimal health decrease. People at age 70 generally require only 70% of the calories that 46-year-olds need. Any excess is stored as fat. As the percent of body fat rises[27] in older people, lean body mass decreases, as do intra- and extracellular body water and bone mass. As a result of these changes, old people have decreased reserves of sodium, potassium, magnesium, calcium, and phosphorus. Nevertheless, the normal aging body functions adequately, although at reduced physiologic capacity. However, the ability to adapt is diminished if chronic disease is superimposed, alcohol is used, or multiple therapeutic drugs are taken, and a cycle of disastrous deterioration can follow.[28]

Alcohol interacts with a variety of sedative and hypnotic drugs and decreases the threshold at which effects occur. It is likely that an older person who drinks alcohol unwisely, and develops an unexpectedly high blood level, will be harmed by concomitant use of barbiturates, benzodiazepines, or chloral hydrate. It is noteworthy that, of the 100 most frequently prescribed drugs, more than half contain an ingredient known to act adversely with alcohol.[29] Since it appears that women use tranquilizers and other psychoactive drugs more than men do,[19] a pattern that continues into advanced age, women are probably at greater risk.[30]

Alcohol abuse harms the central nervous system, a subject that demands special emphasis. Neuropathologic changes in the brain characteristic of chronic alcoholism combine with those of advancing age additively. A frequent result in older drinkers is loss of neurons beyond the threshold of the reserve capacity inherent in all major organs and the consequent failure of intellectual and other brain functions.

Insults to the brain may follow as secondary effects of chronic alcoholism. These include poor nutrition, head injury, traumatic epilepsy, alcoholic confusional states, and delirium tremens. The accelerated decline of cerebral function is not difficult to predict. The cognitive deficits that result include decreased short-term memory, lessened capacity for abstract thinking, hampered ability to carry out complex tasks requiring memory, and disordered visual-spatial relationships.[31,32]

A major concern is the need to distinguish between alcoholism and dementia. Memory loss is often a presenting complaint of older patients. Diagnostic difficulty arises because alcohol abuse is one of many potential causes of memory deficit. Alcohol may cause confusion in older patients who do not appear to be drunk because of the development of tolerance to the drug if they have been drinking for many years, and most dementias in their early stages fluctuate in degree of expression. A pernicious cycle may arise in these situations. Alcohol, ingested to relieve feelings of anxiety caused by memory loss, aggravates the very problem for which it is used. The steps from early dementia of any origin to anxiety and depression and then to drinking are understandable.[33] It is therefore mandatory to consider alcohol abuse as a possible underlying or contributing factor in any older patient who presents with dementia.[34]

In any analysis of these matters, we must recognize that alcohol–aging interactions are putative, not proved. For example, in the various technical studies, nutritional controls are largely absent. Therefore, the distinct actions of alcohol or aging are not easily distinguished when measured against poor nutrition, debility, or concurrent illness.

Treatment

In the sense that each person has his or her own developmental history, so does each generation. Recognition of this cohort effect is essential to an understanding of each older patient's background and has direct implications for individual and group treatment. Furthermore, the cohort effect complicates considerably plans for therapeutic approaches toward alcoholism in the elderly, now and in the future, as do racial, ethnic, and genetic factors.

We must also relate the attitudes of health workers to this complex of biological, social, and societal issues. According to Mishara and Kastenbaum:

> The culturally rooted aversion among mental and public health personnel in general toward devoting themselves to care of the aged does not yield simply and automatically to the call for action, nor should it be expected that geriatricians would readily overcome their resistances to working with alcohol-related problems.[5]

In general, agency personnel in alcoholism programs express a low level of concern about older drinkers.[35] Most organizations focus upon younger alcoholics in trouble with employers, the legal system, or the family. In Alcoholics Anonymous (AA), the preeminent treatment program in the country, only 3% of enrollees are people over 65.[36]

The harmful effects of therapeutic nihilism pervade the field of alcoholism and treatment.[37] As DiClemente and Gordon point out, "The assumption seems to be that children grow, develop and change but that adults only grow older. How much does this pessimistic view color our stereotype of the elderly as either unable to change or too old to have valuable treatment resources wasted on them?"[38]

Goals

The available information suggests abstinence to be a wise and prudent goal for older alcohol abusers.[39] With this in mind, in certain programs it has been shown that almost twice as many patients over age 60 complete the course of treatment as those younger.[40] One explanation offered for this finding is that people who develop alcoholism when they are older have fewer major psychiatric disorders than long-term drinkers.[41]

A major test of success for any treatment program lies in finding the people at risk. Alcoholism, in general, is underreported. As Edith Gomberg[3] notes, "It is estimated that *all* facilities dealing with alcoholism: clinics, hospitals, Alcoholics Anonymous, et cetera, see only about 10% of alcoholics in the United States." The driving force behind the call for help is frequently physical distress or the concern of family members.

Older drinkers are more elusive and less apparent than others. The reasons for this, which directly concern case finding and treatment efforts, include:

- Denial.
- The need to lie, in writing, in order to be accepted by long-term facilities, such as nursing homes.
- Attitudes of agency personnel. Older people rarely fit into treatment categories where successful outcomes, such as return to work, can be demonstrated, so staff members are more easily discouraged about them.
- Problems with transportation and finances, which limit the ability of older people to seek treatment.
- The need to include therapy of other medical illness as part of the plan, a resource often missing in alcoholism programs.
- The paucity of programs directed specifically to the needs of older drinkers.

Therapeutic planning for older alcoholics must incorporate areas of special vulnerability: states of physical and mental health, coordination of tasks, social services needs, and vocational and avocational concerns. Treatment principles must include, as well, the following components:

- Confrontation.

- Clear and transmittable views about abstinence as a measure of success. There are inevitable disputes about this point. AA perceives abstinence as the only goal, without particular concern for other aspects of life. Other efforts seek abstinence but require additional improvements as well. A third view looks basically for life enhancement without the need for abstinence.

- Detoxification, often in the hospital. Close observation is needed to control withdrawal symptoms, which may be particularly hazardous in the elderly.

- Recognition of the risks associated with the use of central nervous system depressant drugs in the detoxification process.

- Rehabilitation and education that include both patient and family.

- Long-term therapeutic contact, individually or in groups; consideration of the involvement of patients with AA.

Methods

Current treatment approaches include the strictly medical, such as drug therapy, social and/or group work, and mixtures of the two.

The logic behind the pharmacological approach to treatment is the assumption that alcoholics suffer from a general state of dysphoria, with anxiety and depression. Since people use alcohol to relieve or suppress their feelings, psychotherapeutic drugs can replace alcohol for this purpose. However, evidence for the efficacy of this approach is lacking. Furthermore, this mode of treatment causes special risks in older people.

The effects of Antabuse (disulfuram), which has been a successful inhibitory treatment for some patients, are completely distinct from tranquilizers and hypnotics. When taken regularly, Antabuse produces a reaction to alcohol that starts with feelings of heat and flushing of the face and body, proceeds to tachycardia with the sensation of palpitation, shortness of breath, and the need to hyperventilate, and culminates in nausea and vomiting.[8] Because of these severe physical effects, Antabuse programs are unwise for older people, whose health may already be marginal.

In psychosocial therapies, the principal approaches to treatment are guidance and counseling. It seems clear that many older alcoholics benefit from a supportive social network in which other people are engaged to help at each stage of treatment and recovery.[42]

Family therapy may be especially useful for older drinkers. It answers the need for social support and works toward resolving isolation and loneliness. In contrast, leaving the family out of the treatment program serves to reinforce disengagement and alienation between patient and relatives.

Individual psychotherapy addresses the patient's main defense mechanism, denial.[33] It may be foolish to pursue this approach in people of advanced age, and psychotherapists in general seem to recognize its lack of pertinence in the elderly. They are often reluctant to accept older alcoholics as patients.

Group therapy, on the other hand, has proven its value.[43] In groups of alcoholics, "the sharing of experiences by similarly afflicted persons promotes the development of meaningful insight."[33] Group work has a secondary value as well. It creates a new social network for its members and relieves the boredom and sense of abandonment that may have led initially to alcohol abuse.

Institutional Programs

Detoxification in acute-care hospitals and psychiatric facilities will work. Then what? Older patients who wish to stay sober may engage in the variety of therapeutic approaches discussed above. However, for those people too frail for independent life, options are slim. Nursing homes tend to reject problem drinkers. They are perceived as unwelcome guests who cause management, health, and social problems. Administrators try to keep their institutions alcohol-free, but alcohol abuse remains a serious, often unrecognized, and untreated disorder in nursing homes.[44] Incarcerated patients may use great imagination to sustain their addiction—an aged amputee in a New York City home kept his bottle hidden in his prosthetic leg.[45]

Model Programs

The four programs discussed below were conceived and designed to address the specific needs of aged alcoholics. They are presented in order of most restrictive (inpatient care) to least restrictive (AA correspondence groups).

Memorial Hospital Medical Center-Chemical Dependency Unit (MHMC-CDU), Long Beach, California

MHMC-CDU is a three-week, two-part, inpatient milieu therapy program that recognizes and addresses the special needs of the older alcoholic. Phase I, detoxification and clearing, has an average duration of 10 to 14 days for the elderly alcoholic, approximately twice as long as for the younger abuser. Phase I may take as long as the full 21 days for an elderly alcoholic who is severely impaired.[46]

The cohort effect is acknowledged and incorporated into the treatment setting. Patients are grouped with their contemporaries and those who have progressed to Phase II visit their counterparts to offer encouragement, serve as models, and acknowledge their own accomplishments achieved on the road to recovery.

Patients proceed to Phase II, daily group therapy, lectures, and educational programs, when the medical care team has ascertained the completion of Phase I. The patient's family is brought in for this last week of treatment in preparation for their role in the patient's life after discharge.

Patients are encouraged to think about their new mode of life—of recovery—from the start. Discharge plans are discussed with a counselor in the social/psychological interview. The counselor selects significant factors from the patient's pretreatment life and redirects them within the treatment plan as reinforcement for the recovery process.

Both phases of the program are designed to restore the older patient's self-image and motivation to live. Emphasis is placed on the development of self-responsibility and autonomy through a support network. Family, friends, and neighbors, or even a volunteer from a senior citizens community program, are an integral part of MHMC-CPU's program and form the foundation for the patient's support network upon discharge from the hospital.[47]

Queen Nursing Home and Treatment Center, Minneapolis, Minnesota

Elderly alcoholics are specifically sought for admission to the Queen Nursing Home in Minneapolis. Until 1973, Queen was a typical long-term care facility, but the staff began to recognize that many residents were alcohol abusers, despite efforts to screen them out. "We were caring for people with a drinking problem anyway, but all we were doing was emptying bottles."[44]

Patients are referred from detoxification centers, hospitals, and occasionally the courts. The personnel include trained alcoholism counselors.

The Queen program begins with efforts to understand the particular problems affecting each patient. Many Queen patients arrive with no support network. Each patient is assigned a counselor who explains the program's policies on money, dress, medication, duration of stay, canteen privileges, room restrictions, and passes for time away from the home.

The patient spends three days under observation and behavior evaluation and then meets with a counselor to map out long- and short-term goals and make plans for group and occupational therapy assignments. The period of treatment typically lasts 3 to 6 months.

As the patient nears the discharge date, the counselor facilitates entry into an AA group and arranges for appropriate living quarters, perhaps with family members, in the patient's own apartment, in a halfway house, or in a general nursing home. It is the counselor's responsibility to arrange for adequate financial assistance. The counselor maintains active follow-up contact with the former patient and there is a Queen alumni group, which functions in much the same way as an AA group. "Their illness is alienation as much as it is alcoholism, and this combination requires a special effort of openness and giving from the staff if the lives of the older problem drinkers are to be made any easier."[44]

Therapeutic Community Care Homes, Winnipeg, Manitoba, Canada

Van de Vyvere, Hughes, and Fish studied types of housing situations frequently used by Winnipeg social service agencies in rehabilitation of elderly alcoholics. Arrangements included family care homes, which offered, in addition to room and board, a warm family environment conducive to maintaining sobriety, a downtown hotel managed by the resident owners, and a downtown boarding home. Certain characteristics were found in each of the settings and are believed to contribute to their success: The absence of an explicit rehabilitation orientation that equates "curing" the chronic elderly alcoholic with absolute sobriety; explicit controls on drinking, although not necessarily to the extent of prohibition; recognition and acceptance of the probability that residents may, from time to time, relapse into former drinking patterns; mechanisms for the restoration of the individual's self-esteem; and uncritical reacceptance of residents into the setting after relapses.

These are more lenient standards than those requiring strict sobriety for successful rehabilitation and may therefore fail to meet current government licensing and funding regulations. Nonetheless, the study recommends that similar housing options be developed as a resource for long-term rehabilitation of older alcoholics.[46]

Helping Hands Program, Long Beach, California

The Helping Hands Program was established as part of the MHMC-CDU (see above) in June, 1976, to help older recovering alcoholics break their cyclic return to the hospital for detoxification.

Any older alcoholic may join the Helping Hands Program, without charge, but referrals are made most frequently from the CDU program, other alcohol rehabilitation services, and senior centers throughout the local area. Groups meet twice a week for therapy and range in size from 14 to 24 persons.

The most important function of the program is the sharing of common aging and alcoholism-related problems, ways to stay sober, and the rewards of sobriety. "The discussion varies according to the make-up of the group but is basically a mixture of an AA Step Study approach, Women for Sobriety philosophy, and a cognitive approach in a peer group setting."[47]

As therapy progresses, patients gain confidence and eventually reach into the community to help others who are recovering from alcoholism. They learn to improve relations at home and become comfortable with people who are not alcoholics. Because participants may range in age from 50 to 90, the focus is on adjusting to life changes and not on old age itself.[47]

Alcoholics Anonymous

Alcoholics Anonymous uses group therapy as its therapeutic mode and is the most effective available resource for large numbers of alcoholics. AA brings together people in trouble and fosters a spirit of understanding and empathy. It encourages development of responsibility for others through one-to-one sponsorships, thereby enhancing feelings of self-worth. The only goal for AA members is abstinence. Excuses, explanations or rationalizations are not accepted.[49–51] AA welcomes all alcoholics, including the elderly, and many members are in mid-life.[50]

Although the elderly are traditionally not well represented at general AA meetings, Alcoholics Anonymous has begun to reach out to the elderly alcoholic. Groups have formed in retirement villages and community centers where the elderly gather. For the homebound, a correspondence program has been formed, and educational materials directed at those over 60 who want to stop drinking are available in large type. More than 125,000 copies were sent out in 1984 alone.[52]

Financing

There are two approaches to financing rehabilitation programs for the elderly alcoholic to make those programs more accessible to the target population: 1) Expansion of current eligibility requirements to include more programs, especially outpatient efforts and those not directly affiliated with a private practitioner or a hospital. 2) Changes in current programs to make them eligible for reimbursement.

Queen Nursing Home, for example, is licensed by the state of Minnesota as both a nursing home and as an alcoholism treatment center.[44] It is also a state-designated skilled nursing facility, which enables it to receive higher support payments for its welfare patients than it would receive as an ordinary nursing home. In addition, it receives payment from private insurance companies which offer alcoholism treatment coverage, a source of revenue expected to increase in the coming years.[53]

While institutional programs, like Queen, may pursue these sources of funding, the need for increased outpatient services demands revision of current reimbursement requirements. Consider:

- Medicare Part A covers alcoholism treatment, along with drug abuse and mental health, under the general category of psychiatric services, which has a lifetime ceiling of 190 inpatient days.

- Alcoholism treatment is not a federally mandated service under Medicaid and therefore falls to the states for coverage. However, many states have not allocated the funds necessary for alcoholism rehabilitation programs.

As a result, in order for necessary programs in this field to develop and thrive, changes in government reimbursement programs are necessary:

- Outpatient treatment programs should be made eligible for 80% Medicare reimbursement after deductible, as are surgical and medical treatments. This would increase utilization of outpatient programs, which are less costly than inpatient care.

- The National Institute on Alcohol Abuse and Alcoholism and the National Institute on Aging should provide grants to develop specialized treatment methods for the elderly.

- Medicaid statutes should be revised to include coverage for the treatment of alcoholism beyond hospital medical and physician-delivered services.

In the private sector:

- Insurance companies should offer expanded inpatient and outpatient alcoholism treatment coverage.

- Demonstration projects should receive funding from private foundations.

- Preretirement counseling should include alcoholism education.[53]

Conclusion

We need to recognize that the origins of alcohol abuse among the elderly are multiple and the consequences varied. Treatment is challenging. For our society to grapple effectively with this issue, a solid plan for action is required. This must include:

- Additional believable clinical studies that clarify the incidence of alcohol use/abuse in older people. Analysis of subgroups within the elderly is also needed.

- Based on this information, policies and programs must be developed that meet the needs of older alcohol users. These should include means for seeking out isolated older people, offering methods for bringing them to appropriate treatment settings, and providing educational forums for patients and their families.

• Means to reverse the spirit of therapeutic nihilism among workers in the alcohol field must be sought. This will be an educational process, to be carried out through professional school curricula, the literature, and other educational methods, such as conferences.

• Financing of program development should be sought through the existing major forms of insurance, such as Medicare, Medicaid, and Medigap coverage. In addition, for the necessary analytic studies, assistance should be obtained through grants from government agencies and foundations.

References

1. Schuckit, M. A. 1977. Geriatric alcoholism and drug abuse. *Gerontologist* 17(2):168–174.
2. Bailey, M. P., Haberman, P. W., Alksne, H. 1965. The epidemiology of alcoholism in an urban residential area. *Q J Stud Alcohol* 26:19–40.
3. Gomberg, E. L. 1980. *Drinking and Problem Drinking Among the Elderly.* Ann Arbor, Mich.: University of Michigan, Institute of Gerontology.
4. Cahalan, D., Cisin, H., Crossley, H. M. 1969. *American Drinking Practices.* New Brunswick, N.J.: Rutgers Center of Alcohol Studies.
5. Mishara, B. L., Kastenbaum, R. 1980. *Alcohol and Old Age.* New York: Grune and Stratton.
6. Schuckit, M. A., Pastor, P. A. 1978. The elderly as a unique population. *Alcohol Clin Exper Res* 2(1):31–38.
7. Bahr, H. M. 1969. Lifetime affiliation patterns of early and late-onset heavy drinkers on skid row. *Q J Stud Alcohol* 30(7):645–656.
8. Goldstein, D. B. 1983. *Pharmacology of Alcohol.* New York: Oxford University Press.
9. Garver, D. L. 1984. Age effects on alcohol metabolism. In *Alcoholism in the Elderly: Social and Biomedical Issues,* ed. J. T. Hartford and T. Samorajski. New York: Raven Press.
10. Vestal, R. E., McGuire, E. A., Tobin, J. D., Adres, R., Norris, A. H., Mezey, E. 1977. Aging and ethanol metabolism. *Clin Pharmacol Ther* 21(3):343–354.
11. Samorajski, T., Persson, K., Bissell, C., Brizzee, L., Lancaster, F., Brizzee, K. R. 1984. Biology of alcoholism and aging in rodents: Brain and liver. In *Alcoholism in the Elderly: Social and Biomedical Issues,* ed. J. T. Hartford and T. Samorajski. New York: Raven Press.
12. Weiss, K. M. 1984. The evolutionary basis of alcoholism: A question of the neocortex. In *Alcoholism in the Elderly: Social and Biomedical Issues,* ed. J. T. Hartford and T. Samorajski. New York: Raven Press.

13. Mayer, M. J. 1979. Alcohol and the elderly: A review. *Health Soc Work* 4(4):128–143.
14. Schuckit, M. A. 1982. A clinical review of alcohol, alcoholism, and the elderly patient. *J Clin Psychiatry* 43(10):396–399.
15. Blose, I. L. 1978. The relationship of alcohol to aging and the elderly. *Alcohol Clin Exp Res* 2(1):17–21.
16. Gomberg, E. S. 1975. Prevalence of alcoholism among ward patients in a Veterans' Administration hospital. *J Stud Alcohol* 36(11):1458–1467.
17. Corrigan, E. M. 1974. *Problem Drinkers Seeking Treatment.* New Brunswick, N.J.: Rutgers Center of Alcohol Studies.
18. Butler, R. A. 1975. *Why Survive?* New York: Harper and Row.
19. Seixas, F. A. 1978. Alcoholism in the elderly: Introduction. *Alcohol Clin Exp Res* 2(1):15.
20. Kafetz, K., Cox, M. 1982. Alcohol excess and the senile squalor syndrome. *J Am Geriatr Soc* 30(11):706.
21. Glatt, M. M. 1978. Experiences with elderly alcoholics in England. *Alcohol Clin Exp Res* 2(1):23–26.
22. National Council on Alcoholism, Criteria Committee. 1972. Criteria for the diagnosis of alcoholism. *Am J Psychiatry* 129(2):127–135.
23. American Psychiatric Association, Task Force on Nomenclature and Statistics. 1980. *Diagnostic and Statistical Manual of Mental Disorders*, 3. Washington, D.C.: American Psychiatric Association.
24. Williams, E. P., Carruth, B., Hyman, M. M. 1973. Community care providers and the older problem drinker. In *Alcoholism and Problem Drinking Among Older Persons,* ed. E. P. Williams, Springfield, Va.: National Technical Information Service.
25. Williams, E. P. 1973. Alcoholism and problem drinking among older persons: community agency study. In *Alcoholism and Problem Drinking Among Older Persons,* ed. E. P. Williams. Springfield, Va.: National Technical Information Service.
26. Rosin, A. J., Glatt, M. M. 1971. Alcohol excess in the elderly. *Q J Stud Alcohol* 32(1):53–59.
27. Forbes, G. B., Reina, J. C. 1970. Adult lean body mass declines with age: Some longitudinal observations. *Metabolism* 19:653–663.
28. Gambert, S. R., Newton, M., Duthrie, E. H., Jr. 1984. Medical issues in alcoholism in the elderly. In *Alcoholism in the Elderly: Social and Biomedical Issues,* ed. J. T. Hartford and T. Samorajski. New York: Raven Press.
29. Lundin, D. V. 1983. Medication-taking behavior and compliance in the elderly. In *Pharmacologic Aspects of Aging,* ed. L. A. Pagliaro and A. M. Pagliaro. St. Louis, Mo.: C. V. Mosby.
30. Mellinger, G. D., Balter, M. B., Manheimer, D. I. 1971. Patterns of psychotherapeutic drug use among adults in San Francisco. *Arch Gen Psychiatry* 25(11):385–394.
31. Flinn, G. A., Reisberg, B., Ferris, S. H. 1984. Neuropsychological models of cerebral dysfunction in chronic alcoholics. In *Alcoholism in the Elderly: Social and Biomedical Issues,* ed. J. T. Hartford and T. Samorajski. New York: Raven Press.
32. Freund, G. 1984. Neurotransmitter function in relation to aging and alco-

holism. In *Alcoholism in the Elderly: Social and Biomedical Issues,* J. T. Hartford and T. Samorajski. New York: Raven Press.

33. Hartford, J. T., Thienhaus, O. J. 1984. Psychiatric aspects of alcoholism in geriatric patients. In *Alcoholism in the Elderly: Social and Biomedical Issues,* ed. J. T. Hartford and T. Samorajski. New York: Raven Press.
34. Peto, J., Skelton, D. 1983. Drug selection and dosage in the elderly. In *Pharmacologic Aspects of Aging,* ed. L. A. Pagliaro and A. M. Pagliaro. St. Louis, Mo.: C. V. Mosby.
35. Brown, B. B. 1982. Professional's perceptions of drug and alcohol abuse among the elderly. *Gerontologist* 22(6):519–525.
36. United States Alcohol, Drug Abuse, and Mental Health Administration. 1981. *Fourth Special Report to the U.S. Congress on Alcohol and Health.* Rockville, Md.: National Institute on Alcohol Abuse and Alcoholism.
37. Vaillant, G., Clark, W., Cyrus, C., Milofsky, E. S., Kopp, J., Wulsin, V. W., Mogielnick, N. P. 1983. Prospective study of alcoholism treatment: Eight-year follow-up. *Am J Med* 75(3):455–463.
38. DiClemente, C. C., Gordon, J. R. 1984. Aging, alcoholism, and addictive behavior change: diagnostic treatment models. In *Alcoholism in the Elderly: Social and Biomedical Issues,* ed. J. T. Hartford and T. Samorajski. New York: Raven Press.
39. Meye, J. S., Largen, F. W. Jr., Shaw, T., Mortel, K. F., Rogers, R. 1984. Interactions of normal aging, senile dementia, multi-infarct dementia and alcoholism in the elderly. In *Alcoholism in the Elderly; Social and Biomedical Issues,* ed. J. T. Hartford and T. Samorajski. New York: Raven Press.
40. Schuckit, M. A. 1976. An overview of alcohol and drug abuse problems in the elderly. Testimony before the Senate Subcommittee on Alcoholism and Narcotics and the Subcommittee on Aging of the Senate Committee on Labor and Public Welfare. Washington, D.C.: Government Printing Office.
41. Ciompi, L., Eisert, M. 1971. Retrospective long term studies on the health status of alcoholics in old age. *Social Psychiatry* 6(3):129–151.
42. Rathbone-McCuan, E., Triegaardt, J. 1979. The older alcoholic and the family. *Alcohol Health Res World* 3(4):7–12.
43. Blume, S. B. 1978. Group psychotherapy in the treatment of alcoholism. In *Practical Approaches to Alcoholism Psychotherapy,* ed. S. Zimberg, J. Wallace, and S. B. Blume. New York: Plenum Press.
44. United States Department of Health, Education and Welfare. 1975. Older problem drinkers: their special needs and a nursing home geared to those needs. *Alcohol Health Res World* pp. 12–17.
45. Brickner, N. Personal communication.
46. Anderson, R. September 11, 1985. Personal communication.
47. Glassock, J. A. 1979. Rehabilitating the older alcoholic. *Aging* (299-300):19–24.
48. Van de Vyvere, B., Hughes, M., Fish, D. G. 1976. The elderly chronic alcoholic: a practical approach. *Can Welfare* 52:9.
49. Alcoholics Anonymous. 1939. *Alcoholics Anonymous.* New York: Works Publishing Co.
50. Alibrandi, L. A. 1978. The folk psychotherapy of Alcoholics Anonymous. In

Practical Approaches to Alcoholism Psychotherapy, ed. S. Zimberg, J. Wallace, and S. B. Blume. New York: Plenum Press.

51. Leach, B. 1973. Does Alcoholics Anonymous really work? In *Alcoholism; Progress in Research and Treatment,* ed. P. G. Bourne. New York: Academic Press.

52. Collins, G. 1975. Elderly alcoholics: finding the causes and cures. *The New York Times,* June 17, C-13.

53. Williams, D. T. 1981. Financing alcoholism services for the elderly. *A Preliminary Report on Aging and Alcoholism of the National Council on Alcoholism.* Mini-Conference on Aging and Alcoholism, 1981 White House Conference on Aging, Washington, D.C.: Government Printing Office.

Twenty

Mental Health in the Elderly

Donna Cohen and Margaret M. Hastings

Recommendations for changes in the delivery and financing of mental health services to the aged must be considered in the context of several other policy domains, including health care, long-term care, rehabilitation, social welfare, and public health, as well as mental health and aging. Each of these categorical areas includes regulations that facilitate or limit mental health services for older persons. Furthermore, each domain uses different diagnostic classifications and treatment modalities as well as separate service-delivery organizations and eligibility criteria. In this chapter we first review the history of previous recommendations to meet the mental health needs of the aged as well as the primary role of states in the evolution and provision of mental health care. Next, we examine three dimensions relevant to understanding mental health and aging policy reform: the needs of the populations to be served, services to be rendered, and financing mechanisms. This strategy allows us to review intersecting issues within the seven major policy domains. We conclude with a summary of emerging aging and mental health policy trends and specific recommendations.

Mental Health and Aging Policy: Past Recommendations

A series of reports over the past 15 years have proposed major policy changes to meet the mental health needs of the aged. The 1971 White

House Conference on Aging recommended that a Presidential Commission on Mental Illness and the Elderly be convened to carry out several specific initiatives, including the establishment of a Center for Mental Health and Aging in the National Institute of Mental Health with authority to fund research, training, and innovative clinical programs. The report also recommended immediate removal of inequities and discrimination in financing of mental health services under Medicare and Medicaid. Several specific policy priorities were identified, including the need to develop options for institutional care, to improve federal supervision of state use of Medicaid funds for mental health services, to support the right of older persons to treatment, and to increase the numbers of quality personnel providing services to the aged.

Seven years later the President's Commission on Mental Health, which had a Task Force on the Elderly, identified a diverse array of policy priorities: outreach and home care, amendments to Medicare, research, more equitable allocation of resources, and revitalization of the Federal Administration on Aging.[1] The report emphasized measures for improving accessibility of services, such as coordination and training at the community level and federal funding for professional training programs in geriatric medicine, psychology, social work, and nursing. The President's Commission report also recommended the removal of barriers to mental health service in Medicare, expansion of home care services, and increased federal resources for research, especially on dementia, through combined efforts of the National Institute of Mental Health, the National Institute on Aging, and the National Institute of Neurological and Communicative Disorders. Similar policy recommendations surfaced in the report of the 1981 White House Conference on Aging.

The recurrent themes in all these reports, which form the historical background for future policy reform, are improvements in Medicare coverage, specialized mental health services, and preservice and in-service training, as well as increased support for prevention programs and research. In the next section we review the primary role of states in the early history of the delivery and financing of mental health care. Mental health policy is unique among health-care policies in that the states, and not the federal government, first took responsibility for its provision and financing.

States as the Historical Agents of Mental Health Care Policy

Care for the mentally ill was once provided by families and local communities, but more than 100 years ago states began developing asylums for the mentally disturbed. As late as 1955 there were 559,000 persons in state-operated institutions, a figure which dropped to 138,000 by 1975 as a result of deinstitutionalization.[2] The evolution of state policy from total institutional care for the mentally ill, including the aged mentally ill, to partial funding and provision of community-based care in the 1960s, reflected shifting responsibilities for care resulting from the advent of Medicaid and other federal entitlement programs, psychopharmacologic advances, and changing public attitudes.

Although deinstitutionalization has been a guiding policy in mental health care for the past 25 years, commitment to deinstitutionalization unfortunately does not include adequate mechanisms at both federal and state levels to develop a responsive community-based service system.[3–4] Medicare does not address the chronic care needs of mentally impaired beneficiaries, and this same pattern of institutional bias prevails in Medicaid expenditures. Both Medicare and Medicaid provide meager and inconsistent funding for adult day care, respite care, and home health and chore services, and they spend little for psychosocial rehabilitation.

State hospitals continue to play a significant role in the delivery of comprehensive services to the most impaired. Since older patients comprise 27% of the resident populations of state and county mental hospitals, state policy decisions surrounding the future of state hospitals and the availability of appropriate services for this severely impaired elderly population will be critical.[5] State facilities have become very expensive to operate due to high labor and plant costs as well as declining patient numbers. About 65% of funds from state departments of mental health still go to institutional funding, although the majority of patients are in the community.

The state hospital population includes not only those who have grown old in state facilities, but also a significant number of new admissions to the state system.[6] Many seriously mentally impaired patients are transferred to state hospitals when Medicare benefits run out and/or when suitable nursing home placement and Medicaid eligibility are not possible. The state hospital focuses increasingly on three groups of patients: those with multiple handicaps or severe behavior management problems and those remanded by the courts. A 1980 profile of admissions to state and county mental hospitals indicates that while 5.4% of all patients admitted to these facilities were 65 years old and older, 66.4% of those patients were admitted involuntarily, presenting mental conditions dangerous to themselves or others.[7] Dementias were the largest primary diagnostic category, followed by affective disorders, schizophrenia, and alcohol- and/or drug-related conditions.

State mental health regulations have focused on the rights of patients within the mental health system, especially on the mental health code, which defines civil commitment standards for patients remanded to a facility because of dangerousness to self or others. These state laws attempt to balance the rights of the patient with the rights of society, a balance that has shifted over time in accordance with public beliefs. In the treatment setting, state mental health codes further define patient rights to receive or to refuse treatment. Laws also regulate the use of restraints, seclusion, and other treatment procedures. To protect older patients and to facilitate legal access to more appropriate geriatric treatment programs, especially in state hospital settings, many state laws now mandate treatment plans and regular review of treatment progress. Continuing concern for patient rights in both state and federal policy was underscored by the passage of the Protection and Advocacy for Mentally Ill Individuals Act by Congress in 1986, a significant policy direction from which the aged mentally ill can benefit. This bill provided grants to states to ensure protection of the rights of mentally ill persons who are residents of treatment facilities and immediately after discharge.

Another unique aspect of state mental health policy has been the development of state-mandated mental health insurance benefits. Since many older persons carry private third-party policies and an increasing number of retirees are carried on corporate benefit plans, increased access to mental health services may result from these state efforts. However, the basic coverage described in state mandates has followed the acute medical model, with an institutional bias and providing limited annual inpatient days and outpatient visit coverage. Little or no coverage is provided for the seriously impaired mentally ill who need rehabilitation help, including housing, life skills training, and an array of medical and social services.

Identifying the Populations to be Served

Older persons who need intensive mental health services include those who have utilized mental health services for a long period, such as long-term residents of state hospitals, nursing homes, or other institutional settings, and those who develop major mental health problems in their later years, including Alzheimer's disease and other dementias, depressive disorders, and paranoid disorders.[8,9]

The assumption that aging is associated with increased risk for mental disorders is a recurrent theme in the literature.[9-11] However, numerous population surveys and studies have produced widely differing results regarding the occurrence of psychiatric morbidity among the aged. Studies using standard screening inventories have shown increased levels of psychopathology among the aged as contrasted with younger ages, whereas the case-identification approach, using diagnostic instruments developed to classify psychiatric disorders in younger populations, have tended to report the opposite. Methodological and measurement problems coupled with high attrition rates among the sick aged account for the inconsistent conclusions regarding the comparative risks of men and women for various mental disorders in middle and later life. Results of the Epidemiologic Catchment Area (ECA) studies did not support the position that persons age 65 and older were at higher risk for psychiatric disorders, with the exception of cognitive impairment.[12] However, these results are not definitive because the ECA studies suffer from significant methodological flaws that complicate the interpretation of the data. If the ECA results are regarded as a low estimate, 12.8% of respondents 65 years and older had either a DSM-III disorder or severe cognitive impairment. Estimates from other studies extend the range to suggest that 15–25% or perhaps more older persons have significant mental health problems.[10,11,13,14]

The number of cases of all mental disorders among the aged will increase as a result of the rapid growth of that population, but the rates for Alzheimer's disease and related disorders will probably increase by a much greater magnitude.[15] The rapid growth of the oldest-old population means that Alzheimer's disease will become an even more pressing problem, requiring appropriate provision of care in a period dominated by the pressures of cost containment. Brody has conservatively projected that by the year 2000 the United States will have more than 4 million patients with Alzheimer's disease and related disorders, and that by the year 2050 we can expect to have over 9 million afflicted individuals.[10] Most will be women, not because women are necessarily more vulnerable to dementia, but because women live longer than men and thus more women enter the risk period. Furthermore, women with Alzheimer's disease live longer than similarly afflicted men, even when rates are corrected for the higher mortality of older men in general.[16]

The treatment and long-term care needs of those with Alzheimer's disease and related disorders have provided the impetus for the most significant policy changes in the 1980s.[17,18] The emphasis on Alzheimer's disease arises directly from the rapid increase in the number and proportion of older people, as well as from vigorous consumer advocacy by family members, especially from within national organizations, such as the Alzheimer's Association, and state associations, such as the Family Survival Project in California and the Alliance for Alzheimer's Disease in Pennsylvania.

Mental health services for the aged must cover a broad spectrum of disorders and conditions, from depression related to life role changes and coping with chronic disease to severe cognitive disorders, such as Alzheimer's disease. Consequently, solutions to better serve the mental health needs of the aged should be crafted from two perspectives: a treatment perspective, focusing on restoration of mental health and rehabilitation; and a public health perspective, focusing on prevention by offering programs to maximize the quality of life and functional effectiveness of older persons, particularly the group 85 years old and older, who are at the highest risk for physical and mental illness, increasing frailty, and loss of independence. Prevention activities, including health-promotion programs, could be targeted to ameliorate the negative effects of growing older. Appropriate preventive mental health services help decrease vulnerability to illness and under certain conditions lower the utilization of other more costly health services.[19]

Delineating the Mental Health Service System

Mental health care for the aged is currently a patchwork of services and financing mechanisms rather than a comprehensive program providing rational and efficacious mental health care.[14] Recognition of the need for a range of services is evident in policy statements developed as a direct result of deinstitutionalization from state mental hospitals over the past 23 years; however, the broad array of services necessary to care for people in the community has not yet emerged.[20]

Mental health services were first defined in federal legislation establishing the comprehensive community mental health centers. The Community Mental Health Center Act was a direct response to President Kennedy's request for a national mental health program to care for the mentally ill. Agencies receiving money under this act were required to provide a coordinated program of five essential types of mental health service—inpatient, emergency, partial hospitalization, and outpatient—as well as consultation and education. Other services recommended but not required included specialized diagnostic services, rehabilitation, preadmission and postdischarge services for state hospital patients, research and evaluation programs, and training and education activities.

Although comprehensive community mental health centers were initially mandated as comprehensive care centers for everyone, a trend toward provision of specialized services for specific populations emerged. In the 1975 amendments to the original legislation, services for children and older persons were identified as essential services. Several other special services were recommended, including assistance to the courts and other public agencies in preadmission screening for state hospitals, follow-up care for those discharged from state hospitals, halfway houses, programs for alcoholism and drug abuse, and public education and consultation activities.

The policy direction for specialized services to the aged was strengthened in 1978 amendments to the Community Mental Health Center Act, in a response to the President's Commission on Mental Health. The Mental Health Systems Act of 1980 also provided special staffing and coordination grants for mental health centers with identified aging programs.[21]

Unfortunately, within a year this specialized aging program policy was superseded by the Alcohol, Drug Abuse and Mental Health Block Grant (ADMBG), initiated as part of the Omnibus Budget Reconciliation Act of 1981, which failed to accommodate the specialized mental health needs of the elderly. The provisions of the ADMBG allowed state discretion in targeting services to the aged, and as a result many community mental health center programs for the aged were discontinued.

As community mental health centers developed, many states passed mental health statutes defining a general community delivery system without specifying specialized services to the aged. For example, Illinois passed statutes ordering that community mental health services be planned, developed, delivered, and evaluated as part of a comprehensive and coordinated system, and the state mental health agency was designated to oversee the programs. The service categories in state legislative policies identified the same range of services as stated in the federal Community Mental Health Center Act. [22]

With the advent of the national Health Planning Law (P.L. 93-641) in 1975, communities began to define essential health services within the geographic area of each Health Systems Agency. Mental heath service planning was specifically identified in amendments to the act, and planning for the aged was subsumed, but not specifically identified, under local Health Systems Agencies and statewide efforts. However, in the fall of 1986 a proposal to eliminate this congressionally mandated national planning program was passed.

Just as the Community Mental Health Center Act was the centerpiece of federal community-based mental health policy, the Older American's Act, passed in 1965, provided a policy fulcrum for a coordinated, comprehensive program of health and social services for all older citizens. There was little emphasis on specialized mental health services for the aged in the Older American's Act, although mental health was identified in the preamble. Mental health services were a priority in a 1981 amendment, the Title IV discretionary demonstration grant program, but few grants were developed. In 1984, families of the victims of Alzheimer's disease and related disorders were made a priority under the services provision section (Title III) of the Older American's Act. Despite these two amendments, mental health services were never emphasized as a core support service in the local aging networks. [21]

The mental health service system and the aging service system evolved as two discrete and uncoordinated systems at federal, state, and local levels. [21] The need for coordinated service planning and implementation was emphasized by a 1982 General Accounting Office report on mental health services that recommended comprehensive case-management strategies to facilitate the interaction of older persons with multiple community-based services and organizations.[23] The report recognized that such services as outreach, home care, and transportation, as well as general mental health services, were essential for quality care.

To achieve an effective care system, a fundamental policy gap between mental health and health and social service systems must be closed, because mentally impaired older individuals usually need services from both systems. Case management evolved as one solution to the gaps between systems, but case management is only effective where services exist to be managed. The lack of appropriate service programs and trained personnel, lack of state leadership in program development, and poor private and public third-party coverage for services have impeded efforts to develop effective case management. In addition, outreach programs necessary to counteract distrust, low self-esteem, and belief systems of many older persons about mental illness have not evolved.

A wide range of service functions has always been recommended to provide appropriate mental health care for the aged, including prevention, emergency and crisis services, assessment, intensive care treatment, skilled and intermediate nursing care, nonmedical community residential alternatives, home health and respite care, case management, and family support. These generic service functions address the needs of different patient groups and therefore provide a comprehensive system of caring to support the aged or any age group in the least restrictive setting and provide the optimum potential for rehabilitation. Furthermore, the absence of a full set of components leads to overutilization or inappropriate utilization of one or two services. For example, nursing homes often have been used inappropriately because of a lack of community adult day care and of residential alternatives for mentally ill older persons.

Given the prevalence of treatable mental health problems in the aged, significant utilization of outpatient service might be anticipated. However, use of community mental health centers rose only slightly between 1971 and 1982, from 3.4% to 6% of the populations served.[24] Even lower rates of utilization were found among racial and ethnic minorities, especially when services were not modified in the context of cultural beliefs, living patterns, and the unique problems of the minority aged. Many existing barriers may explain these findings. Professional ageism has restricted service availability. Psychiatrists, psychotherapists, and other mental health professionals have been pessimistic about the treatability of older persons or have not felt the relationship to be rewarding or gratifying. These professional barriers underscore the need for policies that mandate better training and education of mental health personnel. Training must be directed toward changing attitudes, disseminating knowledge, and developing clinical diagnostic and treatment skills. At least one survey of community mental health centers suggests that when specialized services and trained staff are available, utilization by older persons increases.[24]

Professional ageism is not the only possible explanation for poor service utilization. The aged themselves have been barriers. The need for independence, fear or suspicion, passivity, poor self-image, concern about costs, disbelief in the value of mental health care, and the stigma of mental illness are all significant issues for the older consumer. Public education of our aging population will be important in shaping future policies.

Policy for Financing Mental Health Services

Perhaps the most significant barrier to utilization is financing policy. Historically, funding responsibilities have shifted between levels of government and between the public and private sectors. To better understand the current flow of funds available to produce mental health services for the aged, we need to review funding sources as well as federal, state, and local funding policies. Resources utilized in the specialty mental health sector for services to all populations may clarify the critical sources of revenue.[25,26] The estimated mental health revenue base in 1980 was $30.5 billion, and the payment sources for personal mental health expenditures were: 25% from federal sources, 35% from private sources, 28% from state and local revenues, and 12% from insurance. In 1980, personal mental health care represented 14% of national medical expenditures. Sixty-three percent of that mental health total was for institutional care.[25] Nursing homes accounted for approximately 30%, while state public mental hospitals accounted for an additional 23%.[27] The nursing home figure was larger because of Medicaid payments related to deinstitutionalization. In 1982 nursing home expenditures were equally divided between public and private sources and totaled $27 billion, more than four times the annual expenditures of all state mental health authorities together.[28]

Mental disorders are expensive,[29,30] ranking third in overall health-care spending, behind diseases of the circulatory and digestive systems. When personal health-care expenditures were analyzed by age and sex, mental disorder expenditures for persons 65 years old and older ranked fifth for men and second for women. Institutional care continues to dominate mental health expenditures. Among males of all ages, hospital care represents the largest personal mental health care expense. For women over 65 years old, the largest expenditure in mental health services is for nursing home care, probably reflecting the greater longevity of women.

Federal Financing

The largest potential funding sources for mental health services for the aged are entitlement programs, including Medicare, Medicaid, Supplemental Security Income, Old Age and Survivor's Insurance, and medical services from the Veterans Administration (VA). Although a substantial proportion of its 30 million enrollees look to Medicare financing for care of mental disorders, there are major funding limitations for mental health services. Lifetime coverage is restricted to 190 days of inpatient care in a psychiatric facility. There is also a limit of $250 per year for outpatient services, and this minimum outpatient financing also requires a 50% copayment. In 1981 Medicare reimbursements for psychiatric care and substance abuse treatment was $995 million, or 2.4% of Medicare reimbursements. Although inpatient psychiatric services are temporarily exempt from Medicare diagnosis-related groups, it is anticipated that when the prospective payment system is implemented, it will further limit mental health inpatient benefits.

Medicaid is the single largest mental health program in the country. Medicaid finances a variety of mental health services, mandatory and optional, that must be made available to the mentally ill on the same basis as for other persons receiving general health-care services under Medicaid. Mandatory mental health benefits include inpatient services in the psychiatric unit of a general hospital, outpatient hospital services, physician services, and services at skilled nursing facilities. Optional mental health services that states may include are inpatient care for those 65 and over in a psychiatric institution, day care and partial hospitalization, intermediate care for those 65 years and over in an "institute for mental disease," and services rendered by mental health professionals other than physicians under certain conditions.

At first glance, Medicaid appears to offer the potential for financing mental health services for the aged. However, states are free to set limits on the amounts and scope of coverage for mandatory and optional services. As a result, mental health benefits for the aged vary significantly from state to state. In 1981, through the Omnibus Budget Reconciliation Act, a Medicaid waiver for home- and community-based services was offered to states that was aimed at funding community services as an option for those needing institutional care, such as the mentally ill aged. Thus, states accepted into the waiver program have been able to provide an alternative to the institutional benefit bias in Medicaid.

The VA is a major federal funding source for mental health benefits to the aged. Both its pension and medical programs provide significant services to the aged mentally ill. In 1983 total medical care expenditures for the VA system were $8.3 billion.[31] The mental health benefits were substantial, including extensive inpatient, outpatient, and long-term care. Most VA care is provided through vertically integrated programs in 172 hospital centers and outpatient clinics and 101 nursing home units. Long-term care services are provided under contract in community nursing homes or subsidized state veterans' facilities. Acute psychiatric care is available at 128 hospitals. Eighty thousand beds are utilized daily, with approximately 30% devoted to psychiatric care and nearly 30% used for extended care.

By 1990, veterans 65 years old and older will comprise over 60% of the male population of that age. As a result of this demographic projection and increasing unemployment, Medicare restrictions, and lack of long-term care capacity nationally, pressure is increasing on VA services, especially for nursing home beds for the mentally ill aged. A major advantage for older persons in gaining access to VA services is the absence of the spend-down policy found in the Medicaid program. Thus, older men are in a favored position for access to intensive mental health services.

Other federal funding sources for support of services to the aged with mental health problems are categorical and block grants to states which then distribute funds through the relevant state agency. Categorical funding targets programs for specific population groups; for example, the Older Americans Act provides grants to states for support of older persons at the community level. The Alcohol, Drug Abuse and Mental Health Block Grant provides funds to states for community-based services, with an emphasis on the chronically mentally ill and the mentally ill aged. Appropriations nationwide in 1986 were approximately $490 million, a small amount compared to the more than $6 billion appropriated annually by state mental health departments.

The Social Services Block Grants program is the largest of the Health and Human Services block grant programs to the states, having an annual federal appropriation of $2.8 billion. This federal initiative has the greatest potential to help older persons at risk for significant mental problems. In most states the aged receive a significant percentage of these funds, which primarily provide support services to prevent institutionalization, rather than health and medical procedures provided under other federal entitlement and state programs.

State and Local Financing

State governments finance services for the mental health needs of the aged through several programs: departments of mental health and aging, rehabilitation services, social welfare, and the state Medicaid program. At the state level, mental health funding responsibilities are disbursed by type of service provided and population served. Federal block grant and categorical funds are also received and administered by designated state agencies. The most critical roles in state financing policies for mental health services to the aged include planning and promoting interagency coordination at the state and local level. States determine which populations and services will receive the funds under the state's control.

Certain mental health services for older persons may receive local tax dollars raised by townships, municipalities, and counties. Since local public funding is inextricably linked with state and federal funding policies, the degree of local funding responsibility and service-delivery decision making vary substantially from state to state and even among local governments within a single state. Local governments serve as an important administrative arm of the state in the mental health care service-delivery system. Not only do they raise funds, but many counties are responsible for administering state funds for certain services. Counties and cities often operate hospitals, provide senior citizen services, and operate specialized in-home and respite services for the aged mentally ill. The role of local government will probably expand with increasing pressure on state and federal funding sources.

Changes Needed in Financing Policy

Changes in financing policy are needed to create a comprehensive system of services that responds effectively to older persons with mental health-care needs. Coordinated state planning is an essential first step in bringing disparate financing mechanisms together. Until this occurs, service fragmentation related to diffused financing responsibilities will continue to complicate the delivery of comprehensive care.

Changes in service capacity are also needed, but important questions remain about whether increased capacity can be developed to prevent the most expensive forms of institutional care. Payment systems for older persons must relate to level of disability, rather than focusing on payment rates for a setting or specific unit of service. More innovative financing mechanisms should be implemented, including capitation systems and private long-term care insurance.

The emergence of an accessible system of mental health-care services depends on a balanced public–private partnership. Unless substantial improvement in service delivery and cost control are carried out thoughtfully by both sectors, services may simply become less available. Current private mental health insurance coverage has not developed from a rational sense of the system of services needed; rather, it has developed incrementally, in and around an existing publicly financed pattern of care. However, private mental health insurance coverage has had a significant effect on the distribution of care by providing services and priority access to those who may need the services least. Those who are most impaired tend to end up in the public system, where staffing levels often are low, treatment programs are often limited, and physical facilities are marginal.

One of the major questions in future mental health policy is to what extent the private sector will deal with severely disabled patients. With increased emphasis on competition in the private marketplace, the private provider may compete for the healthier and easier to manage patient who has appropriate insurance or other resources, leaving the older mentally disabled patients to flood public facilities.

Limitations of Prepaid Plans for Psychiatric Care

Although prepaid health-care plans have important advantages, that is, they provide incentives to control costs and to make decisions about more effective resource allocation, they have not led to better and cost-effective care for older populations.[32] HMOs may successfully reduce the rate of hospitalization of Medicare beneficiaries, but treatment of older persons with psychiatric problems is still expensive.[33] Many barriers to mental health care in the fee-for-service and public sector are preserved in prepaid settings.

Fear of the cost of treating the mentally ill and competition from other departments have restricted budgets and services for chronic care. HMOs often require copayments, especially for outpatient care, and the resulting cost of mental health care in HMOs is as large or larger than that in a fee-for-service system.[29] The most common form of cost sharing is limiting coverage, and these limits have the most significant effect on the chronically ill.[34] Mental health care is so restricted in prepaid settings that incentives for institutionalization are increased.[35] Medicare enrollees in HMOs use nursing homes more and home health services less than do fee-for-service populations.[36]

In prepaid plans, incentives shift expensive patients, such as the aged with mental health problems, to other systems of care, which disrupts continuity of care.[37] Since in prepaid plans few incentives exist to maintain contact with patients, chronically ill patients "slip through the cracks."

Prepaid plans have not increased the numbers of mental health professionals trained to care for the aged.

In summary, current evidence suggests that prepaid plans may exacerbate the problems of chronic-care patients and lead to care that is less adequate than that provided in the fee-for-service system. The adverse effects of HMOs on mental health care for the aged suggests that prepaid care, including Medicare vouchers and plans to restructure state mental health systems, requires refinement before it can become a mechanism for policy reform.

The behavior of older consumers also needs to be considered. There are some early reports suggesting that older persons who choose among HMOs are more concerned about acute illness coverage than chronic care.[32] If this is the case, it is likely that a competitive voucher system will eventually reduce mental health care services, because competition to attract enrollees will shift resources from initially available chronic-care services to those that increase enrollment. Therefore, the stigma that older persons attach to mental health services, combined with the bias of medical professionals, suggests that the chronically ill aged will bear the brunt of cost-saving measures. Since prepayment is based on the average cost of services to the aged in the community, there is a financial incentive to screen out the most expensive Medicare beneficiaries. Therefore, the aged with mental health problems will encounter the greatest barriers to enrollment and also will endure the greatest pressure to drop their enrollment. Selective enrollment and disenrollment are not allowed under Medicare regulations, but these practices are difficult to monitor. Selection of enrollees is already occurring, and it is likely that it will be perpetuated by sophisticated marketing techniques.[38]

Although state reforms of the mental health care system are focusing on prepaid arrangements, the disadvantages of prepayment may significantly outweigh its cost advantages.[39] Prepaid capitated care systems that shift decisions about resources away from state legislatures to agencies are likely to work against the costly population of aged with mental health problems.

Recommendations for Action

The major cost-control policies called for in the federal Gramm-Rudman-Hollings legislation will continue to influence the capacity for care and access to care of older persons with mental disorders. Unfortunately, external economic forces constrain the system, precisely when our population is aging rapidly and experiencing increasing demands for mental health care. This reality has two major effects. First, mental health care for the aged, which until now has focused on building service capacity, is turning its attention to serious economic questions and related ethical issues regarding allocation of resources. Second, service demands coupled with limited funding require major efforts to develop prevention policies. Unfortunately, few dollars are currently being spent on prevention programs, in contrast to the billions being spent on treatment and long-term care. Prevention policy for older persons, their families, and the greater community must be strengthened at all levels of government. The demand and need for acute and long-term care services must be controlled humanely by prevention efforts, not just by cost-containment measures, so that resources are available for the most disabled, and early intervention strategies can be employed to reduce the number of severe disabilities. An integrated policy approach is essential for prevention and early intervention strategies.

We offer these specific recommendations:

I. Financing
  A. Remove Medicare discriminatory reimbursement provisions in outpatient and inpatient mental health services.
  B. Expand the types of Medicare outpatient programs and the professional providers covered to increase service accessibility and to reduce utilization of less-appropriate health-care services.
  C. Develop a pilot program, Medicare "Part C," that will provide access to a basic level of flexible long-term care services for those with chronic progressive mental impairments.
     (1) Provide services under Part C that include support and respite services to family caregivers (eliminating the need to spend-down assets to meet Medicaid eligibility).
     (2) Finance Part C through premiums from individuals and premiums paid by Medicaid for indigent persons.
     (3) Focus Part C program coverage on a limited set of services, including adult day care, home care, intermediate care, and respite care.
  D. Under Medicare and Medicaid, expand home-care availability by refining regulations and reimbursement policies so that those with serious mental disorders can receive home-care services.
  E. Expand the Title XIX Medicaid home and community-based waiver program so that more social and support services are available for those eligible older persons with mental impairments who are not in institutional settings.
II. Private Resource Development
  A. Encourage utilization of private resources for long-term care needs of the seriously mentally impaired by developing private long-term care insurance and other private funding, such as home-equity conversion programs.
  B. Include a range of community services as well as nursing home coverage in long-term care insurance offerings.
III. Family Support
  A. Provide incentives and assistance for families who take care of severely mentally impaired elders.
  B. Ensure availability of day care, home care, and respite care.
  C. Plan and develop institutional care facilities so that institutional care can be available when needed.
  D. Provide psychological support services to caregivers.
IV. Leadership and Interagency Coordination

A. Develop advocacy, planning, and oversight capacity in state mental health authorities to facilitate adequate and appropriate mental health services for older adults within the mental health system.
B. Identify points of contact and accountability for these services within state mental health systems.
C. Increase the quality and expertise of personnel who provide services to the aged mentally ill in state hospitals.
D. Achieve greater cooperation between mental health and geriatric service systems at the local level through Area Agencies on Aging and community mental health centers/programs for meeting mental health and psychosocial needs.
E. Require, through state leadership and/or mandate, community mental health boards and/or local planning and service units to expand mental health services to older adults through needs assessment, evaluation of current local services, and initiation of new service programs.
F. Require evidence of coordination among state agencies in meeting the mental health needs of older persons as a condition for receiving funds under federal grants.
G. Promote coordination among federal agencies to enhance basic research initiatives, services research, and service demonstrations; to provide broader, systematic coverage of research needs; and to avoid duplication of effort in mental health and geriatric programs.

V. Public Education
A. Develop national campaigns to educate the public about the mental health problems of the aged. Emphasize the value of prevention and health education.
B. Promote understanding of the symptoms and courses, as well as diagnoses and treatments of severe mental disorders, such as Alzheimer's disease and related disorders.
C. Promote public awareness of the range of services needed in the community for treating mentally disabled older persons, the value of support for those assisting older persons with more severe mental impairments, and the treatability of mental disorders, when they are diagnosed and services are available.

VI. Prevention
A. Provide and support volunteer programs and employment opportunities for older persons at the community level.
B. Develop and expand availability of preretirement and postretirement education programs in cooperation with other community institutions, including junior colleges, universities, industries, and voluntary organizations.
C. Improve the image of aging for the general public and provide education on aging in elementary and secondary schools to combat prejudice, to lessen intergenerational tensions, and to improve community living environments for aging persons.

    D. Provide social support programs and self-help groups for older
       persons who are isolated and/or at high risk for mental health
       problems.
VII. Training
    A. Expand federal and state efforts to include geriatric mental health
       in the core curriculum and basic training of preservice personnel in
       all health, mental health, and social service disciplines.
    B. Provide federal support for regional interdisciplinary geriatric
       training centers that can be utilized by all training programs for
       preservice and in-service education in geriatric mental health.
    C. Require mental health and aging components in state licensure
       qualification and certification and recertification processes for
       health, mental health, and social service personnel.
    D. Initiate in-service training programs in mental health and aging
       for state agencies and departments, as well as joint training sessions
       for local aging, rehabilitation, and mental health services
       networks.
    E. Provide training on mental health problems and severe mental
       disorders for professionals and paraprofessionals at all levels of the
       service system, including those in adult foster care, group homes,
       senior public housing, and nursing homes.

Forces Affecting Policy Decisions

In the future, mental health care for the aged, like the overall health and
human services system, will be caught in the struggle to allocate finite
resources amid increased expectations and demand for service. Difficult
questions will plague policymakers regarding the extent to which resources
should be devoted to the most disabled as opposed to those with better
prognoses. Protected environments will be needed for those who will not or
cannot respond to rehabilitation regimens.

Competition for attractive patients will intensify among service providers and tension will increase between competitive forces and regulatory
powers to control quality in mental health-care services. Consolidation
and collaboration will accelerate among service providers as vertical and
horizontal service integration occurs within the service continuum, enabling providers to gain cost efficiencies and to capture and maintain patients in the midst of a competitive delivery system. Service consolidation
and collaboration will also be driven by the expected introduction of
prospective capitated financing mechanisms for a package of services given
to individuals with more severe mental disorders. The capitated payment
system places the provider at risk, and, at the same time, allows the
provider more flexibility in selecting the most effective set of services at the
least cost.

Forces within an economy burdened by budget deficits and foreign competition will lead to public discussion of major ethical decisions about the distribution of health resources and the extension of life. Ethical dilemmas will become more critical as new medical advances enhance life extension. Resource limitations will place mental health care for the aged in competition not only with other parts of the health system, but also with education, space exploration, defense, and all areas of the public domain. Without shared basic values, these decisions will be difficult, and new ideas and ways of thinking will be needed. Government officials, citizen leaders, researchers, providers, consumers, and taxpayers need a forum where different perspectives can be integrated and plans can be made for the future mental health needs of the aging and aged.

References

1. President's Commission on Mental Health. 1987. *Report to the President.* Washington, D.C.: Government Printing Office.
2. Van Nostrand, J. 1984. Long-term care populations: Demography and projections. Appendices to unpublished presentation. American Health Planning Association-Veterans' Administration Conference, Washington, D.C., September, 1984.
3. Lamb, R. 1984. Deinstitutionalization and the homeless mentally ill. *Hosp Community Psychiatry* 35:899–907.
4. Talbott, J. 1980. *State Mental Hospitals.* New York: Human Sciences Press.
5. National Institute of Mental Health. 1985. *Report on Mental Disorders of Aging.* Rockville, Md.: National Institute of Mental Health.
6. Lowy, L. 1980. *Social Policies and Programs on Aging.* Lexington, Mass.: D. C. Heath.
7. Rosentein, M., Steadman, A., Milazzo-Sayre, L., MacAskill, R., Manderscheid, R. 1986. *Characteristics of Admissions to the Inpatient Services of State and County Mental Hospitals, United States 1980.* Statistical Note No. 177. Rockville, Md.: National Institute of Mental Health.
8. Brody, E. 1985. *Mental and Physical Health Practices of Older People.* New York: Springer-Verlag.
9. Cohen, D., Eisdorfer, C. 1985. Major psychiatric and behavioral disorders in the aged. In *Principles of Geriatric Medicine,* ed. E. L. Biermen, W. R. Hazzard, R. Andres, 867–908. New York: McGraw Hill.
10. Brody, J. A. 1985. The nature of ageing populations. *Nature* 315:463–466.
11. Cohen, G. D. 1980. Prospects for mental health and aging. In *Handbook of Mental Health and Aging,* ed. J. Birren, B. Sloane, 971–993. Englewood Cliffs, N.J.: Prentice Hall.
12. Myers, J., Weissman, M., Tischler, G., Holzer, C., Leaf, P., Orvaschel, H., Anthony, J., Boyd, J., Burke, J., Kramer, M., Stoltzman, R. 1984. Six month

prevalence of psychiatric disorders in three communities. *Arch Gen Psychiatry* 41:959–967.

13. Bollerup, T. 1975. Prevalence of mental illness among seventy year-olds domiciled in nine Copenhagen suburbs. The Golstrup Survey. *Acta Psychiatry Scand* 51:327.

14. Eisdorfer, C., Cohen, D. 1980. *Mental Health Care of the Aging.* New York: Springer–Verlag.

15. Kramer, M. 1980. The rising pandemic of mental disorders and associated chronic diseases and disabilities. *Acta Psychiatr Scand* [Suppl. 285] 382–396.

16. Barclay, L., Zemcov, A., Blass, J., McDowell, F. 1985. Factors associated with duration of survival in Alzheimer's disease. *Biol. Psychiatry* 20:86–93.

17. Cohen, D. 1986. Alzheimer's disease and long term caring. *Pride Inst J Long Term Home Health Care* 5:2–3.

18. Cohen, D., Eisdorfer, C. 1986. *The Loss of Self.* New York: W. W. Norton.

19. Mumford, E., Schlesinger, H., Glass, G., Patrick, C., Cuerdon, T. 1984. A new look at evidence about reduced cost of medical utilization following mental health treatment. *Am J Psychiatry* 141:1145–1158.

20. National Institute of Mental Health. 1982. A network of caring: The community support program of NIMH. 1982. ADAMHA (PHS) 81-1063. Rockville, Md.: National Institute of Mental Health.

21. Fleming, A., Buchanan, J., Santos, J., Richards, L. 1984. *Mental Health Services for the Elderly: Report on a Survey of Community Mental Health Centers.* Washington, D.C.: Department of Health and Human Services Government Printing Office.

22. Hastings, M. 1985. *Financing Mental Health Services.* Rockville, Md.: National Institute of Mental Health.

23. United States General Accounting Office. 1982. The elderly should benefit from expanded home health care but increasing these services will not insure cost reductions. *Report to the Congress by the Comptroller General.* Washington, D.C.: Government Printing Office.

24. Light, E., Lebowitz, B., Bailey, J. 1986. Community mental health centers and elderly services: Analysis of direct and indirect services and service sites. *Community Ment Health J* 22:294–302.

25. National Center of Health Statistics. 1983. *Health, United States.* Hyattsville, Md.: Department of Health and Human Services.

26. ICF 1985. Private Financing of long-term care: Current methods and resources—Final report. Submitted to the office of the Assistant Secretary for Planning and Evaluation USDHHS, Washington, D.C.: unpublished manuscript.

27. United States General Accounting Office. 1983. Medicaid and nursing home care: Cost increases and the need for services are creating problems for the states and the elderly. Washington, D.C.: Government Printing Office.

28. Doty, P., Liu, K., Weiner, J. 1985. An overview of long-term care. *Health Care Financing Rev* 6(3):69–78.

29. Sharfstein, S., Muszynski, S., Myers, E. 1984. *Health Insurance and Psychiatric Care: Update and Appraisal.* Washington, D.C.: American Psychiatric Association.

30. Waldo, D., Lazenby, H. 1984. Demographic characteristics and health care use and expenditures by the aged in the United States: 1977–1984. *Health Care Financing Rev* 6:1–49.
31. Congressional Budget Office. 1984. *Veterans Administration Health Care: Planning for Future Years.* Washington, D.C.: Congressional Budget Office.
32. Schlesinger, M. 1986. Chronic care in prepaid settings. *Milbank Memorial Fund* 64:189–215.
33. Greenlick, M., Lamb, S., Carpenter, T., Fischer, T., Marks, S., Cooper, W. 1983. Kaiser-Permanente's Medicare Plus Project: A successful Medicare prospective payment demonstration. *Health Care Financing Rev* 4:85–97.
34. Levin, B., Glasser, J., Roberts, R. 1984. Changing patterns in mental health service coverage within health maintenance organizations. *Am. J Public Health* 74:435–458.
35. Boaz, J. 1985. Managerial criteria for evaluating a mental health service, Part I. *HMO Ment Health Newsletter* I:1–2.
36. Weil, P. 1976. Comparative costs to the Medicare program of severe prepaid group practices and controls. *Milbank Memorial Fund* 54:339–364.
37. Bonstedt, T., McSweeney, J. 1985. Interpretation of psychiatric exclusions in HMO's. *HMO Ment Health Newsletter* 1:5–8.
38. Iglehart, J. 1985. Medicare turns to HMO's. *N Engl J Med* 312:132–137.
39. Mechanic, D. 1985. Mental health and social policy: Initiatives for the 1980's. *Health Aff* 4: 75–88.

Twenty-one

Prevention and Early Intervention

William R. Hazzard

The tragedy of a stroke, of a fall and accompanying fracture of an osteoporotic bone, or of heart failure after a myocardial infarction is a painful reminder that prevention should be the ultimate goal of health and social care. However, even allowing for the triumphs attributable to specific immunization, the fabric of firm scientific evidence does not unequivocally justify aggressive preventive intervention strategies beyond childhood. The lack of convincing data has been translated into conservative, even nihilistic, attitudes toward the prevention of disease, especially of chronic disease, and hence especially among elderly persons. Dealing with these attitudes requires a critical review of their scientific basis, recognition of the barriers to effective preventive health maintenance among the elderly in the current United States health-care system, assessment of a widely recommended program of preventive health services for the aged, and formulation of proposals to improve preventive health care, especially among the elderly.

Preventive Gerontology*

Preventive medicine is usually defined in three stages: primary, secondary, and tertiary prevention. Primary prevention does not permit a disease to

*Preventive gerontology is the phrase coined to describe strategies, varying differentially

cross the clinical horizon. Secondary prevention does not permit recurrence of the first episode of clinical disease (e.g., prevention of a second myocardial infarction while maintaining function after the first). Tertiary prevention stresses recovery of function and its preservation at a higher level (e.g., rehabilitation of the stroke patient). Although much of preventive medicine in the elderly is clearly tertiary and secondary, primary prevention remains the ultimate goal. Ironically, however, our health-care system is specifically targeted toward the diagnosis and treatment of disease and is most obviously lacking in primary prevention of such disease. The resolution of this paradox is the purpose of this chapter.

In order to place preventive gerontology and specifically primary prevention in the elderly in their proper perspective, it is useful to review the concept of social and physiological homeostasis: the maintenance of homeostasis across the human life span; the respective effects of time, disease, and aging upon homeostasis; and the implications of these phenomena for preventive medicine.

Homeostasis may be defined narrowly as the maintenance of an optimal physiological steady state. It includes the ability to react to internal and external stimuli appropriately and in a timely manner, usually with compensatory mechanisms that tap physiologic reserves. These reserves are not constant across the life span, generally increasing during infancy and childhood, peaking during young adulthood, and declining gradually thereafter. Age 30 is often used as a benchmark age of maximum efficiency,[1] although some functional capabilities peak earlier and others later. Assessing the onset and rate of decline in physiologic and psychological competence has occupied a large proportion of gerontological research in "normative aging" to date. General observations proceeding from this research have included: 1) the great individual variation in the time of onset and rate of decline in competence among different persons and among different physiologic systems within a given person, and the generally greater variance among persons of comparable age with advancing chronological age; 2) the amplification of potential defects in measures of physiological reserve when perturbing stimuli are great, when the *time* of return to baseline or *rate* of task performance is a parameter under study, or tasks to be performed are complex and involve multiple interacting systems; and 3) the importance of cohort effects and differential survival in interpreting this research, which is most evident when cross-sectional studies are contrasted with longitudinal studies.

Of special importance to preventing dysfunction in the aged are at-

---

by age, designed to retard time-related disease processes so that they will not cross the clinical threshold during the normal life span. Preventive geriatrics, therefore, is the subset of preventive gerontology that deals with preventive medicine in the elderly.

tempts to dissect the effects of reversible disorders and disease from those of aging per se (primary aging). Primary aging is thought to be immutable; what is potentially changeable is defined as secondary aging. Of special note are certain attributes of declining physiological reserve that have been long accepted as inevitable concomitants of aging but are being questioned in contemporary research. For example, the decline in cardiac function that occurs with age may reflect only the effects of atherosclerosis, a potentially preventable disease process.[2] Even in the absence of atherosclerosis, age-related changes may reflect the effects of reduced physical activity with aging rather than primary aging: diminished sensitivity to neurotransmitters, such as epinephrine and norepinephrine, and hence decreased heart rate response during exercise, may be attributable to increased sedentariness and may be amenable to alteration through exercise training in the elderly. Such interactions make the segregation of primary aging and secondary aging difficult indeed. Nevertheless, the possibility of overcoming actual or potential limitations through conscious alterations in lifestyle, such as exercise programs for the elderly, has raised the hope of "rectangularizing" the relationship between age and physiological function (Figure 21.1) in a manner analogous to the "rectangularization" of the human survival curve, which has proven so attractive in the work of Fries (Figure 21.2).[3] His thesis suggests that premature mortality can be virtually eliminated by individual and collective changes in lifestyle notably through alterations in diet, exercise, and patterns of self-induced toxic exposure (principally alcohol and tobacco). This would result in a shift of the survival curve upward and rightward toward a rectangular shape, given the "barrier to immortality" represented by the fixed upper limit of the human life span (ca. 120 years).

Perhaps less obvious in issues of primary versus secondary aging is the role of time per se in the progression of disease processes from the subclinical to the clinical level. Two examples clearly illustrate this concept. Atherosclerosis may become a universal process in humans if they survive long enough, reaching clinical significance in the form of myocardial infarction, stroke, or peripheral vascular disease (Figure 21.3). Similarly, osteoporosis might progress to the point where spontaneous fractures would develop in all persons if they were allowed adequate longevity. A third example is more problematic: Alzheimer's disease or a related cognitive disorder might prove to be universal should survival beyond 100 or 110 years become the norm. Thus, a byproduct of longer mean survival is an increased incidence of clinical disorders that are time-, and not necessarily aging-, dependent.[5]

Another clear precept is the multifactorial nature of most disorders in old age, as opposed to the prominence of unifactorial, often monogenic, disorders in childhood. For example, atherosclerosis occurring in child-

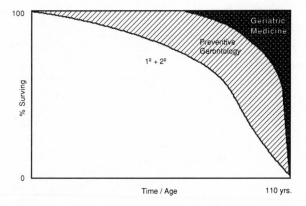

Figure 21.1. Preventive gerontology as the area between the realms of primary (immutable) and primary + secondary (mutable) aging. Decrements that occur with aging today are a blend of preventable and unpreventable changes. In the future, as the principles of prevention are applied, geriatric medicine will deal increasingly with the support of persons in preterminal decline.

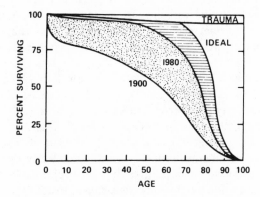

Figure 21.2. Human survival curves for the United States in 1900, 1980, and an (ideal) point in the future (circa 2050), when premature deaths will have been reduced to the minimum possible. *Source:* Data from Ref. 3.

hood is usually attributable to a single major defect, homozygous familial hypercholesterolemia. At the other end of the age scale, atherosclerosis is never unifactorial, and even the common risk factors for coronary heart disease are relatively weak predictors in the elderly. For example, total plasma cholesterol and a positive family history are no longer predictive after age 60.

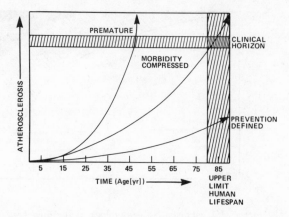

Figure 21.3.   Vectors describing the time course of atherosclerosis. Premature morbidity and mortality result when the disease takes an accelerated course, morbidity and "natural death" are compressed if it takes a gentler course, or prevention is accomplished when death from alternative causes supervenes. *Source:* Ref. 4.

One key to preventive medicine in the elderly is the recognition that psychological and social variables are as important as physical status in determining functional capacity in the aged. Thus the multifactorial nature of illness in the elderly (or its mirror image, health and independence) has at least three dimensions—the socioeconomic, the physical, and the psychological—and perturbations in any of the three may trigger a cascade of problems. As the person's limited reserves become exhausted, further declines may prove irreversible, leading inexorably to death (we have sometimes called this the "slippery slope phenomenon"). While the basic nature of the aging process is still widely debated[6], the concept of a species-specific maximum lifetime potential[7] is clearly established from studies of comparative biology. Since the age-specific decline in no single parameter of physiologic competence is sufficient to account for irreversible loss of homeostatic control, it is the synergism among declines in multiple systems and, moreover, among physical, psychological, and social forces, that truly specifies the upper limit of the human life span.

A probabilistic approach to human survival thus leads to the conclusion that death is virtually inevitable in all persons by 120 years. Not surprisingly, therefore, the shape of the human survival curve in very old age is consistent with the possibility that death occurs largely in random fashion among the extremely aged.

Recently, the figure of 85 (±4) years has been advanced by Fries[3] as the mean and median age of death at some point in the future (ca. 2050), when premature death will have decreased to an irreducible minimum. This estimate has been vigorously challenged,[8,9] with opponents pointing out that death rates have recently been declining most rapidly among those age 85 and older. Nevertheless, even if the figure is closer to 95 or 100 years and the standard deviation is not as low as 4 years, it is clear that homeostasis— physical, psychological, social—becomes progressively precarious in old age in a fashion that exponentially increases the risk of collapse as the upper limit of the human life span is approached.

The implications of these realities for preventive gerontology are clear:

1. Given the fixed upper limit of the human life span, the more closely that limit is approached, the less is the benefit of any mode of prevention as measured in person-years; conversely, the earlier the intervention, the greater the potential benefit as measured in person-years.

2. Given the precarious state of homeostatic balance in old age, physical, social, or psychological alteration is potentially hazardous, and the benefit:risk margin of any intervention may frequently be very narrow in the elderly (which may not have been the case at an earlier stage in life) or even adverse. For example, restriction of dietary fat of animal origin, indicated by national consensus to reduce serum cholesterol levels and attendant cardiovascular disease risk in young adulthood and middle age, may not have sufficient time to retard atherogenesis if started in old age. Furthermore, instituting such a diet in old age risks malnutrition because of the diet's decreased palatability and the body's earlier satiety with low-fat foods, especially among older persons who have diminished taste perception and decreased appetite.

3. The later the intervention, the more proximate must be the benefit; moreover, given the disastrous cascade that may follow even a trivial challenge to homeostasis in the elderly, interventions are most effective when targeted toward the "trigger phenomena" that may initiate that cascade. For example, effective interventions include immunization to prevent influenza, prevention of falls by improving lighting or removing barriers to free access to toilet facilities, and encouragement of liberal fluid intake during a heat wave. Furthermore, efforts at therapy and rehabilitation may yield dramatic recovery of function in the most vulnerable (scrabbling up the slippery slope).

4. The benefits of preventive interventions in old age should not be measured only in traditional, quantitative terms (i.e., survival). An additional six months of life in a vegetative state or restricted environment may be less desirable than two more weeks of independence; therefore, an element of risk-taking must be incorporated in preventive geriatrics, and an evaluation of the quality of the life potentially extended must be factored into any intervention strategy.

Thus, conventional wisdom regarding prevention in the population as a whole may not apply to the elderly, and much humility and much more research regarding the principles of prevention in the elderly are in order.

On a practical level, these tenets translate into a complex equation for assessing the risks and benefits of preventive and therapeutic interventions in the elderly (Table 21.1). Furthermore, estimating the net benefit:risk ratio in the individual elderly patient is notoriously imprecise. The variance in individual homeostatic reserve increases with age; social and psychological factors, difficult for the clinician to quantify, play a greater role in determining outcome; and virtually no research has been performed on specific interventions *among the elderly* themselves. For example, the Coronary Primary Prevention Trial of the Lipid Research Clinics had an upper age limit of 59 years at entry. Moreover, such research as has been performed has almost invariably studied subjects who are atypical among the elderly, that is, those who are taking no medication and have no major life-limiting conditions. Furthermore, although persons who have survived into their seventies and eighties are likely to possess physiologic, social, and psychological characteristics that promote longevity, few such factors predicting longevity have been specifically identified. Hence, estimation of risk is difficult at best.

One biological parameter that has been identified is the low-density lipoprotein cholesterol (LDL-C):high-density lipoprotein cholesterol (HDL-C) ratio. Cholesterol is transported in the blood bound to specific proteins. That carried in the LDL is positively correlated with risk of atherosclerosis, while that bound to HDL is inversely related to such risk; hence the ratio between the two expresses the net effect of both risk indices. This ratio increases in predictive power (notably in its denominator) in old age and appears to be strongly genetically determined.[10] However, the search thus far has proved elusive for a sociopsychological analogue of the HDL-C, which would be a measure of the resilience that so clearly determines function in the elderly, often in the face of astounding handicaps. This has led to a plethora of assessment "instruments," publications on assessment, and a geriatric subdiscipline in and of itself.[11-13] Thus, assessment of the elderly patient is an imprecise art at best, challenging the astute clinician to the maximum.

In the face of these uncertainties, it might be tempting to abandon an aggressive approach to prevention in the elderly. Reinforced by the negative financial incentives to preventive medicine, physicians have generally adopted an expectant if not frankly nihilistic attitude toward preventive geriatrics. Compounding the problem, the difficulties of rigorous research and practice of preventive geriatrics invite uncritical acceptance of fads or pseudoresearch, most often in such broad areas as behavior ("stress"), exercise, and nutrition. The elderly, especially the healthy elderly who are aware of their increasing vulnerability, are therefore susceptible to advice that is unfounded and possibly frankly dangerous. Therefore, geriatric

Table 21.1. Factors that Relate Directly or Inversely to the Efficacy of a Given Intervention as Part of a Strategy of Preventive Gerontology as Applied to Hypertension

Factor	Example
Factors Directly Related	
Power of intervention over risk factor	Certain drugs in treatment of hypertension
Synergistic effect of intervention on other risk factors	Simultaneous increase in HDL cholesterol with use of alpha blockers
Duration of effect of intervention	Upper limit of life span minus sum of age at which blood pressure is reduced and F-factor,* i.e., life span − (age + F-factor)
Factors Inversely Related	
Risks of intervention (including those of diagnostic procedures)	Syncope or falls with hypotensive drugs; dehydration from renal angiography
Costs of intervention	
Economic	Physician and hospital costs
Noneconomic (quality of life)	Loss of palatability of certain foods attributable to sodium restriction
Antagonism between risk reductions from specific intervention in one sphere and risk increases in another	Increased LDL and decreased HDL cholesterol with use of thiazide diuretics and beta blockers
Existing disease and end-organ damage	Myocardial scarring from previous infarction
Competing causes of morbidity and mortality	Malignancy, immunocompromised status, COPD

Source: Ref. 5.
Note: COPD = chronic obstructive pulmonary disease. HDL = high-density lipoprotein. LDL = low-density lipoprotein
*F-factor is the time to maximal effect of reduction (time at which the risk associated with lowered blood pressure becomes equivalent to the risk of an individual who has been at that blood pressure all along).

practitioners, physicians and nonphysicians alike, are well advised to apply their keenest scientific and clinical powers to the formulation of sound preventive strategies while retaining an appropriate humility toward the crudeness and limitations of this craft.

The focus on cardiovascular disease that has been undertaken in many programs is rationalized by estimates of the potential gain in life expectancy if deaths attributable to atherosclerosis were reduced (Table 21.2) and by the recent decline in cardiovascular morbidity and mortality that suggests the potential for change in the risk of coronary heart disease (Figure 21.4), a change attributed by most experts to a decrease in cardiovascular risk factors proceeding from changes in behavior.[15,16] Although much has been gained from interventions instituted long before old age,[17,18] it is noteworthy that the percentage declines in cardiovascular mortality have been consistent across the entire adult life span, including those beyond

Table 21.2.   Gain in Life Expectancy from Eliminating Specified Causes of Death and Chance of Eventually Dying from These Causes: 1969–71

	Gain in life expectancy, yrs		Chance of eventually dying	
Causes of death	At birth	At age 65	At birth	At age 65
Major cardiovascular and renal diseases	11.8	11.4	.588	.672
Diseases of the heart	5.9	5.1	.412	.460
Cerebrovascular diseases	1.2	1.2	.122	.149
Malignant neoplasms*	2.5	1.4	.163	.145
Motor vehicle accidents	0.7	0.1	.020	.006
All other accidents	0.6	0.1	.026	.018
Influenza and pneumonia	0.5	0.2	.034	.037
Diabetes mellitus	0.2	0.2	.020	.021
Infective and parasitic disease	0.2	0.1	.007	.005

Source: Ref. 14. National Center for Health Statistics, U.S. Public Health Service, "U.S. Life Tables by Cause of Death: 1969–71," T.N.E. Greville, "U.S. Decennial Life Tables for 1969–71," Vol. 1., No. 5., 1976.
* Including neoplasms of lymphatic and hematopoietic tissues.

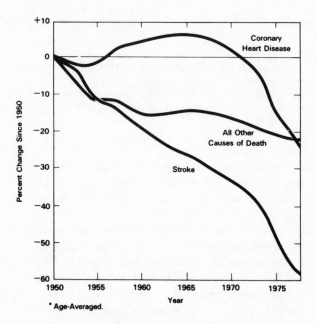

Figure 21.4.   The decline in the U.S. mortality rate since 1950. While mortality from stroke has declined progressively, deaths from coronary heart disease increased initially but have decreased progressively since the mid-1960s. Source: Ref. 16.

age 85. Thus it may never be too late to decrease cardiovascular risk through alterations in behavior, and the principle that preventive strategies in the elderly should focus on "trigger phenomena" (classically a fall or infection) may be overdrawn, perhaps applying best to the minority of the older population who are teetering at the edge of collapse.

The dilemma of preventive medicine in the elderly is perhaps best illustrated by hypertension (Table 21.1). First, the prevalence of hypertension increases progressively with advancing age in all industrialized societies; when blood pressures of 160 mm Hg systolic and/or 95 mm Hg diastolic are used for the diagnosis of hypertension, it is found in 46% of women and 41.7% of men age 75–79.[17] Second, a recent reevaluation of the Framingham Study data clearly confirms the strength of hypertension as a risk factor in coronary heart disease and stroke among the oldest cohort.[18] (The Framingham study, an ongoing observational study of the population of Framingham, Massachusetts, progressively affords insights into health issues of geriatric relevance as that study group enters old age.) Third, the means, largely pharmacologic, are readily at hand to reduce systolic and diastolic blood pressure in persons of all ages, and many elderly appear to respond to even low doses of inexpensive thiazide diuretics.[17] These factors, together with the clearly positive results of clinical trials in younger hypertensive subjects, would suggest that extrapolation to treatment of the elderly would be justified. However, no rigorous clinical trial of the treatment of hypertension in the elderly has yet been completed. While a major multicenter trial of the treatment of isolated systolic hypertension in the elderly—the Systolic Hypertension Project in the Elderly (SHEP) Study—has recently been mounted in the United States, many clinicians are adopting a cautious therapeutic stance pending the outcome of that study, treating only severe systolic hypertension in the meantime. Perhaps most conservative are geriatricians, who are all too familiar with the disasters that may befall the overtreated elderly hypertensive: postural hypotension, syncope, falls, and even strokes. At the other end of the spectrum, geriatricians are equally familiar with the risks associated with untreated hypertension in the elderly: stroke, myocardial infarction, or sudden death. Thus the horns of this dilemma will remain sharp for the time being, at least until the completion of the SHEP trial, which is the *only* formal clinical trial of just one of the many unresolved issues in preventive geriatrics.

A Preventive Health-Maintenance Program for the Elderly

In the absence of clear guidelines for prevention of disability and death in the elderly, a twofold approach appears most rational: a mass and an individualized strategy.

The mass strategy offers safety and low cost. The physician's role in this program is primarily leadership—by example and by advice disseminated through the media (Table 21.3). The content of this strategy is largely the same for the elderly as for younger people. The primary emphasis is upon prevention of cardiovascular disease and malignancy through alterations in diet and "hygienic" behavior. The strategy espouses nonpharmacological interventions that are to a large extent in the realm of practical advice. ** It features seven common-sense attributes of hygienic living, which have been demonstrated by Belloc and Breslow[19] to be associated with lowest mortality across the entire adult life span: getting 7–8 hours of sleep nightly, eating breakfast regularly, avoiding between-meal snacks (later studies suggest, however, that this seems of little real benefit), avoiding cigarette smoking, avoiding excessive alcohol intake, maintaining a reasonable body weight, and engaging in regular physical activity. While inherently attractive, such a program cannot be defended by the most rigorous approach to clinical epidemiology. For instance, how could one conduct a double-blind trial of the effect of number of hours sleep in the prevention of disease? Nevertheless, given the relatively innocuous nature of the advice and the negligible cost of communicating it in mass media, it is hard to fault such a common-sense approach. At the same time, it is important for the clinician, the patient, and the family not to expect too much of this advice, since the benefits of a change in behavior by many will accrue to but a few. On balance, however, this program can have a major aggregate beneficial effect, given the number of persons at risk. On a more individual level, the program can provide reassurance to older persons that they are minimizing risk in a participatory manner, and its implementation in groups of elderly persons may enhance socialization, another preventative especially applicable to the elderly.

The attenuation of time- and/or age-related disease processes through hygienic behavior modification across the adult life span has received publicity in the writings of Fries in the scientific[3] and lay[20] literature. The concept of slowing a disease such as atherosclerosis to the point where it becomes clinically manifest only at about the time of "natural death" (from a concatenation of multiple system collapse) is appealing. The amplification of this concept of prevention to apply to a long list of age-related diseases (Table 21.4), and its nonapplication to a shorter list of trivial age-related phenomena, such as hair greying, has been widely promulgated without uniformly rigorous scientific evidence. As a result, almost all segments of the scientific community have felt obligated to repudiate nearly

---

**Part of the sheer fun of geriatric medicine is in discovering the wisdom of our elders passed along by oral tradition, often by grandparents. These seven common-sense rules of hygienic living are clear examples of the validity of traditional family advice.

Table 21.3. The Physician's Role in Prevention of Chronic Disease

Personal evaluation of the (imperfect) data base; development of a consistent philosophy
Supportive role in community prevention programs
   Source of technical expertise
   Figurehead in intervention campaigns, where advocacy is honest and justified
   Role model in personal lifestyle, avoiding "Do as I say, not as I do"
Development of a consistent pattern of professional practice
   Individualize intervention strategies to given patients
   Interpret discrepancies between mass and individual risk and disease outcomes for both patient and support persons
   Treat the sick, avoid iatrogenesis, give comfort

Source: Ref. 5.

every individual component, casting doubt upon the validity of the entire concept in the process. Nevertheless, many of the precepts of Fries's approach, sharing with those of Belloc and Breslow the untestability of most components, can be incorporated into mass programs of disease and dis-

Table 21.4. Nonmodifiable Aspects of Aging

Arterial wall rigidity
Cataract formation
Graying of hair
Kidney reserve
Thinning of hair
Elasticity of skin

Partially Modifiable Aspects of Aging

Aging Marker	Personal Decision(s) Required
Cardiac reserve	Exercise, nonsmoking
Dental decay	Prophylaxis, diet
Glucose tolerance	Weight control, exercise, diet
Intelligence tests	Training, practice
Memory	Training, practice
Osteoporosis	Weight-bearing exercise, diet
Physical endurance	Exercise, weight control
Physical strength	Exercise
Pulmonary reserve	Exercise, nonsmoking
Reaction time	Training, practice
Serum cholesterol	Diet, weight control, exercise
Social ability	Practice
Skin aging	Sun avoidance
Systolic blood pressure	Salt limitation, weight control, exercise

Source: Ref. 20.

ability prevention across the life span at low cost, with little risk, and with the potential of great benefit throughout much of later life.

Notable in this multipronged approach to health promotion is the leverage of multiple benefits gained through a relatively simple regimen. For example, regular aerobic exercise may improve cardiovascular fitness, attenuate atherosclerosis (possibly by raising HDL levels), reduce bone mineral loss, enhance joint function, and improve morale and confidence. Avoidance of cigarette smoking reduces risk of atherosclerotic disease, chronic obstructive pulmonary disease, and various kinds of cancer. Furthermore, a diet low in saturated fat may reduce the risk of both atherosclerotic disease and cancer.

On the other hand, the simplicity of such a program risks its uncritical application to persons of all ages. Thus it is important to identify those aspects that may not be appropriate among the elderly and to add those that may be especially applicable to them. Notable among the factors that are not constant with age is relative body weight, or obesity. The controversial recent work of Andres[21] suggests that underweight is associated with at least as great a risk of premature mortality as overweight, and minimum mortality is associated with average weight, not a "desirable" relative body weight as defined by the (1959) Metropolitan Life Insurance tables (which have generally equated the leanness of youth with the optimal). Andres has recently redefined recommended weight for height on the basis of minimal mortality rates by *age*. His analysis suggests that the tables for recommended relative weight, even as liberalized in 1983, are too permissive at younger ages and still too stringent at older ages: upper limits for weight are too high among those 20–29 years old and too low among those 60–69. Although these data do not include many of the elderly, their logical extrapolation to the very old suggests that retention of adipose mass in old age is a positive attribute of health and carries a good prognosis. Certainly clinical experience documents the inverse: underweight, and especially weight loss, represents an ominous sign in patients of all ages, especially the elderly, and attempting to redress nutritional (notably caloric) deficiency in the sick elderly patient constitutes a major, common theme in geriatric practice.

A related corollary is also worthy of note.[22,23] Hyperlipidemia is not a major cardiovascular risk factor in the elderly, since total cholesterol levels do not correlate with risk above age 60. Thus dietary alteration to reduce weight or lower lipid levels is rarely indicated in the elderly, sick or well. Given the myriad factors that discourage adequate nutrition in the elderly, encouragement of dietary intake, including group eating programs, should be promoted by all means possible.

Beyond these relatively traditional, biomedically defensible attributes of mass strategies to promote health in the elderly are those aspects of a more

social and psychological nature. Here the data to support specific intervention strategies in the individual elderly patient or "prepatient" are especially scanty. Nevertheless, social and psychological research, especially
on the "macro" level, has clearly documented the high prevalence of
mental disorders among the independent elderly, few of whom receive
specific treatment. Moreover, functional disabilities assume a dominant
role among the elderly (Figure 21.5), but few functional disorders are
amenable to specific, single medical therapies. Therefore, in primary as
well as secondary and tertiary prevention, emphasis is placed upon complex regimens of medical, psychological, and social therapies, with significant synergism among the three to promote optimal function. Regimens
might include treatment of hypertension, support group therapy at a senior
center, and involvement in community affairs. A critical precept of geri-

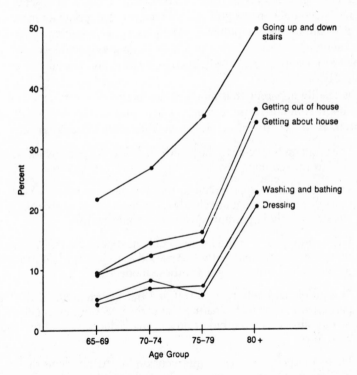

Source: Reprinted with permission from R. C. Benedict and R. Hoke, *Caring for Elderly Persons,*
April 1973 (mimeographed).

Figure 21.5.   Elderly persons reporting difficulty in household mobility.
Source: Ref. 24.

atrics is also relevant here: "Support the supporters." Thus, strategies to assist family members, friends, and neighbors in their care of elderly persons, sometimes through relief, such as day care and respite care, constitute a major component of preventive strategies for the elderly.

The Lifetime Health Monitoring Program

The concept of differential intervention strategies across the life span has received increasing interest and support in the last decade, first with the definition and growth of primary care medicine and recently with the new interest in geriatric medicine. A specific impetus toward formalizing these strategies was the publication in 1977 of the Breslow-Somers Lifetime Health Monitoring Program (LHMP).[25] This program divides the human life span into 10 periods based upon the characteristics of these different portions of life. The last two periods were those of the older adult (ages 60–74) and old age (75 years and older). The LHMP defines a brief set of goals and specific components of professional services appropriate for incorporation into care of the asymptomatic older person, such as a screening physical examination focused upon problems of greatest incidence and relevance to function in the elderly, such as hearing and dental assessments (Table 21.5).

It is readily apparent that much of this program is very practical and based upon common sense as much as upon justification through formal research. However, the principles upon which it is based are specific:

- The program is specific to the health goals of older persons and acceptable to this group.

- The procedure is appropriate to the treatment or prevention of diseases or problems that are clearly identified and jeopardize the quantity or, equally important, quality of remaining life.

- The natural course of diseases or problems that might be identified in this program are sufficiently understood as to justify identification of problems and intervention via those modes.

- The problems likely to be identified by this program in the older participant are of such a nature that early detection, especially in the asymptomatic premorbid state, can reduce mortality and/or morbidity.

- There are specific modes of intervention for the problems that might be identified by this program, and the risks, costs, and benefits of such intervention are sufficiently known and favorable that treatment by these means will be indicated.

- The prevalence and seriousness of the problems that might be dis-

Table 21.5. Lifecycle Preventive Health Services Study
Recommended Services for the Well Elderly Population at Annual Health Visits

Services	Older adults 60–74	Old age 75+
History and Physical Examination with Referrals as Indicated		
Height and weight	+	+
Blood pressure	+	+
Hearing screening	+	+
Breast examination (women over 50 annually)	+	+
Mammography (women over 50 annually)	+	+
Rectal examination	+	+
Complete examination including physical, social, and psychological function	+	+
Dental examination	+	+
Laboratory Examination		
Stool for occult blood (annually)	+	+
Blood glucose	+	
Immunizations		
Tetanus (booster every 10 years)	+	+
Influenza vaccine	+	+
Pneumococcal vaccine (once)	+	+
Counseling with Referrals as Indicated		
Nutrition	+	+
Accident prevention	+	+
Physical activity and exercise	+	+
Alcohol, other drug use	+	+
Cigarette smoking	+	+
Obesity	+	+
Teaching breast and skin self-examination	+	+
Retirement	+	+
Daily oral hygiene	+	+

Source: Ref. 26.

covered are sufficient to justify the economic and noneconomic costs of such intervention.

• The program is relatively inexpensive and can be administered readily, preferably by nonphysicians, with little discomfort to the client.

• The resources exist to diagnose more fully or treat conditions likely to be identified by this program.

Attractive as this program appears, it has not yet been validated through specific research. However, many experiments and demonstrations currently in progress are testing this or closely related programs of health screening in the asymptomatic elderly. Some of these are targeted toward cost-benefit analyses, with the specific goal of reducing overall cost of care of a given elderly population. Rationalizing and projecting a favorable outcome for these seem particularly difficult. First, given the traditional reluctance of elderly persons to seek medical care, the widespread application of this program is almost certain to detect previously untreated disorders and, at least in early phases, increase the cost of care of those persons in whom such disorders are identified. Simply screening an unselected elderly population will identify many instances of cardiovascular disease, osteoporosis, malignancies, and hearing, visual, foot and dental problems, among others. Second, the efficacy of even the most narrowly defined forms of intervention has been difficult to prove even in younger persons at high risk.[27–30] Furthermore, a much-publicized program of balanced, multifaceted treatment of nonelderly at increased risk (the Multiple Risk Factor Intervention Trial, or MRFIT program, designed to reduce cardiovascular disease incidence through individualized regimens of diet, smoking cessation, and blood pressure control) did not demonstrate reduced mortality, an outcome attributable to unanticipated complications of the intervention in a specific subgroup,[31] Moreover, such studies were performed at high cost, and the forms of treatment tested were themselves relatively costly. Clearly the specificity of LHMP as applied to the elderly is far less focused than even the MRFIT protocol. Also, the risk of an inappropriate conclusion being drawn from studies that focus upon cost is very great. If cost is not reduced, should such a program specifically *not* be instituted? Finally, the "window of opportunity" for these studies, even if not directed toward cost issues, is almost certain to close before they are completed and their outcome rendered moot by other forces, chiefly politicoeconomic, that are likely to determine the future of such programs. Hence decisions will have to be made at both the micro level (in a given elderly patient) and the macro level (in the elderly as a group) in the absence of clear answers from rigorous research.

Economic Issues Influencing Preventive Health Programs for the Elderly

Economic forces related to issues of supply and demand and cost and financing currently present major barriers to the widespread application of programs of disease prevention, notably among the elderly. One factor is the traditional bias against preventive services in third-party reimbursement, specifically in the Medicare program. Section 1862 of Title XVIII of the Social Security Act, upon which Medicare is based, specifically prohibits reimbursement for preventive services, including "routine physical check-ups, eyeglasses or eye examinations for the purpose of prescribing, fitting, or changing eyeglasses, hearing aids or examinations there-for . . . immunization . . . or orthopedic shoes or other supportive devices for the feet."[12] Given the obvious relationship to present or near-term functional disability of eye, ear, and foot problems in the elderly, this policy can only be interpreted as aversion of major costs by not reimbursing out-of-pocket outlays by older people (i.e., expenditures borne by older persons themselves for the treatment of health problems, once detected). Moreover, the design of the recent HCFA-sponsored demonstrations to test the efficacy of a "package" of preventive services with cost as a primary analytical endpoint (see Harrington, Chapter 2) is almost certain to confirm this bias. Screening community-dwelling older persons will disclose health problems previously unknown to the patients, or more likely, accepted as inevitable concomitants of aging and so left untreated. However, once detected, such problems (e.g., of hypertension, gum disease, and hearing loss) will lead to treatment and its associated cost and will not necessarily prevent later, higher-cost diseases and disabilities. Therefore, physicians or other health-care providers who have wanted to incorporate preventive services into their geriatric practice have had to be clever, dedicated, or both, to remain financially viable. Toward that end, conscientious practitioners have incorporated the LHMP or variations on its theme into visits for conditions that do permit reimbursement.[32] After all, what elderly patient does not have a minimum of one treatable condition justifying at least an annual evaluation? Nevertheless, if preventive medicine is to be incorporated into the mainstream of health care of the elderly, Medicare, Medigap, and other insurance mechanisms must alter their orientation fundamentally (most likely at the expense of coverage for high-cost hospital care and last-dollar, catastrophic costs). In the absence of such a fundamental change in reimbursement mechanisms, however, even programs as attractive and inexpensive as the LHMP are likely to be practiced sporadically or as a "loss leader" to help save programs, particularly those tied to hospitals, that are currently in financial jeopardy.

In that vein, with considerations of cost and control of inflation in the health-care sector of primary contemporary concern, the elderly are being discovered as "the new . . . market"[33] and potentially the salvation of the business of health-care delivery. Central to this industry in the United States have been hospitals, with their high fixed costs and major role as employers in many communities, particularly in inner cities where the public sector has been primarily responsible for the health-care costs for the poor. Caring for the growing number of poor elderly who are concentrated in these neighborhoods may thus be viewed as an opportunity to preserve the hospital enterprise.

In these competitive times, hospital administrators may be willing to underwrite the costs of speakers on health for senior citizen groups and health fairs, and even to provide funding for individualized screening programs to attract and identify persons who may be candidates for hospitalization and high-cost treatment. Physicians, not necessarily attuned to the special aspects of preventive gerontology, are likely to collaborate in this effort, responding to their professional and altruistic responsibilities and their competitive entrepreneurial instincts. Group practices may employ revenue-sharing schemes to underwrite the program costs by pooling income among primary, secondary, and tertiary care physicians. Therefore the potential risk of exploitation of the elderly, in the name of prevention and health maintenance, must be recognized and considered by planners and regulators as well as by providers who, like their patients, may become caught up in the momentum of a movement beyond their control.

In a perfect world, the resolution of this dilemma of too much versus too little prevention would appear to lie in some form of prepaid or otherwise capitated health-care financial scheme. In this circumstance, *all* the relevant costs of caring for the elderly would be shared over a very broad base, ideally including the future elderly as well, and would incorporate institutional and noninstitutional, "medical" and "social" long-term care. The expense of this effective prevention program would be absorbed easily into the overall plan, representing a very small fraction of the total, yet reducing substantially the aggregate cost of health care for the elderly. The elderly are heterogeneous with respect to health care, as in all other areas. This heterogeneity (particularly when viewed cross-sectionally) is reflected in the emergence of various terms such as the "70–9" phenomenon: 70% of Medicare costs are concentrated in 9% of the elderly.[34] The cost of preventive services concentrated in the other 91%, if formulated along the eight principles enunciated by Somers, is certain to prove almost negligible relative to costs of treatment and support of the dependent, sick, and, grim experience would suggest, largely preterminal 9%. Should such prevention programs prove truly cost-effective, the savings thus accrued could be utilized to enrich other programs and reward the practitioners involved. Thus there appears to be no rational basis for legislative or bureaucratic impediments to widespread implementation of the social health maintenance organization, an expanded HMO focused on the elderly that incorporates long-term care and social services. Will the ultimate HMO, an American equivalent of the National Health Service plus a social services component, prove to be the ultimate answer?

Summary

Preventive health care has traditionally suffered relative neglect in the treatment-oriented, hospital-based American health-care system. This neglect has been most notable in the approach to care of the elderly, for whom Medicare has specifically prohibited reimbursement for provision of such important requisites to function as eyeglasses and hearing aids.

The development of individualized preventive health programs for the elderly is especially complex, given the great variation in levels of function and homeostatic reserve among older persons of comparable age and between the healthy, generally younger elderly and the oldest, most disabled, sick or dying elderly. Moreover, the contribution of social and psychological forces to functional status in the elderly is clear to all health practitioners. Thus, no blanket formula of preventive health maintenance can be applied to the elderly as a group, and detailed physical, psychological, socioeconomic, and, most important, functional assessment represents a major component of the art of geriatrics.

Nevertheless, recent reductions in mortality among the very oldest segment of the population (85 and older), who share decreases in cardiovascular deaths with their younger cohorts, promise further benefits from hygienic approaches to risk-factor reduction across the entire life span. These programs of aerobic exercise, a diet relatively low in fat— especially saturated fat—and the avoidance of cigarette smoking derive as much from common sense as from scientific research, and formal evaluation research on such programs may never be sufficiently rigorous to prove their efficacy in the elderly. The mass media and group education programs may promote these approaches, and physicians caring for the elderly may translate them into individualized regimens as part of routine evaluations. Although current reimbursement schemes do not permit payment for individualized programs applied in isolation, they can be readily incorporated into routine primary care for specific problems.

The rapidly changing health-care marketplace may also make these programs attractive to health-care providers, since they enhance identification and recruitment of present and future patients for hospital care. Thus in some instances prevention programs may represent a double-edged sword to today's elderly: By identifying treatable health problems they impose the risk of hospitalization, which ironically is a major factor in morbidity and institutionalization. Therefore, the real benefits of preventive health maintenance programs for the elderly will be realized only through capitation or other arrangements that contain incentives to limit hospitalization and other high-cost care to what is necessary for optimal patient welfare.

References

1. Shock, N. W. 1980. Physiological and chronological age. In *Aging: Its Chemistry*, ed. A. A. Dietz. Washington, D.C.: American Association for Clinical Chemistry.

2. Weisfeldt, M., Gerstenblith, B., Lakatta, E. 1984. Alterations in circulatory function. In *Principles of Geriatric Medicine*, ed. R. Andres, E. Bierman, and W. Hazzard. New York: McGraw-Hill.

3. Fries, J. 1980. Aging, natural death, and the compression of morbidity. *N Engl J Med* 130–135.

4. Hazzard, W. R. 1984. Atherosclerotic cardiovascular disease: Differential prevention strategies across the lifespan. In *Arterial Disease in the Elderly*, ed. R. W. Stout. Edinburgh: Churchill Livingstone.

5. Hazzard, W. R. 1983. Preventive gerontology: Strategies for healthy aging. *Postgrad Med* 74:279–287.

6. Hayflick, L. 1984. Theories of biological aging. In *Principles of Geriatric Medicine*, ed. R. Andres, E. Bierman, and W. Hazzard. New York: McGraw-Hill.

7. Cutler, R. G. 1984. Evolutionary perspective of human longevity. In *Principles of Geriatric Medicine*, ed. R. Andres, E. Bierman, and W. Hazzard. New York: McGraw-Hill.

8. Schneider, E. L., Brody, J. A. 1983. Aging, natural death, and the compression of morbidity: Another view. *N Engl J Med* 309:854–856.

9. Manton, K. G. 1982. Changing concepts of morbidity and mortality in the elderly population. *Milbank Memorial Fund Q* 60(2):183–245.

10. Gleuck, C. J., Gartside, P. S., Steiner, P. M., Miller, J., Todhunger, T., Haaf, J., Pucke, M., Terrana, M., Fallat, R. W., Kashyap, M. L. 1977. Hyperalpha- and hypobeta-lipoproteinemia in octogenarian kindreds. *Atherosclerosis* 27:287–406.

11. Fillenbaum, G. G. 1978. Validity and reliability of the multidimensional functional assessment questionnaire. In *Multidimensional Functional Assessment: The QARS Methodology. A Manual.* 2nd ed. Durham, N.C.: Duke University Center for the Study of Aging and Human Development.

12. Bergner, M., Bobbitt, R. A., Pollary, W. E., Martin, D. P., Gilson, B. S. 1976. Sickness impact profile: Validation of a health status measure. *Med Care* 14:57–67.

13. Kane, R. A., Kane, R. L. 1979. *Assessing the Elderly: A Practical Guide to Measurement.* Lexington, Mass.: Lexington Books.

14. Brock, D. B., Brody, J. A. 1984. Statistical and epidemiological characteristics. In *Principles of Geriatric Medicine*, ed., R. Andres, E. Bierman, and W. Hazzard. New York: McGraw-Hill.

15. Stern, M. P. 1979. The recent decline in ischemic heart disease mortality. *Ann Intern Med* 91:630–640.

16. Levy, R. I. 1981. Declining mortality in coronary heart disease. *Arteriosclerosis* 1:312–325.

17. Whelton, P. K. 1984. Hypertension in the elderly. In *Principles of Geriatric Medicine*, ed. R. Andres, E. Bierman, and W. Hazzard. New York: McGraw-Hill.

18. Kannel, W. B., Brand, F. N. 1984. Cardiovascular risk factors in the elderly.

In *Principles of Geriatric Medicine,* ed. R. Andres, E. Bierman, and W. Hazzard. New York: McGraw-Hill.

19. Belloc, N. B., Breslow, L. 1972. Relationship of physical health status and health practices. *Prev Med* 1:409–421.

20. Fries, J., Crapo, L. 1981. *Vitality and Aging.* San Francisco, Calif.: W. H. Freeman.

21. Andres, R. 1984. Mortality and obesity: The rationale for age-specific height-weight tables. In *Principles of Geriatric Medicine,* ed. R. Andres, E. Bierman, and W. Hazzard. New York: McGraw-Hill.

22. Hazzard, W. R. 1984. Drug therapy of hyperlipidemia and obesity in the elderly: When therapeutic ratio dips below unit. In *Drug Treatment of the Elderly,* ed. R. E. Vestal. Sidney, Australia: ADIS Health Science Press.

23. Hazzard, W. R. 1984. Disorders of lipoprotein metabolism. In *Principles of Geriatric Medicine,* ed. R. Andres, E. Bierman, and W. Hazzard. New York: McGraw-Hill.

24. Benedict, R. C., Hoke, R. 1973. Caring for elderly persons. (Mimeograph.) In *Hospitals and the Aged: The New Old Market,* ed. S. J. Brody and N. W. Persily. Rockville, Md.: Aspen Systems Corp.

25. Breslow, L., Somers, A. R. 1977. The lifetime health monitoring program: A practical approach to preventive medicine. *N Engl J Med* 266:601–608.

26. Somers, A. R. 1984. Preventive health services for the elderly. In *Principles of Geriatric Medicine,* ed. R. Andres, E. Bierman, and W. Hazzard. New York: McGraw-Hill.

27. Lipid Research Clinics Program. 1984. The lipid research clinics coronary primary prevention trial results. Part I: Reduction in incidence of coronary heart disease. *JAMA* 251:351–364.

28. Veterans Administration Cooperative Study Group on Antihypertensive Agents. 1970. Effects of treatment of morbidity in hypertension. Part II: Results in patients with diastolic blood pressure averaging 90 through 114 mm Hg. *JAMA* 213:1143–1152.

29. Hypertension Detection and Follow-up Program Cooperative Group. 1982. The effects of treatment on mortality in "mild" hypertension. *N Engl J Med* 307:976–980.

30. Fries, E. D. 1982. Should mild hypertension be treated? *N Engl J Med* 307:306–309.

31. Multiple Risk Factor Intervention Trial Research Group. 1982. Multiple risk factor intervention trial. *JAMA* 248:1465–1477.

32. Kennie, D. C. 1984. Health maintenance of the elderly. *J Am Geriatr Soc* 32:316–323.

33. Brody, S. J., Persily, N. A. 1984. *Hospitals and the Aged: The New Old Market.* Rockville, Md.: Aspen Systems Corp.

34. Hersch, B., Silverman, H., Dobson, A. 1982. *Medical Summary: Use and Reimbursement by Person, 1976–1978.* HCFA Pub. No. 03137.

Part Five

Ethical and Political Dimensions of Reform

As a result of medical breakthroughs, innovative financing techniques, new sources of care, and novel conceptual frameworks, the horizons of health services for the elderly seem to expand almost daily. As in most periods of great ferment, these upheavals herald great opportunity and grave risk. With wisdom, vision, and careful thought, bold and effective new strategies can emerge from turmoil; policies implemented without sufficient attention to their ethical and political consequences, however, are likely to be disastrous.

The Gordian knots tied by ethical conundrums and political dilemmas are difficult to unravel. While technology makes life-sustaining intervention possible, it also becomes tangled in a web of connections involving the rights of patients to mediate their own care, the pressure to conserve diminishing resources, and the conflict between traditionally aggressive medicine and personal autonomy. Who will disentangle that web? Who is empowered to allocate scarce medical care? Who is allowed to pull the plug on a patient?

From their detached vantage point, policymakers and financial wizards may conclude that the cost of a particular source of care does not justify its widespread use. But who will have access to a medical procedure others are denied? Someone with the most political clout, or someone with the greatest need? A wealthy old-old patient with few years left to live who can

pay any costs of care, or an indigent younger patient who has many productive years ahead but depends on public resources? Alas, no definitive
answers exist to these and countless other complex moral questions, and
this section offers no packaged solutions. What follows, instead, is a framework in which to view the ethical and political dimensions of health care
for the elderly.

Unless it respects its target population, geriatric care can be neither
ethical nor equitable. Yet, charges Terrie Wetle, blatant and subtle ageism
often warps health policies. By usurping the decision-making rights of their
elderly patients, health professionals have sometimes smothered personal
autonomy with paternalism. Wetle warns that the autonomy of the institutionalized elderly is particularly at risk and cautions against too readily
invoking the "common good" as a justification for circumventing a patient's will.

When public policy involves itself with life and death issues, its decisions should be subjected to ethical scrutiny, claims Monsignor Charles J.
Fahey, who writes that moral solutions must carefully balance individual
and societal needs. The author analyzes the interconnections among ethics, demographics, culture, moral theology, and public policy and calls for
more deliberate planning to enable the elderly to realize a productive and
fulfilling "third age."

Cost containment may exacerbate present rationing of health care based
on ability to pay, according to Robert H. Binstock, in his analysis of the
political environment in which the nation's health and welfare agenda is
being shaped. Binstock discredits the conventional notion of a powerful
old-age lobby that wields great political clout and scrutinizes the effect of
popular perceptions, misconceptions, and stereotypes about old age on the
political climate.

Twenty-two

Ethical Issues and Value Conflicts in Geriatric Care

Terrie Wetle

Autonomy and the Elderly

American society values the autonomy of the individual. The concept of individual autonomy is the foundation of informed consent and underlies the relationship between the individual and his care providers. As the noted utilitarian, John Stuart Mill, stated more than one hundred years ago, "Neither one person, nor any number of persons, is warranted in saying to another human creature of ripe years, that he shall not do with his life for his own benefit what he chooses to do with it."[1]

Bodily integrity, religious freedom, and individual self-determination have each been used to support the concept of personal autonomy. Liberty is a fundamental principle, either as an inalienable right or simply as a rational necessity, and it is an essential part of the social covenant for founding a moral system.[2] Autonomy is the individual's right to self-determination, which means that decisions are voluntary and intentional, and not the result of coercion, duress, or undue influence.[3] Technically, few, if any, decisions are truly autonomous.[4] The individual is constrained by available choices, his own strengths and weaknesses, and the wishes of others.

An earlier form of much of this chapter appeared in Wetle, T. 1985. Ethical issues in long-term care of the aged. *J Geriatr Psychiatry* 8(1):63–73.

For the elderly, however, the available choices are fewer, and the wishes of others are more likely to take precedence. Assaults on the autonomy of elders may be subtle. A physician may give an elderly patient less than complete information regarding the purpose or risks of a diagnostic procedure or may automatically include adult children in discussions of test outcomes and treatment options. On the other hand, assaults on autonomy may be blatant. Health-care professionals may choose not to include an elderly person in treatment decisions and may ignore expressed wishes regarding treatment or placement, involuntary hospitalization, or institutionalization in a nursing home. One might also argue that the existing institutional bias in reimbursement and gaps in the service continuum constitute additional assaults on autonomy, since autonomous decisions depend not only upon the right to make a choice but also upon a reasonable range of options from which to choose.[5]

Assaults on Autonomy: Paternalism and the Common Good

Erosion of an elder's autonomy may often be paternalistic. Paternalism, the interference with an individual's liberty of action, is "justified by reasons referring exclusively to the welfare, good, happiness, needs, interests or values of the person being coerced."[6] At times, however, a facade of paternalism may cover motivations that have less to do with the good of the individual than with some perception of what is good for the family, for the institution, for the care provider, or for society. Paternalism usually is practiced when the individual for whom decisions are being made is unable to make decisions for himself because of cognitive impairment, lack of consciousness, or extreme physical disability. Unfortunately, a paternalistic approach is often taken with older persons even when there is no evidence that their decision-making capability is compromised. It is likely that this practice is based on the ageist assumption that to be old is to be incompetent. Interestingly, with younger adults, competence to participate in decisions is assumed unless there is considerable evidence to the contrary.

Paternalism toward the elderly may result, in part, from the wish to protect older citizens. However, this protection carries with it the potential to harm. Not including the older person in the decision process may mean that decisions are made without complete information about the client's wishes, fears, expectations, financial situation, circumstances at home, or even symptoms of disease. An elderly woman who says, "I don't want an operation for this breast cancer," may be saying that she is fearful of the pain of surgery, that she couldn't tolerate the disfigurement of such a surgery, or that she doesn't believe the operation would make any difference for comfort or survival. She may also be saying that she doesn't believe that she is "worth" the surgeon's time and effort. Each meaning requires a different action. The only way to understand the individual's unique message is to interact with and include the elder in the decision-making process. Noninclusion of the elder in the decision process may also result in "learned helplessness": an individual who is treated as helpless may well become helpless, meeting our limited expectations.[7]

As trained professionals, we believe that our advice is valuable. We are disturbed when patients or families make choices that go against our judgment. Not surprisingly, efforts to seek adjudication of incompetence are virtually always triggered when an individual chooses not to take our advice. Justifications for this type of assault on autonomy are frequently based on the argument that the substitute decisionmaker knows better what is good for the patient. Furthermore, these justifications may be strengthened by arguments that personal autonomy may be compromised in favor of the common good. Widely acknowledged circumstances in which the common good supersedes personal autonomy include the quarantine of patients with highly contagious disease or the confinement of individuals who are a threat to others. This argument has also been used to justify the placement of frail elders into nursing homes, with the reasoning that resources are scarce. When it becomes more expensive to maintain the individual at home than in a care facility, it is argued that the patient should be transferred to a nursing home so that more people can benefit from these scarce resources. Some managed care programs have spending targets that limit the amount to be spent on home care for individual clients to some proportion of average nursing home costs.[8]

The "common good" argument has also been raised in refusal-of-treatment cases. A brief case study provides one such example:

> Mrs. G, a 76-year-old woman with a below-the-knee amputation resulting from complications of long-standing diabetes, had a good recovery from surgery, had learned to use a prosthesis, and had returned to her own apartment where she lived alone. When similar complications developed in her other leg, Mrs. G refused an amputation, stating that "once was enough." After two long hospital stays for sepsis and other complications, Mrs. G was brought to the hospital in a coma, and, after discussions with a distant niece, the surgery was performed. Mrs. G recovered and, with rehabilitation, adjusted well to a second prosthesis. Medicare billings for services *prior to* the last hospitalization and surgery totaled more than $62,000.

Some would argue that this case represents an avoidable expenditure of public funds, and that the common good would have been better served if Mrs. G's refusal of surgery had been overridden earlier in the process, thus avoiding the costs of at least one of the hospitalizations.

In these times of budget austerity, how do we weigh Mrs. G's right to refuse treatment, when such a refusal results in large and quite likely *avoidable* expenditures of public monies? Given current efforts to limit Medicare and Medicaid spending, close scrutiny of cases like Mrs. G's is likely. Furthermore, as more elders enter capitated health plans, such as health maintenance organizations (HMOs), efforts to minimize expenditures are likely to put the autonomy of individuals at even greater risk.

Clarification of Values

Discussions of individual autonomy in health-care decisions often focus on the patient-physician relationship. The public and the courts generally respect the expertise of the physician to make diagnoses and intervene in matters of health.[9] However, a much broader range of actors should be considered, including nurses and allied health professionals, social workers, clergy, the legal profession, family members and other care providers. Each has a part in the decision-making process and provides special and often conflicting professional philosophies, practices, and ethical codes.

Another example illustrates the problems that may arise among different types of care providers.

> Miss B, an 84-year-old, had lived many years with her brother who had a history of multiple hospitalizations for schizophrenia. Because of frail health and problems with mobility, Miss B had not been out of their apartment for more than five years, and she depended totally on her brother for shopping and errands. When her brother was hospitalized once again because of his bizarre behavior and assault of a neighbor, the landlord began eviction proceedings and called a local agency to seek assistance with Miss B, expressing concern that there were garbage smells coming from the apartment, and noting that no one had been in or out of the apartment in more than a week. A social worker was dispatched to evaluate the situation. At first Miss B refused even to talk with the social worker, insisting that she did not need any help. On the third visit, however, Miss B allowed the social worker into her apartment but refused to accept a homemaker or any other intervention except for a Legal Aid attorney to assist her in fighting the eviction. A week later, Miss B was found on the floor of her apartment, having fallen at least two days before. She was hospitalized. The hospital physician, alarmed at her physical condition, recommended a nursing home placement.
>
> Miss B's social worker was angry with the Legal Aid attorney for not fighting institutionalization of Miss B and with the physician for not considering community-based alternatives. The attorney was angry with the physician for not consulting her regarding the placement, and believed that the social worker had violated confidentiality by sharing information with community agencies in seeking care for Miss B. The physician was angry that the social worker had so blatantly neglected Miss B's needs by not bringing her into the hospital after their first conversation.

Each of the professionals involved in the case had a different perspective and approach to Miss B. The social worker, trained to act as an advocate in seeking assistance for the client even when the client refused such assistance, hoped that early intervention would forestall a more serious and perhaps irreversible crisis. The attorney perceived that her role was to execute the client's wishes as the client expressed them. The physician, believing that the patient's competence was compromised, wanted to protect her from further harm. Each person was acting within the ethical code of his or her profession, attempting to do what was "right" for the patient.

What is the most productive course of action when professional values come into conflict? Ordinarily, decision making rarely involves explicit discussion and consideration of the values at play. We assume that the various decisionmakers hold common values, with priorities similar to our own. Because these assumptions are rarely given voice, confusion and anger are likely to occur as action is taken. A first step to avoid such confusion is careful clarification, in relatively simple statements, of assumptions, values, and ethical perspectives held by each participant in the decision-making process. Discussions can, of course, be on a case-by-case basis, but they may be more productive when multidisciplinary teams of service providers discuss the values and ethical considerations of their work in a more general way, separated from the emotions of a specific case at hand. Clarification of values within and between professional disciplines and among providers, families, and clients provides a framework for discussion when conflicts do arise, as well as a common language for approaching resolution of those conflicts. Central to such discussions should be the expressed wishes of the client, keeping in mind the many factors that influence the exercise of autonomy.[4]

Impediments to Autonomous Decision Making

The major assumption underlying the exercise of autonomy is that the individual has been provided adequate information with which to make a decision and is free of undue influence or coercion. However, ageism among professionals, society, and even elders themselves can alter the presentation and interpretation of relevant information. First, well-documented gaps in the professional training of physicians, nurses, social workers, and others providing care to elderly patients lead to mistaken beliefs and negative assumptions regarding the appropriateness and efficacy of treatment for elders. Clinical experiences in caring for older clients may reinforce these negative attitudes and practices. Thus, the information about diagnosis, treatment, and prognosis provided to the patient may be incomplete, biased, or just plain wrong. Furthermore, societal and individual ideas about what constitutes a life worth living may influence those presenting options to older persons or their families. Statements like "She's already lived a full life, why make her suffer through surgery?" would never be made about a 20-year-old, and may indicate devaluation of the later years as well as a bias against intervention.

Certainly, elders are more likely to be financially or physically dependent on others than are younger adults. An individual who is not self-sufficient may well choose different treatment alternatives than one who is independent. Those who are financially dependent on children may, for example, feel constrained to choose treatment options that are less expensive, just as elders who are dependent on their families for personal care may choose less desirable care options that reduce family dependency. Independent elders often express a greater fear of becoming dependent on others for their care than of death itself, and they reflect this fear of dependence in treatment decisions. Moreover, because a large percentage of elders is likely to be dependent on others, care providers often assume dependency to be a characteristic of all aged persons. This assumption influences individual treatment decisions as well as distribution of resources among care options on a broader level. The institutional bias in public support of services to the elderly interacts directly with the perception of dependency.

The elderly in *institutional* settings are at particular risk of compromised autonomy in decision making. The very nature of the institutional setting reinforces negative feelings of dependence, encourages helplessness, and takes away from the individual all but the most trivial of decisions. Furthermore, few nursing home residents actually choose the physician responsible for their care. The lack of regular involvement of physicians with institutional residents makes it unlikely that either will even know the other, let alone develop a knowing, trusting relationship. [10] Compounding these barriers to autonomy is the fact that many residents have some impairment of cognitive function. This has two major effects on clinical decision making. First, cognitive impairment makes it difficult to determine the patient's wishes. Second, because many nursing home patients are cognitively impaired, caregivers tend to treat *all* residents as if they were impaired.

Nursing home resident/patients' rights groups continue to struggle to teach the administration and staff of institutions that many residents are competent and able to pursue meaningful and active lives, to maintain contact with the outside world, and to make decisions regarding treatment and care.

The Elderly and the Family

Shifts in dependency relationships often occur as an older person becomes progressively functionally impaired. These shifts change patterns of interaction within the family and call into question long-accustomed styles of decision making and power relationships. Furthermore, changing societal patterns of family interaction and labor force involvement will continue to decrease the availability of women, the traditional family-care providers. A confusion of values affects the determination of the appropriate level of support to expect from families for their older members. The view that the aged should be cared for at home within an extended, multigenerational family relies heavily on the "good old days" myth that such an arrangement was once the norm in the United States. Although records are spotty, rates of institutionalization of the elderly have remained constant for a century and a half. Moreover, contrary to popular opinion, families are not rushing to dump their elder members into nursing homes. It has been estimated that family members provide as much as 80% of home care and, although it is not reimbursed by Medicaid, it has considerable costs.[11,12] Studies of informal home care show that family providers are likely to be suffering a variety of stress-related problems, including alcohol and drug abuse, depression, divorce, and physical problems such as ulcers and cardiac disease.

The issue of family care is directly related to the broader question of intergenerational responsibilities.[13] What does one generation owe another, or, more generally, how do we distribute scarce resources among generations?[14] Will we enter a period of intergenerational warfare, as the dependency ratio between supporters and those being supported decreases and as suggestions to limit resources for the old become more public?[15] These unanswered questions shadow the formulation of health policy for this country.

The Health-Care System: Allocation of Resources

The current distribution of resources in the health-care system is biased in a variety of ways. First, public monies are more likely to be spent for medical/technical services than social services, are more likely to pay for institutional services in hospitals and nursing homes than for services that keep elders in their own homes, and are more likely to pay for later, more intrusive interventions than earlier interventions that support elders, their families, and other informal caregivers.[8] Public monies for nursing home care are available only to those who have exhausted virtually all of their personal resources (via Medicaid "spend-down"), or who have had the foresight and professional guidance to divest themselves of such resources. Despite state efforts to apply the ethic of equity, public reimbursement for nursing home care for two individuals with identical needs living in the same state may vary by as much as $50 per day.

Fragmented, incremental decision-making processes have resulted in our current patterns of allocation. However, policymakers have begun to seek methods for making more systematic allocation decisions. One increasingly popular approach is cost-effectiveness or cost–benefit analysis. Cost–benefit analysis reduces the costs and benefits of particular health programs to monetary values, allowing comparisons across programs. This approach is difficult to apply to social programs. For example, how does one assign monetary values to improved quality of life or freedom to stay in one's own home? Furthermore, the methods used to assign values to even the seemingly more "objective" measures systematically discriminate against the old. For example, measures of the value of a program that saves lives use life expectancy to determine "life years saved," but also use expected productivity and discounted future earnings to determine the value of those life years. The elderly, who have shorter life expectancies than the young and who are not working because of retirement policies, tend to fare poorly in such analyses. In fact, if public program costs, such as Social Security and Medicare, are factored into the equation, the elderly may actually end up with negative values assigned to each year of life saved! Cost-effectiveness analysis has a useful place in the allocation of health resources. When it compares the costs of programs in relationship to given outcomes, it offers a powerful tool for selecting effective approaches to specific health-care problems. However, such analysis should make explicit the values it uses in the decision process.

The Health-Care System: Organization and Responsibility

Apart from the allocation of resources, several value issues arise in the organization of geriatric health care. Ideally, the future system of care will more closely reflect commonly held values, such as the frequently stated preference that elders remain in their own homes for as long as possible. Future health-care planners may ask how social planning might develop supports for family members to encourage the care of elders. Which services are most cost-effective in maintaining elders at home? When is an institutional placement the most appropriate choice?

A companion value is that elders be cared for in the least restrictive, most appropriate environment, both for quality-of-life considerations and for cost-effectiveness. The current system makes this difficult. Inadequate public reimbursement for heavy-care patients, lack of nursing home beds, and gaps in community care systems result in elders' being cared for in settings that are more restrictive than is needed. The numbers of patients kept for "administrative days" in acute-care hospitals provide evidence of the lack of placement alternatives. Contributing to the problem is the lack of case managers to assist the elder and the elder's family in care planning and in negotiating the system.

A final value for consideration is the affirmation that society does indeed take responsibility for the care of elders.[14] A variety of public programs recognize that responsibility, and yet current and future cohorts of elders fear a continuing erosion of these programs. The service system as it stands is fragmented, confusing, and difficult to negotiate. However, the quality of scientific knowledge of health care for the elderly continues to improve, as do the attitudes of care providers.[16] The current demographic and financial crises provide the incentives to build a cost-effective yet humane care system that results in a better quality of life, not only for the elderly but also for the providers of geriatric care.

References

1. Mill, J. S. 1859. *On Liberty.* 2nd ed. London: John W. Parker and Sons.
2. Veatch, R. M. 1981. *A Theory of Medical Ethics.* New York: Basic Books.
3. Dworkin, G. 1971. Paternalism. In *Morality and the Law,* ed. R. A. Wasserstrom, 104–126. Belmont, Calif.: Wadsworth.
4. Collopy, B. J. 1988. Autonomy in long-term care: Some crucial distinctions. *Gerontologist* 28:10–17.
5. Wetle, T. 1988. The social and service context of geriatric care. In *Geriatric Medicine.* ed. J. W. Rowe and R. W. Besdine, 52–74. Boston: Little, Brown.
6. Dworkin, G. 1972. Paternalism. *Monist* 56(1):64–84.
7. Avorn, J., Langer, E. 1982. Induced disability in nursing home patients: A controlled trial. *J Am Geriatr Soc* 30:397–400.
8. Fox, P. 1981. *Long-Term Care: Background and Future Directions.* HCFA Pub. No. 81-20047. Washington, D.C.: Health Care Financing Administration.
9. Dyke, A. 1973. Ethics and medicine. *Linacre Q* 40(3):182–200.
10. Besdine, R. W. 1983. Decisions to withhold treatment from nursing home residents. *J Am Geriatr Soc* 31:602–606.
11. Brody, S. J., Poulshock, W., Masciocchi, C. 1978. The family caring unit: A major consideration in the long-term support system. *Gerontologist* 18(6):556–561.
12. United States General Accounting Office. 1979. Entering a nursing home: Costly implications for Medicaid and the elderly. *Report to the Congress by the Comptroller General.* PAD-80-12. Washington, D.C.: Government Printing Office.
13. Daniels, N. 1982. Equity of access to health care: Some conceptual and ethical issues. *Milbank Memorial Fund Q* 60(1):51–81.

14. Kingson, E. R., Hirshorn, B. A., Cornman, J. M. 1986. *Ties that bind: The interdependence of generations.* Washington, D.C.: Seven Locks Press.
15. Callahan, D. 1987. *Setting Limits: Medical Goals in an Aging Society.* New York: Simon and Schuster.
16. Lutsky, N. 1980. Attitudes toward old age and elderly persons. *Annu Rev Geriatr* 1:287–336.

Twenty-three

The Ethical Underpinnings of Public Policy

Charles J. Fahey

Questions about life, death, and medical interventions, especially questions about public investments in health care and about the beginning and end of life, always stimulate a high level of debate interest. Unfortunately, a systematic approach to the ethical underpinnings of these questions has not kept pace with the number and complexity of the issues.

Medical ethics has traditionally been identified with decisions about the treatment of individuals, which indeed is an area for ethical reflection but does not exhaust the scope of the term. The behavior of groups, of society, and of government is subject to ethical analysis as well.

Ethics itself is a systematic way of dealing with the "oughtness" of things. There are many approaches to this inquiry, but they all can be characterized by an attempt to establish principles and a disciplined way of looking at the behavior of individuals and of groups. Ethics borrows from many different disciplines in its examination of human experience. At its heart is an attempt to deal with the relative goodness or badness of human acts.

Therefore, in a sense, everyone is an ethicist. Everyone makes value judgments every day. However, the basis for judgments may be more or less carefully developed in different individuals.

In our complex society, we are in constant interaction with others.

Virtually everything we do affects someone else, just as we are profoundly influenced by others. Ethics is the stuff of all these relationships.

The Older Person, the Law, Ethics, and Medicine

The reality that average life expectancy at birth has increased 60% since 1900 has outstripped our ability to understand and cope with it. Attitudes, behavior, values, policies, and structures appropriate for another period and different demographic realities are inadequate to deal with current and future population patterns. The decrease in mortality in every age cohort has resulted in greater numbers of older persons, with the most dramatic growth in the numbers of old-old. Even more significant are the quality-of-life improvements among older persons.

The typical 65-year-old of today is healthier, is better educated, and has more personal and social resources than his age-mate of a generation ago. While there still are sickness, disability, and poverty among the old, the general picture is more favorable than that of even just a few years ago.

Older persons are more than statistics. They are family members, consumers, voters, patients, club members, congregants, and educators. They influence and are influenced by every sector of society, so the "graying" of society generates a new ethical agenda and changes culture itself. It profoundly affects family life and, most importantly for this discussion, public policy. There is no facet of public policy that is more interactive with changing demographics than health care, which contributes to the prolongation of life and is, in turn, profoundly influenced by it.

Definitions

Public policy is articulated in statutes, rules, regulations, reimbursement techniques, tax provisions, and court decisions. One of our most important social vehicles is government. The hopes and dreams as well as the concerns and fears of individuals, families, and groups find expression in public policy. This policy is developed through the political process, in which joint decisions are made about things that we must face together; yet every public policy decision involves some compromise and some loss of individual autonomy.

While *law* is related to ethics, the two are not the same. Law, by nature, is broad and often crass, and although it affects our behavior it does not necessarily affect our convictions. Law itself must stand ethical scrutiny. Ideally, legal structures are built on the presumption that the majority of human interactions will be carried out without appeal to legalities. *Ethics*, in contrast, embodies personal, internalized principles and precepts that affect our entire outlook on life and relationships. Thus, law can impose sanctions but it cannot invade our consciences. It can constrain us or demand things but it does not govern our every act. Our ethic does.

Since health care involves life itself, it is no wonder that it is subject to both legal and ethical scrutiny. This scrutiny extends not only to the behavior of a physician with a patient, but also to the behavior of agencies and institutions and to the allocation of resources. The latter becomes particularly important in a period of economic austerity, real or apparent. The "oughtness" of things, the degree of equity supported by decisions, and the relative importance of different courses of action become significant when it is perceived that not everything can be done nor can everyone be served in the same way.

Value refers to the worth of a thing. In the area of the social sciences, value is the perceived utility of an action. Actions that are in tune with human dignity are considered better or good, and those that are inimical to human dignity are considered less desirable, bad, or evil. Social sciences observe people's values, or preferences, by listening to what we explicitly "call things" or by measuring the way we behave.

Culture embodies all the traditions, beliefs, and values that a certain people, bound together by geography or some other tie, consider central to their common life. Although culture is constantly changing, it is a powerful force in our personal and shared lives.

Ethics, in prescribing what ought to be, constitute a review of people's acts and institutions whereby a value is put on them. Ethics are therefore a set of principles in accord with which persons and groups can judge the appropriateness of actions. Inevitably, ethical judgments involve balancing what enables an individual to achieve fullness as a human being and what is needed by the group (society) to ensure that all persons, today and tomorrow, will have an equal opportunity for a decent existence.

Morality focuses on the religious experience, in contrast to ethics, which appeal to human reason. All religious traditions provide a perspective on the human condition, both that of the individual and that of the collective human experience. Inevitably, these perspectives contain dictates regarding the behavior of individuals. This is the stuff of moral theology.

Culture, ethics, moral theology, and public policy are all challenged by the new demographic imperative. Each is influenced by it, and each influences it. In addition, they all influence one another, because personal and social values are inherent in each. Health issues are inextricably bound up with each of these realities. Health care is inevitably the personal and social area in which difficult, sometimes excruciatingly difficult, choices must be made by society and by individuals.

One final definition is in order here. It is the distinction between technology and values. As a society we have benefited from an explosion in knowledge and its application to our daily lives. In no sector of society is this more evident than in the development and delivery of health care.

Generally, we have cause to celebrate these advances in science and technology. However, no advance is value-free, and each must be evaluated regarding both its intrinsic merit and its value within the total human enterprise.

The truth of this assertion is illustrated by several tragic examples of well-intentioned technological advances, such as in drug developments that have ultimately caused much human suffering. Too often, focus on the immediate gain from a technological advance can obscure the unintended, secondary effects. The application of knowledge is never value-free, and rarely does the institution within which the knowledge has been developed and applied have adequate perspective to evaluate its effect on the whole human condition. Obviously, it is the role of ethics and morality to provide this perspective in health care.

Pluralism and Change

America is a pluralistic society committed to personal freedom, but this ideological pluralism is a source of both strength and weakness. Some societal values, such as a concern for the poor, seem to be deeply embedded in our culture. However, there are increasingly evident signs that a free marketplace, economic approach is dominating the distribution of goods and services.

While we celebrate the Declaration of Independence, the Constitution, and the Bill of Rights, it is unlikely that they could be crafted today. "We hold these truths to be self-evident, that all Men are created equal, that they are endowed by their Creator with certain inalienable Rights . . ." It is questionable whether the philosophic concept underlying these sentences would evoke a consensus in contemporary society.

Our commitment to freedom makes us distrustful of outside activity that may inhibit individual initiatives. The call of the Reagan Administration for deregulation and less governmental intrusion strikes a responsive chord.

Change

Fortunately, democratic institutions offer us the opportunity to evaluate our corporate activities and make midcourse corrections. As we close out the twentieth century, we are in the midst of a period of reevaluation whose breadth and depth we have only begun to realize. Growing international interdependence is governed by many important vectors, all of which are intensified by the improving communication and increased mobility of people. Domestically, the future of the American economy, the role of taxation, and the reciprocal responsibilities of various levels of government are all part of the equation. The graying of the population and its influence on the health-care system inevitably are part of this process.

Currently, debate about Medicare, Medicaid, and Veterans Administration health activities has centered on such issues as cost-containment measures and other "technological fixes" that beg the value questions underlying these programs. The real issue in this debate is the interaction of society with its older citizens. Thus, emerging health issues, which are so closely coupled with difficult public policy issues, demand that the ethical agenda triggered by the graying of society be carefully examined, now.

A New Agenda

The gray revolution affects individuals, family life, the political system, neighborhoods, the marketplace, and the church and synagogue, in addition to the health-care system. The magnitude of these effects has yet to be realized, but clearly they constitute a new reality, involving all persons and institutions.

The reality that many, if not most, persons in the developed world will live into their eighties, with varying degrees of independence and productivity, raises a fundamental moral/ethical question about the obligation that a prolonged life puts upon the individual and society. For the individual, lifestyle choices made in youth will influence health in old age, and today's economic choices will help determine the availability of resources in the less productive and more dependent periods that may be associated with age. For government and other societal structures, there is the consideration of responsibility for such areas as health-care costs of those who voluntarily assume risks that can lead to them being in need. These obligations call for a new agenda in dealing with the increasing number of us who can expect to live fully into a third age.

The Meaning of the "Third Age"

It is useful to consider life as having three ages. The first part of life is associated with the role of a "learner." It is a time of growth in "wisdom, grace, and age." While this growth is life-long, it is the primary task of the first age. The second age is marked by autonomy. In this age, persons make fundamental choices about careers, special friends, marriage, children, and where to live. These choices having been made, the many other choices of one's life tend to be subordinated to maintaining the fundamental choices and fulfilling the roles inherent in these fundamental choices. In the past, and for many persons in less developed countries today, death would intervene before this phase of life was completed.

However, in the developed countries, many have a chance to complete the tasks, fulfill the roles, and enjoy the status associated with the second age, often with a significant amount of life, often 20 or 30 years, still ahead. These last decades are the challenging third age.

Currently, the third age tends to be organized around a twofold paradigm: work/retirement and family life, but there are an increasing number of indicators that these organizing factors are inadequate for this new stage of life.

Fordham University's Third Age Center is forwarding the notion that this period of life should be marked by consciousness and intentionality. Having exhausted the primary roles of the second age, the individuals in their third age have time to examine their youthful decisions about values, lifestyle, friends, work, where one lives, one's use of leisure activities, and the importance of money to life, and to affirm or modify these decisions. Unfortunately, for all too many older individuals, a kind of inertia sets in that precludes this creative approach to the rest of their lives. To counteract this tendency, individuals need organizing principles for the third age, as there were for the first and second ages.

The Family

Public policy often recognizes the fact that the family is central to life. Yet profound changes are occurring in American family life that are not fully understood. The family's role and function have been modified by reason of decreased emphasis on the nuclear family, increased divorce rates and remarriage, the changing role of women, and the mobility of families. Society has not yet addressed the role of this changing family, particularly with regard to its disabled elderly members (even in families where the elderly are not disabled, the effect of the change from a norm of four generations to an anticipated norm of five generations must be examined).

Traditionally, a woman, either a spouse or a daughter, has been the caregiver for the older disabled person, but changing lifestyles and expectancies give rise to questions concerning the future of such informal support. It has been part of our societal ethos that children care for their frail parents, but in the new reality of the multigenerational family subject to divorce and remarriage, the order of priority among family members can change radically.

These changes make it necessary to undertake both new ethical reflections concerning rights and responsibilities within families and renewed public policy discussions that consider the person at risk and the effect of policy on individual and family behavior. For example, although other administrations had consistently interpreted Congressional intent as well as the Medicaid statute itself as precluding states from seeking the participation of children in paying for services for their otherwise eligible parents, the Reagan Administration reversed this policy. Discussion of the implications for family relations was overshadowed by fiscal considerations, and there has been virtually no debate about the equities involved.

A particularly poignant problem is presented by the example of an elderly couple, one of whom needs extensive long-term care services. In most instances their resources are considered to be jointly owned, and thereby available for the care of the disabled spouse. The "well" spouse, usually the wife, is then faced with a spend-down period in which the couple's savings are depleted, leaving little for her needs.

The Corporate Ethic

For purposes of ethical analysis, persons who have come together to perform services for others in a corporation can be considered to have formed a new entity that is analogous to an individual, morally and legally. The corporation is capable of acting like an individual and it must exercise the same responsibilities as an individual. As a person acts in an ethical or an unethical way, so does a corporation.

Human service agencies serving older persons should be especially aware of their corporate ethic. Unfortunately, many tend to be totally reliant on outside agencies for standards of behavior. As is true of law generally, regulatory processes are generic and minimalist. No matter how detailed and pervasive they may be, they exhaust the relationship between the person served and the institution.

Therefore, each institution has to make explicit its convictions by translating them into corporate values operationalized in policies, practices, and procedures. It should hold itself accountable for its behavior. It should develop techniques of reflection and means of continual value renewal.

Society and Risk

The sharing of risks is a hallmark of American society, informally on a neighbor-to-neighbor basis, and formally in institutionalized social structures. Therefore, although we value the centrality of the family's role in meeting human need, we also recognize that all of us are at risk for illness, accidents, and disability, and that most families, no matter how prudent and frugal they are, cannot bear the costs associated with some of these events. Some risks are so high or so much part of the overall economy of the country that society has developed insurance mechanisms, such as Social Security, Medicare, and unemployment insurance, to provide protection to all persons against financial catastrophe while spreading the costs broadly. These measures are a recognition of our interdependence. While they contain an element of self-interest, they also appeal to our consciences.

However, we have yet to make definitive societal decisions about the risks associated with old age. There are many publicly supported programs for older persons. Some are universal in their coverage, while others are means-tested, but neither individually nor collectively do they constitute insurance protection against the catastrophic effects of frailty and disability in elderly people.

The Public Policy Agenda

Samuel H. Preston's widely published presidential address, presented at the Population Association of America's annual meeting in Minneapolis, Minnesota on May 3, 1984, discusses the implications of the growing share of the federal budget that is being devoted to the elderly. He forwarded the thesis that through a "set of private and public choices" we "have dramatically altered the age profile of well-being." He further noted "Let's be clear that the transfers away from the working-age population to the elderly are also transfers away from children, since the working ages bear far more responsibility for childrearing than do the elderly."[1]

He further noted "The reorientation toward the elderly is consistent with the declining share of the GNP that is represented by savings and with dramatically rising debt service burdens on future generations."[1]

His address concluded with the observation that a move toward increasing familial responsibility may be based not on the premise of families' strength, but on their very weak voice in the public dialogue.

His argument, while buttressed by substantial empirical data, is profoundly value based. He asks if we have become selfish and asserts that one can read self-interest for interest in the elderly.

The Senate Special Committee on Aging noted in its information paper, "America in Transition: An Aging Society," that increased federal spending for health care has not reduced health costs to older Americans. "The elderly pay nearly a third of their total health care bills out of pocket, a percentage that has remained constant in recent years."[2] The Senate report continues: "Today, rising health care costs rather than spending for retirement income, are the greatest source of increase in public spending on the elderly. . . . generally, the share of the Federal budget going to the elderly is expected to remain fairly stable for the next two decades, as declines in retirement income spending offset increases in health spending. Only then should overall spending on the elderly rise as a proportion of the budget, and then only if health costs have been allowed to rise unchecked in the interim."[2]

It seems unfortunate that efforts to protect the elderly from the increased cost of health care are construed as an inappropriate policy decision. Furthermore, any discussion that pits one population group against another in the policy arena without consideration of other expenditures is flawed.

Ethics and Policy

In initial efforts to deal with the federal budget deficit, economic and political considerations have dominated the public discourse; there has been little discussion of the "oughtness" or ethic of our public acts.

In biomedical ethics, discussion tends to focus on the decision-making process. The patient's freedom to make decisions is emphasized, not the fundamental "oughtness" of the treatment proposed.

As difficult as it may be, we must attempt to delineate an ethical agenda for these discussions. We must address the issues: our expectancies for individuals in the light of a prolonged life span and for families as they are changed today and will change tomorrow; the role of the private sector, including the so-called mediating structures and informal interactions; and the role and responsibility of government at all levels in helping us all share the burdens of those who are the poorest and most vulnerable among us.

References

1. Preston, S. H. 1984. Children and the elderly: Divergent paths for America's dependents. *Demography* 21(4).
2. United States Senate, Special Committee on Aging. 1985. *America in Transition: An Aging Society*. Washington, D.C.: Government Printing Office.

Twenty-four

Aging and the Politics of Health-Care Reform

Robert H. Binstock

This chapter focuses on the political effects that aging, as well as perceptions of old age and age relations, may have on the reshaping of American health care. In the context of population aging, or as some have termed it, "the aging society":[1] Will older persons and old-age organizations have a significant political role in shaping health care for the elderly? What is the political environment in which the present agenda of health and welfare policies toward aging is being addressed? What roles do current perceptions of old age and age relations play in the politics of policy issue framing? In turn, what are the potential consequences of the issues that are now framing the choices that lie ahead in shaping health care for the elderly? Finally, are there alternative constructs for framing the politics of such issues that can provide us with different—and perhaps more useful—choices for shaping the future of health care in an aging society?

Population Aging and the Distribution of Political Power

An axiom of public rhetoric purveyed by journalists, leaders of aging-based organizations, and partisans of a variety of social causes is that older persons

Some portions of this chapter draw upon the author's article "The Oldest Old: A Fresh Perspective or Compassionate Ageism Revisited?" 1985. *Milbank Memorial Fund Q* 63:420–451.

wield significant political power—as it is frequently termed, "senior power"—in shaping policies affecting aging.[2,3] Moreover, the conventional expectation is that further increases in the numbers and proportions of older persons will substantially enhance their political influence on decisions about Medicare, Medicaid, Social Security, and a variety of other issues that appear to be highly salient to the self-interests of aging persons. This point of view implies that older persons and their organized representatives will have a major influence in shaping health care for the elderly.

Despite this conventional wisdom, there has been no evidence to date that so-called senior power has played a significant role in shaping major policies toward the aging, such as Medicare and Social Security. In fact, the enactments and amendments of such policies have been attributable largely to the initiatives and preferences of public officials in the White House, Congress, and the bureaucracy who have been focused on their own agendas for social and economic reform.[4–8]

There is no sound reason to expect that population aging will bring about a major redistribution of power to older persons for shaping health-care reform or other purposes. To be sure, persons 60 years of age and older already constitute about 15–17% of Americans who vote in national elections, and this proportion can be expected to grow in the years immediately ahead.[9] Furthermore, the number and membership rolls of aging-based interest groups has grown exponentially in recent decades.[10–13] However, the sources of power available through these modes of political participation are limited in the context of the American political system. The basic reasons for these limitations are briefly summarized here.

The Larger Context of the American Political System

If one conceives of modern democratic systems as being arrayed upon a continuum ranging from centralized to fragmented power, the American system is located among those characterized by extreme fragmentation.[14] Public power is dispersed among 80,000 distinct governments, semi-autonomous structures within those governments, and tens of thousands of quasi-governmental entities, such as Health Systems Agencies and Area Agencies on Aging. In addition, significant power is dispersed among innumerable private entities—economic, social, professional, and religious elites; industrial, commercial, and trade organizations; political action groups; and organized citizen constituencies—all of which have influence in governmental and nongovernmental spheres of decision making. Moreover, our political parties are loose, relatively undisciplined coalitions that hardly begin to pull together these fragments of power in any concerted fashion.

In this context the two main sources of power that might be available to large, mass constituencies like older persons—voting and mass-membership interest groups—are only tenuously and tangentially linked to the processes of policy decision making. Much more important in the processes that determine public policy are such factors as the preferences and initiatives of public and private elites [often pursued through economically and professionally based interest groups], structural changes in the economy and a variety of social institutions, the diffusion of ideas, technological innovations, and goods and services, and the predominant political culture and ideology.[15]

Even within the limited context of the power that is potentially available through voting and mass-membership interest groups, older persons and aging-based advocacy groups have had little political significance and are unlikely to in the future. This is apparent from evidence to date, as well as from basic understandings of political behavior.[7]

Old Age and Voting Behavior

Older persons do not vote in a monolithic bloc, any more than do middle-aged persons or younger persons. Consequently, the aged do not wield power as a single-issue voting constituency.

As Table 24.1 should make clear, election exit polls have shown repeatedly that the votes of older persons distribute among candidates in about the same proportions as do the votes of other age groupings.[16–18] Although men and women can be seen to have distributed their votes differently from each other, persons 30 years of age and older cast their ballots in these elections in a similar fashion. Examination of properly sampled exit polls from other national elections shows these same phenomena.

None of this should be surprising, since there is no sound reason to expect that a cohort would suddenly become homogenized in its political behavior when it reaches the "old age" category. Diversity among older persons may be at least as great with respect to political attitudes and behavior as it is with respect to economic, social, and other characteristics.[7]

The very assumption that mass groupings of the American citizenry vote on the basis of self-interested responses to single issues is unwarranted. Candidates, not issues, run for office. In the context of choosing between candidates, a voter's response to any one issue is part of an overall response to a variety of issues in a campaign and to many other campaign stimuli that may have little to do with specific issues or the presumed "self-interest" that might be implied by a single issue.[19] Moreover, within a heterogeneous group, such as older persons, self-interested responses to any single issue are likely to vary substantially. The best available studies show that even in the context of a state or local referendum that presents a specific issue for balloting—such as propositions to cap local property taxes or to

Table 24.1. Vote Distribution, by Age Groups and Gender, in Presidential Elections

	1980			1984		1988	
	Reagan	Carter	Anderson	Reagan	Mondale	Bush	Dukakis
Percent of All Voters	51	41	7	59	41	53	45
Percentage of Men							
18–29 years old	47	39	11	61	37	55	43
30–44 years old	59	31	4	62	37	58	40
44–59 years old	60	34	5	63	36	62	36
60 years and older	56	40	3	62	37	53	46
Percentage of Women							
18–29 years old	39	49	10	55	45	49	50
30–44 years old	50	41	8	54	46	50	49
44–59 years old	50	44	5	58	41	52	48
60 years and older	52	43	4	64	35	48	52
Percentage of Adults							
18–29 years old	43	44	11	58	41	52	47
30–44 years old	54	36	8	58	42	54	45
44–59 years old	55	39	5	60	39	57	42
60 years and older	54	41	4	63	36	50	49

Sources: Refs. 16, 17, and 18.

finance public schools—old age is not a significant variable associated with the distribution of votes.[20]

The Power of Old-Age Interest Groups

Similarly, the power available to mass membership interest groups "representing"[21] older persons is limited. As implied by the preceding discussion of electoral behavior, such organizations have not been able to cohere or even to shift marginally the votes of older persons. For example, in the 1980 presidential campaign, the leaders of several major aging-based organizations endorsed President Carter in his bid for re-election. Nonetheless, a majority of older persons voted for his opponent, Ronald Reagan, and in the same proportion as voters in younger age groupings.[16] Experience in other modern democratic states has been comparable. When attempts have been made to organize the votes of older persons to affect the fate of a particular candidate, party, or proposition, they have not been notably successful.[22]

Some forms of power, however, are available to old-age interest groups. In the context of what Lowi has characterized as American "interest-group liberalism,"[23] the old-age mass-membership organizations—as well as other organizations that are involved in dealing with older persons as consumers, clients, and subjects for study—have a role in representing "the interests of the aged." While the inherent distortions of such forms of representation are well known,[21] the normative position that has evolved for interest groups in American politics provides these organizations with sufficient credentials to participate in most formal and informal policy processes that are relevant to aging. Indeed, in the classic pattern of American interest-group politics, public officials find it both useful and incumbent upon them to invite such organizations to participate in policy activities. In this way, public officials are provided with a ready means of having been "in touch" symbolically with millions of constituents, thereby legitimizing subsequent policy actions and inactions. A brief meeting with the leaders of these organizations can enable an official to claim he or she has duly obtained the represented views of a mass constituency.

The legitimacy that old-age organizations have for participating in interest-group politics gives them several forms of power. First, they have easy informal access to public officials—to members of Congress and their staffs, to career bureaucrats, appointed officials, and occasionally to the White House. Consequently, they can put forth their own proposals—regarding Medicare, nursing home regulations, and a variety of other matters—and work to block the proposals of others. To be sure, their audiences or targets may be unresponsive, but access provides some measure of opportunity. Second, their legitimacy enables them to obtain public platforms in the national media, Congressional hearings, and national conferences and commissions dealing with old age, health, and a variety of subjects relevant to policies affecting aging. From these platforms the organizations can exercise power by initiating and framing issues for public debate and by responding to issues raised by others. A third form of power available to these groups might be termed "the electoral bluff." Although these organizations have not demonstrated a capacity to swing a decisive bloc of older voters, no politician wants to offend "the aged" or any other latent mass constituency if he or she can avoid doing so. In fact, the image of senior power is frequently invoked by politicians when, for one reason or another, they desire an excuse for doing nothing or for not differentiating themselves from their colleagues and electoral opponents.

These forms of power, while minor in comparison to the power available to organizations that are based upon major economic interests, do appear to have some impact. Historically, as indicated earlier, the aging-based interest groups have not played an influential role in shaping Medicare, Medicaid, Social Security, and the Employee Retirement Income Security Act. Rather, the influence of these organizations has been confined largely to the creation and maintenance of relatively minor policies that have primarily distributed benefits to professionals and practitioners in the field of aging, not directly to older persons themselves.[10,12,24]

Today, as policies affecting old age have taken top position on the agenda of domestic policy issues, the old-age interest organizations seem to have become one of what Heclo has characterized as antiredistributive veto forces in American politics.[25] The limited power these organizations have available to them is being applied in a defensive effort to maintain the existing distribution of benefits and privileges among older persons, as well as among the many professional and practitioner interests that have emerged and flourished in relation to the growth of the elderly population.

In waging a defensive battle against changes in existing old-age policies, the aging-based interest groups promote the image of senior power. In doing so they have attempted to define as "politically unfeasible" any changes in the existing framework of policies that would appear to be against the self-interests of the artificially homogenized elderly constituency for which they purport to speak.

Despite such efforts by old-age interest groups, many public policy decisions adverse to older persons have proved to be politically feasible in recent years through changes in Medicare, Social Security, and other programs. Medicare deductibles, copayments, and Part B premiums have increased continuously. Old Age Insurance (OAI) benefits have been made subject to taxation. The legislated formula for Cost-Of-Living-Adjustments (COLAs) to OAI benefits has been rendered less generous, and the implementation of COLAs has been postponed. The redistributive mechanism of "minimum benefits" under Social Security was eliminated for new OAI eligibles at the outset of this decade (under the Omnibus Reconciliation Act of 1981), and the Tax Reform Act of 1986 eliminated the *extra* personal exemption that all persons 65 years of age and older have been receiving for years as they have filed their federal income tax returns.

Such adverse changes are relatively minor, of course, in comparison to more drastic reforms in old-age programs, put forward as proposals by public officials and discussed by policy analysts, that would restructure policies toward aging more fundamentally.[26–27] Furthermore, the defensive efforts of old-age interest groups, through the limited forms of power available to them, may have had some effect in "containing the damage." But, as is argued below, the relatively minor character of these changes is more likely attributable to ways in which the underlying American penchants for political incrementalism and pragmatism are being expressed in response to the policy challenges of an aging society.

Population Aging and the Agenda of Public Policies

Over many decades, through disparate threads of public action that have not been guided by a master design, American society has woven a large and complex tapestry of programs on aging. Today, for a variety of reasons, that tapestry seems to be unraveling, and issues involving aging are at the

center of most the controversies in contemporary public policy. Our predominant societal response to these controversies has been to reinforce or
to replace specific weakened threads in the tapestry; we do not seem to be
willing to step back to gain some perspective for viewing the tapestry in its
entirety and to envision the potential implications of preserving it through
the decades ahead.

The Construction of an "Old-Age Welfare State"

American policies toward older persons have been adopted and amended
in substantially different social, economic, and political contexts throughout the past half-century. Widely variant interpretations have been made
of the reasons why each policy was originally enacted and subsequently
altered. In the 50 years since passage of the Social Security Act of 1935,
innumerable explanations for its enactment have been put forward.
Among them are: a desire to provide immediate financial assistance to
millions of older persons who had no other significant source of income; an
attempt to get older workers out of the labor market to make room for
younger workers; a response to political pressures from large, grass-roots
old-age pension organizations; and a far-sighted construction of the first leg
of a "three-legged stool" [consisting of Social Security, pensions, and sav-
ings] that would ultimately provide adequate retirement income.[28] Similarly, among the interpretations applied to the enactment of Medicare in
1965 have been: a way to make health insurance available to retired
persons who could not obtain it once they were no longer eligible for
employee group insurance plans, a mechanism for income redistribution,
and an intentional "first step" toward the eventual establishment of a
universal national health insurance program.[4,6]

Regardless of interpretations of the "original intent" of any of these and
other policies toward aging, by the mid-1960s a common theme was taking
shape. Through the cumulative effects of many separate legislative actions,
American society had adopted and financed a number of old-age benefit
programs and tax and price subsidies for which eligibility is not determined
by need.

This theme was strengthened as old-age-based interest groups, which
had begun to develop a national presence in the 1960s, repeatedly articulated compassionate stereotypes of older persons.[10] For nearly two decades
these "advocates for the aged" were telling us that the elderly were poor,
frail, socially dependent, objects of discrimination, and above all *deserving.*
Through the late 1970s virtually every issue or problem that could be
identified by these organizations as affecting some older persons became a
governmental responsibility toward older persons in general. Programs
were established to provide nutritional, legal, supportive, and leisure ser-

vices; housing; home repair; energy assistance; transportation; help in getting jobs; protection against being fired from jobs; special mental health programs; a separate National Institute on Aging; and on, and on.[12,29] American society had learned the catechism of compassionate stereotypes very well and expressed it through a variety of governmental programs and objectives implying that virtually all older persons have a common set of characteristics that require public intervention.

These perceptions of older persons, and the old-age categorical arrangements that express them institutionally, have reflected an underlying *ageism*, which consists of the attribution of the same characteristics, status, and deserts to an artificially homogenized group labeled "the aged," and the assumption that many of the biomedical, behavioral, economic, and social characteristics we conventionally associate with older persons are inevitable conditions of old age.

The intents and effects of ageism—unlike those of racism—have not been wholly prejudicial to the well-being of its objects, the aged.[30] Until recently, many elements of ageism have been impelled by compassionate concerns for the welfare of elderly individuals and have been expressed through a great many policies providing benefits and protection to older persons solely on the basis of old age.[29]

Because older persons came to be stereotyped as "the deserving poor," they have been exempted from the Calvinist screenings that are applied to other Americans in order to determine whether they are worthy of governmental assistance. Historically, programs for the aged have not been subject to the disdain and stigmatization attached to other welfare programs in American political culture. Indeed, the architects of these old-age programs have developed their own cliché to explain this phenomenon to us: "Programs for the poor make for poor programs." Apparently, compassionate ageism has made a special case of "the aged," creating for older persons a unique sanctuary from the harsh judgments of the Protestant work ethic that is so intricately embedded in American political ideology and culture.

In truth, of course, any of the needs for collective assistance that have been symbolized by old age can be found extensively among persons of all ages. Yet the great bulk of our governmental expenditures on health and social welfare is for benefits to the aged. In effect we have created an "old age welfare state,"[31] and until recently we have seemed largely content with these arrangements.

The Spectre of an Aging Society

Throughout the 1980s, however, the special sanctuary of health and welfare policies that had been created for older persons was threatened. Public resources were viewed as scarce. "Containing health-care costs" emerged as one of the most popular objectives of the day. "Reducing the deficit" became the overriding imperative of domestic politics. Although demographic change has not been responsible for making public resources scarce, for exponential increases in health-care costs, or for the rapid growth of the federal deficit,[32] the aging of our population—or "the graying of America"—is widely perceived as exacerbating, if not creating, these problems. In this contemporary milieu, controversial issues involving old-age programs are virtually pre-empting the present agenda of health and welfare policy debates in this nation. As one economist has put it, the classical metaphor for trade-offs in political economy, "guns vs. butter," has suddenly been replaced by "guns vs. canes."[33]

The spectre of an aging society materialized rather abruptly for Americans at the outset of the 1980s. We were suddenly bombarded by media pronouncements concerning the so-called crises in financing Old Age Insurance and Medicare health benefits through the Social Security payroll tax. Our attention was drawn to the demographic trends that are bringing about unprecedented increases in the number and proportions of older persons in our society. We are becoming aware of the fact that our national government is spending as much on old age benefits as on national defense, about 26% of the annual federal budget.[34]

As we begin to put these pieces together, the prospect of an aging society seems foreboding. Among the many anxieties that have been generated are: the moral dilemmas that may be posed by the allocation of health-care resources on the basis of age; the formidable challenges of financing and developing an adequate and effective range of supportive services for long-term care and rehabilitation of older persons; the labor market competition between older and younger workers within the contexts of age-discrimination laws, seniority practices, and rapid technological change; and a politics of conflict between age groups. Moreover, the long-time dream that biomedical discoveries might dramatically extend the human lifespan now seems to loom as a nightmare because its fulfillment might exacerbate these perceived economic, social, and political problems.

These anxieties, partially based upon extrapolations from demographic trends and current policies toward older persons, have understandably engendered foreboding images of the future, and such extrapolations have rendered increasingly problematic the principles of financing, eligibility, and allocation that are embedded in some of our current policies on aging.[35,36] Doubts about old-age policies have been expressed at a broad philosophical level in debates over whether it makes sense to provide public benefits and protection on the basis of old age rather than need.[27] At a more pragmatic level, issues have been addressed in terms of whether it is politically feasible to replace "universal" and "social insurance" programs for older persons with policies that are more selectively targeted within the older population—and to other population groupings—on the basis of economic need and other forms of need.[37]

These challenges to the ageism expressed in our policies toward older persons are undergirded by the most elementary principles derived from scientific studies of aging and older persons. It is evident that older persons are notably diverse in emotional, physical, behavioral, economic, social, and political characteristics, and that much of our behavior and the conditions that we experience in old age are shaped by the full life course of experience in our youth and throughout our adult years. Nonetheless, American society has adopted many policies that treat all old people as if they were alike. At the same time we are not far-sighted enough to undertake collective actions directed toward children, young adults, and the middle-aged for the purpose of shaping the conditions of our old age.

At the moment, however, we do not seem strongly inclined to confront the problematic principles in our policies toward old age. Rather, we appear to be clinging to both ageism and extrapolation from current arrangements in a fashion that reflects our American penchant for reforming policies through incremental adjustments and pragmatic compromises. Even as we have recently celebrated the anniversaries of major policies toward aging—the fiftieth anniversary of Social Security, the twentieth anniversary of Medicare, Medicaid, and the Older Americans Act, and the tenth for the Employee Retirement Income Security Act—we tend to sanctify them and the principles that they seem to express. We would rather make minor cosmetic adjustments that we can rationalize as "preserving the integrity of the program" than consider if a policy is sound as it functions in a contemporary context. We prefer not to deal with issues that imply drastic reform, such as whether it makes sense to undertake public intervention on the basis of old age rather than need.

The Neo-Politics of Old-Age Stereotyping

As old-age policies have taken top place on the agenda we have found some new ways to deny the diversity among older persons and the life course of experiences that shapes each of us for old age. In turn, these modes of denial have facilitated policy changes that have not disturbed the basic principles upon which we have constructed the old-age welfare state.

Multiplying the Strata of Old-Age Stereotypes

One rubric through which we have made it easier to avoid confronting the problematic principles in our current policies has been to stratify stereotypes of older persons on the basis of multiple old-age categories. In the 1980s it became a widespread practice to label persons 65 to 74 years of age as the "young-old" and to perceive all persons in this age group as healthy and capable of earning income. If retired, they are seen as a rich reservoir of resources to be drawn upon for providing unpaid social and health services and fulfilling a variety of other community roles. In contrast, persons 75 and older are now commonly termed the "old-old" and tend to be saddled with the traditional compassionate stereotypes of older persons as poor and frail.

Ironically, this new set of conventions for old-age stereotyping emerged through distortions of an effort by Neugarten[38] to break down age-based stereotypes. More than a decade ago, to illustrate the growing irrelevancy of chronological age for describing group characteristics, she presented data grouped by conventional and unconventional age markers. However, these illustrative age markers were soon converted by journalists, policy analysts, partisans of various causes, and scholars to establish the young-old and the old-old as new conventions for old-age stereotyping.

More recently the seeds for the growth of an additional stratum of old-age stereotyping have been planted as the National Institute on Aging has launched a research initiative focused on persons 85 years of age and older, described as the "oldest-old."[39] For a variety of reasons that have been set forth elsewhere,[40] it is reasonable to expect that the oldest-old will soon become a common label connoting extreme conditions of poverty, disease, disability, and social dependency among the elderly.

These new stratified conventions for old-age stereotyping have—in effect—staked out a high ground in the politics of compassionate ageism. They have already served politically to legitimate marginal changes in the traditional ages used for old-age categorical policies, without the need to confront the issue of whether old-age categorical policies make sense. For example, the age of initial eligibility for full Social Security benefits is now scheduled to rise gradually from age 65 to 67 early in the next century. Furthermore, many suggestions have been made for moving the age of Medicare eligibility up to age 67, 70, or even 75. In short, a multiplication of strata for old-age stereotypes has made it easier politically to effect minor changes in the ages that are used as very crude markers in public policies for approximating those among the elderly who may need collective assistance of one kind or another.

Reversing Old-Age Stereotypes

The other major rubric that has been used in recent years to deny the diversity among older persons and to avoid violating the political norms of incrementalism and pragmatism, has been to reverse the traditional com-passionate stereotypes of older persons as poor, frail, politically impotent, and "deserving." We now find—in the media, political speeches, public policy studies, and the writings of scholars—a fresh set of axioms of public rhetoric:

- The aged are relatively well off, not poor.
- The aged are a potent political force because there are so many of them and they all vote in their self-interest.
- Because of demographic changes, the aged are becoming more numerous and politically powerful and will be entitled to even more benefits and substantially larger proportions of the federal budget; they are already costing too much and in the future will pose an unsustainable burden on the American economy.[41]

Even as the earlier compassionate stereotypes concerning older persons were partially unwarranted, so are these current ones. They are generated by applying simplistic assumptions and aggregate statistics to a grouping called "the aged" in order to gloss over complexities. If one chooses to compare changes in the median or average income of all older persons with changes in the income of other groupings, one can assert that the aged are relatively well off.[42] If one wishes to ignore abundant evidence to the contrary, summarized above, one can assume that the votes of older persons are determined by issues, particularly an old-age issue above all others, that they will all respond to that issue self-interestedly, and that they will all perceive their self-interests to be the same.[19] If one pretends that outlays for Medicare, Old Age Insurance, and other policies are immutable and mechanistically determined by demographics rather than by legislative and administrative decisions, one can conclude that the aged constitute an unsustainable burden for the American economy.

The seeds of these new stereotypes had been planted through decades of compassionate ageism. It was to be expected that a perceived shrinking of resources would be accompanied by a shrinking of compassion.[43] But the ageism that had been previously constructed remains intact, lumping older persons together in a homogeneous mass.

This reversal of stereotypes—much like the stratification of old-age stereotypes into multiple-age categories—has facilitated many incremental changes in programs affecting older persons, without disturbing the basic principles embedded in policies. On the one hand, the axiom regarding the political power of the elderly makes it seem as if no major or drastic reforms in policies toward older persons would be feasible. On the other hand, the stereotypes portraying older persons as relatively well off and posing an unsustainable economic burden have served as a broad justification for a series of policy changes, such as taxing Old Age Insurance (OAI) benefits for moderate- and high-income older persons, postponement of cost-of-living adjustments in OAI, elimination of the minimum benefit under OAI, and repeatedly increasing deductibles and copayments under Medicare. Such changes have been accomplished without confronting traditional principles of social insurance and age-categorical eligibility or introducing directly the issues of need-based or means-tested mechanisms in the context of Social Security, Medicare, the Older Americans Act, and a host of other policies.

Stereotyping and the Politics of "Intergenerational Equity"

The new forms of old-age stereotyping would not necessarily be pernicious if they simply facilitated minor program reforms while maintaining the facade of policy principles that has been politically acceptable for many decades. But the potential implications seem to be more grave.

On the foundation of these new stereotypes there is a present widespread tendency—among journalists, politicians, scholars, and self-styled advocates for old-age-based interests—to frame public issues in terms of conflicts between age groups. Although there is no systematic evidence of age-group conflict within the American populace as yet, public rhetoric may be fomenting it. Moreover, the very framing of issues in these terms is important in itself, because their structure interferes with our capacity to perceive phenomena in terms of other frameworks that may be more accurate and useful.

The phrase "intergenerational equity" has become a sweeping contemporary label for describing trade-offs in health and social welfare allocations.[44] In turn it has spawned a series of metaphors for more specific dilemmas in the arena of health care and in other sectors of American life.

Justice between Age Groups

"Justice between age groups"[45] has become a metaphor for concern that widespread rationing of acute health care will be brought about by cost-containment measures, such as Medicare's prospective reimbursement on the basis of diagnosis related groups (DRGs) and restraints upon cost shifting from patients who rely upon governmental health insurance. But there is no inherent reason why issues of justice in allocating health-care resources need to be framed on the basis of age. One can just as easily frame trade-offs within age groups, or without regard to age. Better yet, one can frame trade-offs between expenditures in the arena of health care and other arenas.

If the issues of health-care allocations continue to be framed as trade-offs between age groups, it does not take much imagination to envision that a stereotyped group termed the old-old or oldest-old will be assembled in the front row of the trading block. Consider the repeated public discussions of the high proportion of Medicare expenditures on persons who are in their last year of life. In 1983, for instance, Alan Greenspan, now Chairman of the Federal Reserve Board, observed that 30% of the annual Medicare budget is expended on patients who die within the year, and that these persons represent only 5% to 6% of the total number of persons covered by Medicare. There are many spurious elements in the construction of such figures.[46] Nonetheless, Greenspan pointedly asked "whether it was worth it to spend large amounts of money" on such patients.[47] This issue has been stated and restated in one form or another during the past few years. It has usually been phrased in a more refined fashion than the report of a speech by the governor of Colorado in 1984 suggesting that terminally ill old people have a "duty to die and get out of the way."[48] Even with refinements, though, the issue is likely to persist. And it will stay focused on older persons—not on middle-aged persons, youths, or infants who are in their last months of life—because of preoccupation with financing and outlays for the age-categorical Medicare program, the social values implicit in economic theories that undergird policy analyses of the costs and benefits of public expenditure,[49] and continued stereotyping of the aged. Indeed, a noted biomedical ethicist went so far—in a widely publicized 1987 book—as to propose that life-saving health care be denied to persons aged in their late 70s and older, as a matter of public policy in America.[50]

Long-Term Care

"Long-term care" has become a metaphor for health care and social supports for chronically ill and disabled older persons, although the rates of chronic illness and disability and the costs of dealing with them are significant among persons of all ages.[51] Here again, the issue is framed to emphasize the enormous economic, social, and familial burdens of caring for the needs of older persons, without comparable public attention being paid to the implications of such needs and burdens generated within other population groupings. To the extent that attention is given to such needs within younger populations, however, rehabilitation—whether focused on the goals of compensation for or restoration of lost functional capacities—receives a reasonable amount of attention. But only a few[51,52] have given attention to rehabilitation as a dimension of treatment for the chronically disabled elderly, even with the modest goal of maintenance of existing functional capacities. The newer stereotypes of the old-old and the oldest-old are likely to reinforce long-standing tendencies to perceive the challenges of chronic illness and disabilities in terms of caretaking, without rehabilitation, for elderly residual human entities as their functional capacities gradually erode or precipitously decline just before death.

Increasing Dependency Ratios

"Increasing dependency ratios," conventionally expressed as the size of the retired population relative to the productive working population, has become a metaphor for anxieties about the economic burdens of population aging. This construct grossly distorts the issues involved because it is largely an artifact of the existing policy that finances Social Security and Medicare benefits to retirees through a tax based on the paychecks of workers rather than through some other form of taxation.

The most general problem with this construct lies in the use of the number or proportions of workers in a society to assess the productive capacity of its economy. Productive capacity is a function of a variety of factors, including, for example, capital and technological innovation as well as number of workers. Hence, issues involving productive capacity and numbers of workers should be expressed in terms of "productivity per worker," in order to take account of a full range of macroeconomic variables.[53]

More specific flaws in common usage of dependency ratios express the ubiquitous impact of ageism in the framing of issues. Age categories are used to estimate the numbers of workers and retirees—rather than actual and projected labor force participation rates—even though the two approaches can yield substantially different results. Similarly, the focus on retirees as "the dependent population" ignores children and unemployed adults of any age who are economically dependent; for instance, recent research has indicated that a decline in "youth dependency" during the decades ahead may well moderate or even dominate the economic significance of projected increases in "elderly dependency."[54]

Despite such distortions in discussions of increasing dependency ratios, these discussions have seemed to generate several assumptions that may be unwarranted. One is that we will need a far greater number of workers in the decades ahead than can be projected from current age norms for entering and retiring from the labor force. A second is that older persons who would retire under present policies will want to and will be able to work in the future if the incentives to retire and the ages associated with them are marginally adjusted. A third assumption is that there will be employer demand for such workers.

Although these assumptions may be unwarranted, they are being given impetus by the old-old and oldest-old stereotypes. The more that the ages of 75 and over or 85 and over are equated with frailty and social dependency, the easier it is to perceive all persons at younger ages—in their seventies and below—as capable of and obligated to earn their own livings, rather than to view them as exempt from the Protestant work ethic. One can well imagine that policies setting the ages of eligibility for retirement benefits will soon begin to move upward, well before the minor changes that are scheduled to be phased in gradually in the next century. Yet, we know today that two-thirds of current Social Security beneficiaries chose to retire before age 65, even though it meant that they received reduced benefits, and that poor health as well as the availability of pension income is a powerful influence on decisions to retire early.[55]

The Political Power of the Aged

"The political power of the aged" is still another metaphor frequently used to misframe issues in terms of age-group conflicts. As discussed earlier, the political influence of older voters and old-age interest groups is vastly overrated. Nonetheless, the image of so-called senior power persists because it serves certain purposes. It is used by journalists as a tabloid symbol to simplify the complexities of politics.[56] It is marketed by the leaders of old-age-based organizations, who have many incentives to inflate the size of the constituency for which they speak, even if they need to homogenize it artificially to do so. It is called to attention by politicians when they desire an excuse for doing nothing or for not differentiating themselves from their colleagues and electoral opponents. And it is attacked by those who would like to see greater resources allocated to their causes.

In the past decade the image of senior power has been used frequently to frame conflicts between age groups. A notable example was an article by Preston,[3] then president of the Population Association of America, in which he pleaded for more public resources to be devoted to children. He structured his argument so as to draw stark contrasts between children and the elderly with respect to their status and the funds expended on them, and characterized the two groupings as being in direct competition. One of Preston's prime explanations for the comparative success of the elderly was "their political influence," which he attributed to their increased number, their high voting rates, and their self-interested voting behavior on issues. He presented nothing; however, to show that older persons' votes distribute differently from those of persons of any age grouping. All he did to buttress his argument that there is a self-interested homogeneous tendency among older persons was to cite responses to one question in one opinion poll. He did not even begin to deal with the complexities or the realities of voting behavior and its tenuous connections to the processes of policy decision making.

What is likely to happen as stereotypes of the old-old and oldest-old become added ingredients to such caricatures of the American political process? As social welfare and health program cutbacks began in 1981, the children's lobby immediately expressed concern that it would be pitted against the old-age lobby in a struggle over the shrinking pieces of the pie.

Fearing that the old-age lobby would win this struggle, a former deputy assistant secretary for Health and Human Services under President Carter proposed that parents who have children under the voting age of 18 be enfranchised with an extra vote for each such child.[57] Alternatively, why not treat morbid and dependent elders like children? Someone may soon revive Douglas Stewart's proposal, made some 15 years ago, that all persons be "disfranchised . . . at retirement or age 70, whichever is earlier"—a proposal made because its author was disgusted by his perception that the aged were responsible for the election of Ronald Reagan as governor of California.[58] In comparison with age 70, the ages of 85 or even 75 would be easy targets for disfranchisement.

Intergenerational Equity versus Other Forms of Equity

These few examples of current metaphors in the politics of health and social welfare allocations may be sufficient to illustrate that issues are being framed in terms of conflicts between age groups, that the frameworks are frequently constructed from spurious and unwarranted assumptions, and that the emergence of multiple and reversed old-age stereotypes tends to perniciously exacerbate the implications of the issues that have been framed. More important to note, however, is that the very description of issues in terms of age-group conflicts diverts our attention from other ways of viewing trade-offs and options available to us that may be more accurate and more propitious.

Any description of the axis upon which equity is to be judged tends to circumscribe the major options available for rendering justice. The contemporary preoccupation with so-called intergenerational equity diverts our attention from inequities within age groups and throughout our society. Because of the large costs of old-age categorical programs and aggregate statistics on the status of the elderly, the plights of the most seriously disadvantaged persons with the older population are now largely ignored, even though the benefit mechanisms in existing policies do little to substantially alleviate their distress. At the same time, the needs of seriously disadvantaged persons in middle-aged and younger age categories are receiving little attention and emphasis. Through old-age-based programs we spend an enormous amount on health and welfare, but we are not a welfare state in the conventional sense of the term.

It may very well be that we do not want American society to become a welfare state in the broader sense. Viewed in this light, our current expressions of age-group stereotypes and conflicts, and our tendencies to extrapolate, may serve us well. Since the current and projected costs of programs for the aging are perceived as unsustainable, attempts to curtail those costs are dominating our health and social welfare agenda. With our agenda thus occupied by issues of intergenerational equity, we are precluding from serious consideration any substantial health and welfare reforms—involving other issues of equity—that may be badly needed by persons of all ages who are in distress, and for the quality of life in our society.

Whether or not the United States will ever become a broader welfare state, it is certainly becoming an aging society in demographic terms. But the implications of population aging for our society do not need to be simple extrapolations from current perceptions of old age, age relations, and the institutional arrangements through which they are expressed. Extrapolation is only one of many modes of prediction, and it is a relatively inaccurate one because the characteristics of society are dynamic, not static. Yet, our capacities to anticipate and cope with the implications of population aging are being confined to a narrow tunnel of vision where greater numbers and proportions of stereotyped older persons are being viewed within the existing frameworks of policies and institutional arrangements.

To anticipate the health-care and other challenges of an aging society effectively, at least two steps would seem to be essential. One is to inform ourselves continuously about the diversity within current and future cohorts of older persons, and the ways in which life-course contexts are shaping each of us for old age. Even to the extent that age markers are crude approximations for certain statuses, social roles, and societal responsibilities, they change swiftly. A second step, equally important, is to frame issues that express societal health and welfare dilemmas in terms other than conflicts and categorical divisions between age groups. As illustrated earlier, many issues expressing such age-based conflicts are spurious and unwarranted. Moreover, to rely heavily upon extrapolations from today's public policies to predict and plan for the future makes little sense. Generating pragmatic options that express incremental changes in age-categorical policies, in order to preserve the existing tapestry of policies and institutional arrangements, will unduly delay our urgent need to confront fundamental dilemmas that will have to be resolved in meeting the health-care challenges of an aging society.

If we can perceive issues that express equity in terms other than intergenerational trade-offs and conflicts, those issues may generate a series of new practical choices for public and private institutional arrangements in the decades ahead. It is not within the scope of this discussion to set forth a blueprint for such arrangements. But it is feasible to illustrate briefly some of the ways in which health-policy dilemmas that are being expressed in contemporary issues can be viewed in other terms.

Perspectives on Health-Care Rationing

There is no inherent reason why issues of equity in the allocation of acute health-care resources need to be judged in relation to age. In their portrayal of how rationing works in the frameworks of fixed budgets of the British National Health Service, Aaron and Schwartz[59] have shown how older age is but one of the prime criteria involved in rationing decisions there. They have also been careful to note that if extensive and explicit rationing takes place in American health care, it may not take place along the same dimensions that it does in Great Britain.

If rationing does become widespread in the United States, it may very well take place primarily on the basis of the financial status of patients. Some rationing of health care has been taking place for a long time in this country on the basis of economic as well as social and demographic characteristics. The establishment of Medicaid and Medicare in 1965 largely eliminated the phenomenon of "charity cases" by providing public reimbursement for the care of indigent patients and promoting the goals of equal care and equal access to care for all persons. Since then we have had the luxury of pretending that physicians and their associates in the health professions were doing everything they could for everyone. But as cutbacks in Medicaid and Medicare have accelerated cost shifting from the medically indigent to those who have other than governmental insurance or can pay out of pocket—and as insurance companies, insurance premium and out-of-pocket payers, and state governments have reacted—the luxury of the pretense of equal access and care is eroding.

If we can put aside immediate preoccupations with Medicare and the age-categorical principle that it expresses, perhaps we will see that it is the capacity of patients to pay for charges—out of pocket or through third-party reimbursements—that has a great deal to do with the allocation of care. Maybe the concern about old-age-based rationing is justified. But consider what would happen if Medicare coverage became sharply reduced, means-tested, or totally eliminated. Some older persons would be able to pay for extensive and high-quality care out of pocket, and many more would be able to afford to pay premiums that would insure most of the costs of acute care. Near-poor and poor older persons would be left in the same position as medically indigent persons of all ages. In this light we can more clearly see that rationing, and its tacit judgments regarding the worthiness of human lives, might mean the re-emergence of two-class or even three-class medicine.

"Justice between rich and poor" may be a better metaphor than "justice between age groups" for the dilemmas of equity we might confront in the rationing of acute care. With the issue framed on this axis, the specific policy options we might generate and consider would be rather different from those we are contemplating now, and would probably be more accurate reflections of the actual trade-offs in the allocation of health-care resources.

It is also possible that anxieties about extensive rationing are unwarranted because cost containment is not an end in itself. Certainly, none of us is willing to finance what we regard to be wasteful and excessive practices in health care, yet, if steps can be taken to reassure us that physicians, hospital corporations, medical equipment manufacturers, pharmaceutical companies, and medical malpractice lawyers are not receiving more than their "fair share" of health expenditures, then our hunger to contain health-care costs may be satiated. Under such circumstances—which may be extremely difficult to bring about—Americans may very well want the best available care for everyone, even if they have to pay for it through taxes, as well as out of their pockets and by trading off some of their salaries and wages for employee-benefit health-insurance premiums.

As some observers have pointed out,[60] there is no inherent reason why 11%, 12% 13% or more of our gross national product cannot be expended on health care. After 20 years of socialization to the "rights" or "entitlements" provided through Medicare and Medicaid, it could well be that Americans—reassured that they are not paying for waste and excesses— will neither want to impose a ceiling on health-care expenditures nor be willing to accept the rationing practices that such a ceiling would impose.

Walzer has argued that notions of justice throughout history have varied not only among cultures and political systems, but also among distinct spheres of activities and relationships within any given culture or political system.[61] Nothing requires us to devise or accept separate spheres of justice within the health-care arena, either spheres separating age groups or spheres separating the relatively wealthy from the relatively poor. We may prefer to delineate the health-care arena as a single sphere of justice within which no such distinctions are made.

Perspectives on Long-Term Care

Perhaps the best prospects for resolving the challenges of developing and financing long-term care and rehabilitation services lie with adult children—particularly middle-income children—who may be the source of substantial demands for new developments. Many adult children—in their forties, fifties, and sixties—are confronting intractable dilemmas. Faced with the choices of expending more than $40,000 a year for guilt-reducing institutional care, or institutionalizing a parent in a Medicaid warehouse— the Space Age version of the Elizabethan Poorhouse—or absorbing the economic, psychological, social, and other costs of maintaining a chronically ill person in their own homes (perhaps while raising children or

sending them to college), they may push strongly for new alternatives.
One arena in which this demand is being expressed is the private sector market.[62] Many adult children may be only too happy and able to pay for selected components of a continuum of care, not covered by either public or private insurance, that can make community or home-based alternatives to institutions truly viable. This demand may turn into a significant market for private enterprise.

Another way in which such a demand could be articulated is through collective bargaining efforts aimed at reshaping employee group insurance plans. If care for parents and others is becoming a pervasive stress in an aging society, it is certainly conceivable that most of us would like to be insured against the possibility of having to pay extraordinarily expensive bills for long-term care and rehabilitation. Insurance companies would not have to worry about the issue of adverse selection if long-term care insurance is designed as an indissoluble portion of a group health-insurance package. Premiums and benefits for maternity are indissoluble from basic health-benefit plans today, regardless of whether it is possible or probable for a given individual in the group to have a child. If long-term care responsibilities are as pervasive as one anticipates in an aging society, the possibilities and probabilities of such responsibilities would distribute among a labor force grouping in at least a rough approximation of the distribution for maternity benefits.

Still another arena in which the demand for long-term care financing may be felt is national politics. A distinct possibility is a compulsory national insurance program for long-term care,[63] similar to the compulsory program of Old Age and Survivors Insurance. If the demand for long-term care becomes strong enough, compulsory long-term care insurance may be considered as an option to replace Old Age Insurance benefits under Social Security. We may, as a nation, come to consider it more important to insure against the financial catastrophes of long-term care and rehabilitation than against reduced income in retirement. More than half a dozen long-term care bills were introduced in Congress in 1988.

Finally, another way in which the demand for adequate long-term care supportive services may find expression is through the development of locally felt senses of crises, and local government responses that finance such services. Crises generate powerful incentives to those who undertake to solve them, namely the people who directly feel their effects. If we review the history of the United States, we find that fully developed services (beyond the token or symbolic level) have emerged not from national initiatives, but from local crises. It was the extreme impact of sudden and large waves of immigrants from Europe in the latter half of the nineteenth century that led to the development of professional police services, fire-protection services, and public health services. Similarly, development of community-financed services for an ever-growing chronically ill and disabled population may be generated through the crises in the lives of individuals and families that are felt widely and expressed profoundly in local communities.

Even when resources are perceived as scarce, the identification of *essential* services is a dynamic process that continuously brings about different answers, in the form of resource allocations at the community level. Cohesion in values for achieving such answers is always much easier to achieve at the community level than at the level of a mass society of 240 million persons. And in many communities where middle-aged children are coping with the dilemmas posed by caring for their parents and other dependents, there may be substantial cohesion regarding the need to pay local taxes for public long-term care and rehabilitation services, and/or to cut back on other services and facilities.

Conclusion

These are but a few examples of how contemporary health-care dilemmas can be perceived in terms that express neither compassionate and dispassionate ageism nor conflicts between age groups. Whether they are more accurate or even more useful ways to frame issues is certainly open to debate. They have been offered to illustrate that the contemporary politics of stereotypes, policies, and institutional arrangements that reflect current perceptions of old age and age relations divert us from alternative ways of attempting to anticipate and deal with the health-care implications of population aging.

If we are willing to put aside the politics of old-age stereotypes and to perceive the future in terms that transcend the existing tapestry of old-age policies, we may enrich our perspectives and find practicable options that flow from them for coping with and shaping health care for the elderly. The risks are minimal. At worst, such unconventional perspectives may be labeled absurd, and even the half-life of the absurd is very short these days. Ten years ago it would have been outrageous to suggest that Old Age Insurance benefits should be taxed. Today, by virtue of the Social Security Amendments of 1983, they are being taxed by the federal government. Five years ago the notion of extensive and comprehensive long-term care insurance was regarded as impracticable. Today, a variety of initiatives for such insurance are being seriously explored and launched in both the public and private sectors.

Certainly it should be clear by now that the political power of the aged—such as it is—will neither have a significant influence in shaping health care for the elderly nor preclude broader and drastic changes in American health care generally. Since 1981 a great many important

changes have been made in Medicare and other old-age benefit programs—
changes that the conventional wisdom perceived as counter to the self-
interests of "the aged." The so-called old-age lobby did not prevent them.
Indeed, the Medicare Catastrophic Coverage Act of 1988 was endorsed by
the 28-million-member American Association of Retired Persons, despite
the outrage that middle-income older persons have expressed at the new
taxes that this law requires them to pay.[64] If there is a Congressional
response to this sense of outrage, it will probably consist of only a minor
adjustment in the financing structure of the Catastrophic Coverage Act.
The myth of senior power need not limit our perspectives regarding what is
politically feasible.

As we confront the challenges of reshaping health care for the elderly, it
will be especially important for us to examine the principles implicit in the
issues we frame. If we allow our thinking about health-care reform to be
confined by our current policies and the old-age stereotypes they have
come to reflect, we may very well find ourselves engaged in policy debates
based on age-group conflicts that are far worse than those we have experienced to date, openly trading off the value of one human life against
another. The principles of equity that we use to describe our policy choices
will play an important political role in shaping health care for the elderly as
the more general, drastic changes in the financing, organization, delivery,
and allocation of American health-care resources continue to unfold.

References

1. Institute of Medicine, Committee on an Aging Society and National Research
    Council. 1985. *America's Aging: Health in an Older Society.* Washington, D.C.:
    National Academy Press.
2. Malcolm, A. H. 1985. New generation of poor youths emerges in U.S. *New
    York Times* October 20, p. 1.
3. Preston, S. H. 1984. Children and the elderly in the U.S. *Sci Am* 251:44–49.
4. Marmor, T. R. 1970. *The Politics of Medicare.* London: Routledge and Kegan
    Paul.
5. Derthick, M. 1979. *Policymaking for Social Security.* Washington, D.C.: Brook-
    ings Institution.
6. Cohen, W. J. 1983. Securing Social Security. *New Leader* 66:5–8.
7. Hudson, R. H., Strate, J. 1985. Aging and political systems. In *Handbook of
    Aging and the Social Sciences*, 2nd ed., R. H. Binstock and E. Shanas, 554–585.
    New York: Van Nostrand Reinhold.
8. Light, P. 1985. *Artful Work: The Politics of Social Security Reform.* New York:
    Random House.

9. United States Senate, Special Committee on Aging. 1986. *Developments in Aging: 1985*, Vol. 3, 90. Washington, D.C.: Government Printing Office.
10. Binstock, R. H. 1972. Interest-Group liberalism and the politics of aging. *Gerontologist* 12:265–280.
11. Pratt, H. J. 1976. *The Gray Lobby.* Chicago, Ill.: University of Chicago Press.
12. Estes, C. L. 1979. *The Aging Enterprise.* San Francisco, Calif.: Jossey-Bass.
13. Lammers, W. W. 1983. *Public Policy and the Aging.* Washington, D.C.: CQ Press.
14. Binstock, R. H., Levin, M. A., Weatherley, R. 1985. Political dilemmas of social intervention. In *Handbook of Aging and the Social Sciences*, 2nd ed., ed. R. H. Binstock and E. Shanas, 589–618. New York: Van Nostrand Reinhold.
15. Huntington, S. P. 1981. *American Politics: The Promise of Democracy.* Cambridge, Mass.: Belknap Press of Harvard University Press.
16. *New York Times*/CBS News Poll. 1980. How different groups voted for president. *New York Times* November 9, p. 28.
17. *New York Times*/CBS News Poll. 1984. Portrait of electorate. *New York Times* November 8, A-19.
18. *New York Times*/CBS News Poll. 1988. Portrait of the electorate. *New York Times.* November 10, 18-Y.
19. Simon, H. A. 1985. Human nature in politics: The dialogue of psychology with political science. *Am Political Sci Rev* 79:293–304.
20. Chomitz, K. M. 1985. Demographic influences on local public education expenditures: A review of econometric evidence. 1987. In *Demographic Change and the Well-Being of Children and the Elderly*, ed. Committee on Population, Commission on Behavioral and Social Sciences and Education, National Research Council, 45–53. Washington, DC: National Academy Press.
21. Lowi, T. J. 1974. Interest groups and the consent to govern: Getting the people out, for what? *Ann Acad Political Soc Sci* 413:86–100.
22. Heclo, H. 1974. *Modern Social Politics in Britain and Sweden: From Relief to Income Maintenance.* New Haven, Conn.: Yale University Press.
23. Lowi, T. J. 1969. *The End of Liberalism.* New York: W. W. Norton.
24. Lockett, B. A. 1983. *Aging, Politics, and Research: Setting the Federal Agenda for Research on Aging.* New York: Springer Publishing Company.
25. Heclo, H. 1984. The political foundations of anti-poverty policy. In IRP Conference Papers on *Poverty and Policy: Retrospect and Prospects*, 6–8. Madison, Wis.: Institute for Research on Poverty.
26. Binstock, R. H. 1979. A policy agenda on aging for the 1980s. *NatJ* 11:1711–1717.
27. Neugarten, B. L. (ed.) 1982. *Age or Need?* Beverly Hills, Calif.: Sage Publications.
28. Achenbaum, W. A. 1983. *Shades of Gray: Old Age, American Values, and Federal Policies Since 1920.* Boston, Mass.: Little, Brown.
29. Kutza, E. A. 1981. *The Benefits of Old Age.* Chicago, Ill.: University of Chicago Press.
30. Cf. Butler, R. N. 1969. Ageism: Another form of bigotry? *Gerontologist* 9:243–246.

31. Myles, J. F. 1983. Conflict, crisis, and the future of old age security. *Milbank Memorial Fund Q* 61:462–472.
32. Storey, J. R. 1986. Policy changes affecting older Americans during the first Reagan Administration. *Gerontologist* 26:27–31.
33. Torrey, B. B. 1982. Guns vs. canes: The fiscal implications of an aging population. *Am Econ Assoc Papers Proc* 72:309–313.
34. United States Senate, Special Committee on Aging. *Developments in Aging: 1988,* Vol. 1, 11–12. Washington, D.C.: Government Printing Office.
35. Crystal, S. C. 1982. *America's Old Age Crisis: Public Policy and the Two Worlds of Aging.* New York: Basic Books.
36. Nelson, G. 1982. Social class and public policy for the elderly. *Soc Serv Rev* 56:85–107.
37. Binstock, R. H., Grigsby, J., Leavitt, T. D. 1983. *An Analysis of "Targeting" Options Under Title III of the Older Americans Act.* Working Paper No. 16. Waltham, Mass.: National Aging Policy Center on Income Maintenance.
38. Neugarten, B. L. 1974. Age groups in American society and the rise of the young old. *Ann Acad Political Soc Sci* 415:187–198.
39. United States Department of Health and Human Services. 1984. Announcement: The oldest old. *National Institutes of Health Guide for Grants and Contracts* 13(Nov. 9):29–33.
40. Binstock, R. H. 1985. The oldest old: A fresh perspective or compassionate ageism revisited? *Milbank Memorial Fund Q* 63:420–451.
41. Binstock, R. H. 1983. The aged as scapegoat. *Gerontologist* 23:136–143.
42. Quinn, J. 1985. The economic status of the elderly: Beware of the mean. (Mimeographed.) Chestnut Hill, Mass.: Boston College.
43. Binstock, R. H. 1981. The aging as a political force: Images and reality. In *Aging: A Challenge to Science and Social Policy,* Vol. 2, *Medicine and Social Science,* ed. A. J. J. Gilmore, A. Svanberg, M. Marois, W. M. Beattie, and J. Piotrowski, 390–396. London: Oxford University Press.
44. Greenhouse, S. 1986. Passing the buck from one generation to another. *New York Times* August 17, E-5.
45. Daniels, N. 1983. Justice between age groups: Am I my parents' keeper? *Milbank Memorial Fund Q* 61:489–522.
46. Scitovsky, A. A. 1984. "The high cost of dying": What do the data show? *Milbank Memorial Fund Q* 62:591–608.
47. Schulte, J. 1983. Terminal patients deplete Medicare, Greenspan says. *Dallas Morning News* April 26, p. 1.
48. Slater, W. 1984. Latest Lamm remark angers the elderly. *Arizona Daily Star* March 29, p. 1.
49. Kuttner, R. 1985. The poverty of economics. *The Atlantic* 255(Feb.):74–84.
50. Callahan, D. 1987. *Setting Limits: Medical Goals for an Aging Society.* New York: Simon and Schuster.
51. Brody, S. J. 1984–1985. Merging rehabilitation and aging policies and programs: Past, present, and future. *Rehabil World* 8(4):6–9, 42–44.
52. Williams, T. F. (ed.) 1984. *Rehabilitation and the Aging.* New York: Raven Press.

53. Habib, J. 1985. The economy and the aged. In *Handbook of Aging and the Social Sciences*, 2nd ed., ed. R. H. Binstock and E. Shanas, 479–502. New York: Van Nostrand Reinhold.
54. Crown, W. 1985. Some thoughts on reformulating the dependency ratio. *Gerontologist* 26:166–171.
55. Schulz, J. 1988. *The Economics of Aging*, 4th ed., ch. 3. Dover, Mass.: Auburn House.
56. Allport, G. W. 1959. *The ABC's of Scapegoating*. New York: Anti-Defamation League of B'nai B'rith.
57. Carballo, M. 1981. Extra votes for parents? *Boston Globe* December 17, p. 35.
58. Stewart, D. J. 1970. Disfranchise the old: The lesson of California. *New Republic* 163:20–22.
59. Aaron, H. J., Schwartz, W. B. 1984. *The Painful Prescription: Rationing Hospital Care*. Washington, D.C.: Brookings Institution.
60. Schwartz, W. B., Aaron, H. J. 1985. Health care costs: The social tradeoffs. *Issues Sci Technol* 1(2):39–46.
61. Walzer, M. 1983. *Spheres of Justice*. New York: Basic Books.
62. Brody, S. J., Persily, N. A. (eds.) *Hospitals and the Aged: The New Old Market*. Rockville, Md.: Aspen Systems Corporation.
63. Bishop, C. E. 1981. A compulsory long-term care insurance program. In *Reforming the Long-Term Care System*, ed. J. J. Callahan, Jr. and S. S. Wallack, 61–93. Lexington, Mass.: D. C. Heath.
64. Tolchin, M. 1988. New health insurance plan provokes outcry over costs. *The New York Times*, November 2, p. 1.

Part Six

Reconceptualizing the Problem

The authors who have contributed their ideas to this book have made one thing painfully clear—the fabric of health care for the elderly is being torn asunder. If health professionals and planners do not rise to the challenges posed by the convulsions within the system, they risk violating medicine's most cherished principle: First, do no harm.

As long as old methods are relatively workable, there is a temptation to stick with tried-and-true techniques, but if health care for the elderly has truly reached a breaking point, transformation is inevitable. In this section we lay the groundwork for productive change by expanding the conceptual framework within which policies are developed. The search for new ways to think about health care means asking new questions and listening to unexpected answers; it means questioning old assumptions and taking time to think with imagination and vision about new possibilities; it means experimenting with original ideas and accepting a certain percentage of failures.

Like a hamster running in a wheel but moving nowhere, frantic efforts to introduce change are likely to devour energy without producing results. Effective policies, by contrast, are carefully conceived and cautiously implemented. This section is dedicated to the notion that if we begin now to reconceptualize health care for the elderly, we can avoid reaching the point of desperate freneticism.

Health policies inevitably flounder in the absence of sound analysis, writes Eli Ginzberg, whose operating premise is that the definitions used to formulate policy can either strengthen that policy's effectiveness or damage it fatally. He traces some of the shortcomings of today's systems of care to anachronistic approaches and practices, noting, for example, that medical schools still fail to emphasize care for the chronically ill. Ginzberg sees the financing of health care for the elderly as inherently constrained, and believes that long-term solutions ultimately lie in the rationalization of the panoply of government programs designed to support the elderly.

Anne R. Somers surveys the accepted definitions of comprehensive health care for the elderly and concludes that we may simply be unable to afford it. Given that stark limitation, her questions about how much to spend on health care for older people and where new sources of funds should come from are particularly provocative.

The overarching goal of caring for the elderly—maintaining their lifestyle, social independence, and dignity to the maximum extent possible—should always be kept in view when reform is debated, declares T. Franklin Williams. His ideal system of health maintenance would include consumer information, nutritional support, and preventive check-ups, as well as primary, consultative, and rehabilitative care; geriatric assessment, comprehensive home support, and a plethora of institutional options would all be parts of a prime package of long-term services.

The line drawn between the funding mechanisms for acute and long-term care is artificial and inefficient, say authors Robert L. Kane and Rosalie A. Kane, who claim arbitrary divisions do a disservice to the elderly. Drawing upon the Canadian experience, they present the case for an integrated system, criticize the disjointed way in which U.S. health policies have developed, and recommend the management of long-term care as a social service rather than strictly a medical one.

To tinker with the present system of financing long-term care in the United States is to do too little too late, claims Tom Joe, who says that nothing less than a revolutionary change of approach will be adequate to meet new demands. His proposals creatively combine public and private financing, delegate responsibilities to each level of government and to family caregivers, and demedicalize services wherever feasible.

Paul M. Densen, Ellen W. Jones, and Sidney Katz explain the importance of systematically collecting information from practitioners in the field. Questions that identify an agency's target population, the services it receives, and the effect of those services generate baseline data indispensable for measuring how well policy is being translated into practice and for minimizing guesswork when systemic changes are proposed.

Twenty-five

How to Think about Health Care for the Elderly

Eli Ginzberg

This chapter examines the many complexities involved in thinking about health care for the elderly, on the ground that conceptual weakness will inevitably result in poor policy. True, sound policy requires a second ingredient—a commitment to humane values—but in the absence of sound conceptualization and analysis, policy will flounder.

Two terms in the title of this chapter, "health care" and "the elderly," are critical. Consider the concept of "health care": A homebound person receives assistance three times a week for several hours from a home health aide who does the shopping and helps the disabled person take a bath. Is this health care? Or: Many persons are maintained in nursing homes that do not employ registered nurses around the clock or schedule regular physician visits for assessment of the changing health status of the residents. Is this health care?

What about the concept of "the elderly"? Is it an arbitrary designation that covers all persons over the age of 65, or should it be reserved for a narrower band, say the group 75 years and older or even 85 and older? For example, in some respects, including their pattern of utilization of health-care services, the "young-old," persons between ages 65 and 74, more closely resemble persons between 55 and 64 than they do the "old-old," persons over 85.

There is evidence of considerable uncertainty and disagreement in the selection of chronological age criteria for dealing with the elderly. The Social Security legislation was amended several years ago to raise the age of entitlement to full benefits from 65 to 67; several states have moved to eliminate age as a factor in terminating employment, and it is increasingly common for surgeons to operate on patients who have passed their eighty-fifth, even their ninetieth, birthday.

This dilemma has far-reaching implications. In the absence of chronological determinants it is difficult, often impossible, to establish objective criteria for societal and organizational decisions, such as the time that the chief of surgery of a teaching hospital should be asked to step down, or the time that an individual should become eligible for his or her pension. Furthermore, reliance on such "objective" criteria leaves much to be desired. In an effort to resize, more and more American corporations have resorted to an early retirement strategy that encourages executives to leave at age 55, and sometimes even earlier. Social Security provides for retirement benefits to begin anywhere from the age of 62 to age 70, with payments adjusted to age.

How do we take account of variations in vitality and performance among members of the same age group, as well as between the young-old and old-old? A significant minority of the old-old keep working or are engaged in other purposeful activities until they die, and they remain substantially free of disease and disability, suffering no loss of function other than a reduction in physical vigor. At the opposite extreme are individuals whose health has so deteriorated that they are housebound or bedridden and require constant care. These contrasting conditions are found among the old-old, but to a lesser degree also among the young-old.

It is therefore important to avoid gross generalizations about the health status of the elderly. Although aging is associated with an increase in chronic illness and other disabilities, most people are able to continue the activities of daily life independently or with modest support from others. Even among the old-old, only a minority are in nursing homes, and some are substantially free of impairment.

Furthermore, during the last two decades, the elderly in the United States have made marked gains in income and access to health-care services, as a consequence both of federal programs and of increases in personal assets. Significant improvements in federal programs include substantial increases in benefits received from Social Security, the indexing of these benefits to compensate for inflation, the introduction of Supplemental Security Income for the needy elderly, the growing proportion of persons retiring at age 62 or 65 who are entitled to partial or full benefits, and special provisions for those below the age of 62 who are permanently disabled. Further improvement in the economic position of the elderly has resulted from increases in private pensions, home ownership, and savings.

In terms of cash income alone, the proportion of persons 65 and older who fell below the poverty level declined from over 35% in 1959 to 12.6% in 1985.[1] In recent years, the federal government has also introduced and enlarged transfers in kind—medical and nursing care, food, housing, and related benefits. When these are taken into account, the proportion of the elderly below the poverty line in 1985 dropped, according to the lowest of several estimates, to 3.2%. Only one in thirty of all elderly persons was living in poverty.[2]

As other chapters of this book make clear, the period since the early 1960s has seen important advances in the income, health services, and social supports that have been made available to the elderly both by federal and state governments and by private pension plans and enhanced personal savings. The absolute and relative improvements in the position of the elderly have outpaced those of any other demographic group, notwithstanding the continued shortfalls in income, health care, and social services for particular subgroups of this population.

Unresolved Problems

The generally upbeat assessment of the improved economic position of the elderly must not obscure severe deficiencies in various dimensions of their lives. A small minority continue to live in poverty, even after receiving various services in kind. In addition, there is a much larger number who escape the definition of poverty but who have incomes less than twice the poverty ceiling. Half of all the elderly are found within this income range. The most vulnerable group are women living alone: about 2 million, or more than one in four, live in poverty. Among the aged who live alone, five times as many women as men subsist below the poverty level. These unattached women account for more than half of all the elderly living in poverty.[2]

Furthermore, despite the broad entitlement and coverage provided by Medicare, a small number of the aged, those who encounter catastrophic illness, remain financially vulnerable. This explains the recent amendments adding catastrophic insurance to Medicare.

By all accounts, the two most serious shortcomings in the present structure of health-care financing for the elderly relate to nursing home services and home health care. Skilled nursing home care costs in excess of $100 per day. Although Medicare has eliminated the requirement of prior hospitalization for admission to such care, reimbursement is limited to 150 days; Medicaid pays only for those who are without financial means. As a result, elderly persons who do not qualify for Medicaid because their income and assets exceed the ceiling must pay for their care themselves or look to their children to cover their nursing home costs. Obviously, only the wealthy and those on the upper end of the income scale can afford an annual bill of $25,000 or more for nursing home care that may run for several years.

Many of the elderly can remain in their own homes, provided they have assistance in the performance of daily activities, such as shopping, cleaning, and bathing. Here, too, the Medicare program is very restrictive, providing services only to persons who require concomitant nursing or other professional care for a defined medical condition. Again, persons who are not eligible for Medicaid must cover such outlays themselves or seek financial assistance from their children. Annual expenditures of $5,000 to $10,000 for part-time assistance and of $25,000 for full-time care represent a financial burden that only a small minority of families can meet, especially when help is required not for a few weeks or months but for several years.

In summary, a small minority of the elderly lack even the minimum income that would make their last years bearable, and a great many more—about half of all those over 65—subsist close to the margin of poverty. This means that they can live reasonably well so long as they are not confronted with a basic change in their circumstances, such as the need for assistance in the performance of their daily activities or admission to long-term nursing home care.

Professionalism and Consumer Choice

In the United States, the individual states long ago devolved onto the medical profession a high degree of responsibility for self-regulation, which in turn, enabled physicians to play key roles in determining how health-care services, both in-hospital and ambulatory, were delivered to the public. For example, President Lyndon B. Johnson concluded that it was the better part of political wisdom to reach an agreement with the American Medical Association specifying that Medicare would not alter the traditional physician-patient relationship. Accordingly, the federal government agreed to reimburse physicians for the care of the elderly on a fee-for-service basis, with rates determined by the UCR standard—usual, customary, and reasonable.

For Medicaid, the states were not required to follow federal policy on physician reimbursement, and many of them soon placed a low ceiling on the amount that they would pay for an office visit. As a result, a substantial proportion of physicians, especially those in large cities, overtly or covertly refused to accept Medicaid patients, or at most were willing to treat only a selected few. This forced many of the indigent to seek care from the emergency rooms of neighborhood hospitals or from "shared practices" (Medicaid mills), usually staffed by physicians with the least training and competence.

The practice of home visits by physicians was largely discontinued with the onset of World War II. Although Medicare Part B (SMI) will pay for house calls, until recently most of the elderly have found it very difficult to be treated at home. The rationale offered by physicians has been that adequate medical assessment cannot be made without the use of the sophisticated, nonportable equipment found in their offices or in the hospital. The marked increases in hospitalization of the elderly in the post-Medicare period reflect this style of practice, and the trend is reinforced by the ability of physicians to see more patients and bill at a higher rate when services are performed in the hospital.

On any one day, almost double the number of patients are found in nursing homes (roughly 1.4 million persons) than in acute-care hospitals (750,000).[3] Nevertheless, except in the best of the long-term care facilities, physicians are conspicuous by their absence. Many of the residents do not receive a medical examination from one month to the next, sometimes from one year to the next, and failing proper diagnosis and treatment, many deteriorate unnecessarily.

Medical school training in the United States concentrates on diagnosis and treatment of the acutely ill, with little emphasis being given to care of the chronically ill. Thus, professional bias among care providers and the absence of suitable reimbursement for nursing home visits go far to explain the low level of medical care received by many of the institutionalized elderly.

Furthermore, until recently, since Medicare paid hospitals on a cost-reimbursement basis (which even for a few years included a 2% override to help finance innovations), hospitals became the principal beneficiaries of the much-enlarged flow of federal funds. As more elderly patients were admitted and their treatment was intensified, federally covered hospital expenditures increased rapidly.

Nursing homes, most of them under private ownership and management, attracted a large part of the funding made available through the Medicaid program. As owners opened new homes or expanded existing ones, beds were rapidly filled by elderly persons, who themselves sought to be admitted or whose families urged their admission in order to be relieved of the continuing burden of their care.

Decisionmakers concerned with Medicare and Medicaid have always been reluctant to approve a broad program of reimbursement for home health care on the grounds that, once they started down this road, the substantial contributions made by the patient, members of his or her family, and neighbors would be withdrawn in whole or in part, and large additional costs would be shifted to the public purse. In recent years Medicare has increased its reimbursements for home health-care services but it has kept tight controls over such payments so that they continue to represent only a small percentage of total Medicare outlays.

Organizations that lobby for the elderly have been pressing for reforms in the structure and financing of health-care services that would permit the deployment of public funds to help aged individuals remain in their own homes rather than be forced to enter nursing homes. However, despite growing interest in and out of Congress, only minor adjustments have been made to expand Medicare. Understandably, the spokesmen for the elderly have been unwilling, except in the case of hospice care, to "trade off" a lower level of reimbursement for acute care in favor of alternatives. Congress is concerned that, without such trade-offs, broadening entitlements for nonhospital care will be additive, not substitutive, and, in the face of large out-year deficits, it is unwilling to take the risk. Congressional caution has been reinforced by recent reports from the General Accounting Office (GAO) that found no clear-cut evidence of net savings from the experimental programs it reviewed. The GAO suggests there may even be the risk of higher total costs from an expansion of alternatives to hospital care. [4]

The critical issue is that no societal mechanism currently exists to rationalize the flow of expenditures for health services for the elderly among the complementary settings of home, nursing home, hospice, and acute-care hospital and to provide the optimal amount of care for the available dollars, giving due consideration to the elderly's preference for remaining in their own homes as long as is feasible. The search for a rationalizing mechanism has been inhibited by the strong resistance, overt and covert, of influential providers and funders, such as federal and state governments, acute-care hospitals, nursing homes, and physicians, to serious experimentation that could threaten their entrenched interests.

Organization, Financing, and Resource Use

Unfortunately, the difficulty of altering the present flow of resources for the provision of health and related services to the elderly goes beyond the resistance of interested parties. To begin with, health care must be delivered to people where they reside. This means that the federal government can never ensure that all beneficiaries will obtain the services to which they are entitled under the law, because it cannot ensure that a physician will be available to treat them, much less that he will not overcharge them.

Although the federal government pays between 50% and 78% of all Medicaid costs, state governments regulate such critical matters as the capacity of nursing homes, methods of copayment by families, and the fee schedules of physicians. Recently, in order to reduce expenditures, the Department of Health and Human Services has authorized waivers giving state governments greater latitude to control expenditures while maintaining or improving the quantity and quality of care. In areas of the country where local government plays an active role as funder, gatekeeper, and provider of services to the citizens who are dependent on public dollars, responsibility is divided between the state and local bureaucracies.

These organizational complexities extend beyond the interrelations among the several levels of government. The great majority of nursing homes are under private ownership and management: of the almost 26,000 nursing homes in the United States, over 21,000 are privately owned.[5] Even allowing for the fact that the facilities that are under public and nonprofit auspices have, on the average, larger capacity, the private sector controls over two-thirds of all nursing home beds.[5]

The tensions arising out of the division of responsibility among those who finance, provide, and control health-care services for the elderly are reflected in the recent actions of many state governments to limit the expansion of nursing home beds through the use of certificates of need. State governments have discovered that available nursing home beds invariably become filled. Hence, one way to limit the state's costs for nursing home care is to control bed capacity.

Another source of tension between state governments and private providers of nursing home care has been the reluctance of most states to make use of their licensing authority to control effectively the quality of care that is provided. Aside from the costs of inspection, which are high when homes are inspected annually, many states have hesitated to decertify and close nursing homes that fall below acceptable standards, especially in areas with long waiting lists. Politicians believe that the citizenry generally prefers a lower level of care to the absence of care.

Complexities also arise in dovetailing the responsibilities of the individual patient and his or her family with government's responsibilities for the financing of care. The issue is directly joined in the case of patients who can remain in their own homes on the condition that they receive assistance in performing their daily activities. Medicare will reimburse for such personal care services only if they are required in conjunction with a recognized therapeutic service, such as nursing care and/or physical therapy. As a further example of these complexities, recent revisions in the Medicaid regulations of several states, including Massachusetts, Maryland, and New York, mandate a larger contribution by the family to the costs of nursing home care for individuals who require it.

Most governments have been unwilling to broaden eligibility under Medicaid to include personal care services because they recognize that such care is currently paid for by the patient or members of the patient's family or is voluntarily provided by family and friends. Municipal government in New York City is the outstanding exception. With support from New York State, it has put together funds from several sources (including Medicaid) to provide home health care for 40,000 persons, at a cost of approximately

$800 million annually. In Britain, greater flexibility in commingling public and private funds for the care of the homebound elderly permits local authorities to pay for relief workers or for the short-term transfer of patients into residential facilities to provide a respite for family caregivers.

Equity and Ethics

Under contributory pension systems, many individuals who die prematurely or soon after they retire receive less from the system than they have paid in. Others who live well into their seventies or longer receive much more in benefits than they have contributed. This situation has not led to conflict in most countries because the younger generation recognizes that if government did not cover the minimum needs of their parents, the residual responsibility would fall on them. They realize further that sooner or later they will be among the elderly and will have to depend on the system for some part of their support. Potential conflict has been further attenuated because economic productivity has risen, and the total pool of goods and services available for distribution has increased during most of this century. The elderly, who have contributed to enlarging the stock of human and physical capital, the basis of productivity gains, have an indisputable right to share in the enlarged income available for current consumption.

However, conflicts have arisen and will arise in the future about the appropriate share of national expenditures that should be allocated to meet the income and health-care needs of the elderly. The long bout with inflation and the recent retardation in the rate of economic growth have contributed to these conflicts. A related problem has been the fiscal integrity of the public pension systems. In many European countries, legislatures are aware of growing strains in the financing of pensions. Nevertheless, politicians, loath to unleash the wrath of the elderly, have sought to delay taking corrective actions. In the United States, Congress only recently (1983) amended Social Security to reduce current and prospective benefits. It remains to be seen whether these changes will provide the long-term financial solution that has been claimed for them.

The American social welfare system was structured with a major concern for equity. The initial Social Security legislation was intentionally skewed in favor of the elderly, who would be most in need of government assistance to maintain even a minimal standard of living. In the succeeding decades, many amendments to the system have been particularly sensitive to the needs of those who leave the labor force without adequate retirement income. As noted earlier, major progress has been made to ensure that through entitlements and means-tested transfers, all of the elderly will be able to live above the poverty level.

However, favorable evaluation of Social Security in the United States and of most public pension systems abroad should not obscure the tensions that exist between entitlements and means-tested transfers. Many persons who have supported themselves throughout their adult lives are loath to seek "charity" in their later years. For example, a significant proportion of the British elderly do not claim the supplementary grants to which they are entitled, and many people in the United States who could qualify for Medicaid or other means-tested benefits do not apply.

Since almost all public pension systems include a wage-related component in the determination of benefit levels, those who have held low-level jobs and have an intermittent employment record—notably women—are likely, once they retire, to receive an amount that is insufficient to maintain them at a reasonable standard of living. There does not appear to be any way of ensuring that all persons receive an adequate pension without means testing. If the economies of the developed countries experience a period of sustained growth, it may be possible in the future for all persons to receive an adequate pension at retirement. In the interim, however, means testing cannot be avoided.

Many developed countries have long operated a national system of medical insurance that provides access to hospital treatment for all persons, the elderly as well as those of working age. However, law or custom often limits the amount and quality of medical care provided the elderly. In the United Kingdom, where hospital financing has been most constrained, the elderly have been subject to two types of rationing. Those who do not require emergency treatment must join a queue and wait their turn for elective procedures. Since many of the elderly suffer from chronic rather than acute conditions, they account for a high proportion of those in the queue. Furthermore, in the United Kingdom, as in many other European countries, expensive interventions, such as open-heart surgery, renal dialysis, and hip and knee replacements, are not uniformly available to the elderly on the grounds that these costly procedures should be limited to persons in the younger age groups who are likely to benefit the most from them.

Once a society explicitly restricts the total amount of its resources allocated to therapeutic medicine, it is difficult to fault a rationing policy that favors the younger age group, but this does not put the matter to rest. A question of equity remains: Does a civilized society with a reasonable command of resources have the right to deny the elderly life-extending and pain-reducing treatment while still spending large sums on defense, recreation, or cultural activities?

An acceptable policy is difficult to formulate and to carry out, even when the society, such as the United States, has made a commitment to furnish the full panoply of modern medicine to all persons, including the elderly. Yet the question arises: How sensible is it to engage in heroic interventions to keep alive patients, including the elderly, who are unlikely to regain a significant degree of functionality or the ability to care for themselves? Those who favor the present practice of maximal care for all argue that one can decide only retrospectively, not prospectively, whether medical intervention is justified. On the other hand, a growing number of questions have been precipitated by the finding that approximately 25% to 30% of all Medicare expenditures are incurred by patients who die within 12 months.[6]

The formulation of standards and procedures for determining whether and when to institute or discontinue life-prolonging interventions for moribund patients, the elderly and nonelderly represents a major challenge that will not be readily overcome. This does not mean, however, that the issue should be ignored. The growth of "right to die" movements reflects the concern of many citizens that they, or their legally responsible relatives, be consulted in the decision to institute or continue a life-prolonging procedure.

Emerging Pressures

Skeptics who argue that recent revisions of Social Security will not ensure its long-term financial stability may prove to be right, if the American economy is plagued once again by a combination of rapid inflation, slow economic growth, and a sustained high level of unemployment. Even barring this unfavorable constellation, the Trust Fund may not have the necessary resources to meet its obligations to the large number of beneficiaries who will become eligible after the year 2010, when the baby-boom generation begins to reach retirement age. The prospective rise in the retirement age to 67 will help to moderate the financial pressures on the system so long as there is no increase in longevity, which would work to offset these gains. However, unless the world economy—of which the United States remains the leader—should collapse, unfavorable economic conditions are not likely to undermine the Social Security system for the remaining years of this century.

The outlook with respect to health care for the elderly, however, is less propitious. The Reagan Administration early on signaled the Congress that programs for the elderly needed major changes in policy and financing, and its record during its years in office showed some successes and some failures. In seeking to moderate federal outlays for Medicare patients, the administration's major success was the establishment of prospective reimbursement for inpatient hospital care, which has been associated with substantial declines in hospital utilization (although it was not the cause of these declines). However, it is too soon to predict whether reimbursement by diagnosis-related groups (DRGs) will in fact enable government to control effectively its outlays for medical care. The most recent projections of the Health Care Financing Administration give no basis for optimism. Although the rate of increase in Medicare Part A expenditures has moderated somewhat, outlays for Part B have increased significantly in recent years, reflecting the expanding utilization of ambulatory care.

The Reagan Administration also moved to encourage health maintenance organizations (HMOs) to enroll Medicare patients, and it is in the process of altering the payment systems for physicians' services, graduate medical education, and capital costs. However, its proposals to substantially increase copayments by Medicare beneficiaries were defeated and it was unable to win Congressional approval to place a ceiling on the federal contribution to Medicaid.

During these same years, many states took the initiative to cut back their Medicaid programs, but the plight of many of the poor and near-poor in obtaining essential health-care services and the more buoyant economy since 1983 have led to a reversal of this policy; in fact, many state governments have actually expanded the number of Medicaid-eligibles. However, states continue to limit the expansion of nursing home capacity, with the result that many of the sick and frail elderly experience increasing delays in gaining admission.

As of late 1989, the overall picture relating to health care for the elderly is neither rosy nor gloomy. There is no new money in sight to underpin a large-scale expansion of nursing home capacity or a significant improvement in the quality of nursing home care. Furthermore, there is no significant new money in sight to broaden Medicare (or for that matter Medicaid) entitlements to effect a major increase in home health care. Both are likely to expand, but only with private, not governmental, dollars. There may conceivably be some new governmental funds available for nursing home and home health care if current expenditures for hospitalization of Medicare beneficiaries can be redirected although in the current budgetary stringency this seems unlikely.

Directions for Future Health-Care Policy for the Elderly

Total expenditures for health-care services for the elderly amounted to almost $120 billion in 1984. In descending order of importance, the major categories of expenditure, hospital care, nursing home care, and physician services, accounted for approximately 85% of the total. The remainder went for dental services, other professional services, drugs, and insurance. Thus, for a population of almost 27 million persons age 65 or over, the per capita health-care expenditure amounted to $4200, which is about equal to the average sum that each retired person receives from Social Security. [7]

Admittedly this is a large outlay, probably in excess of $180 billion in 1989. The critical questions are: What can be done to improve the prospects for more and better services for the sick and feeble elderly, and what should be avoided in order not to worsen the problems that they face?

On the positive side, it is important to maintain the elderly's broad access to acute-care hospitals so that they will be able to receive the benefits of therapeutic medicine. There may be opportunities, however, to avoid heroic interventions, not only to reduce dollar outlays but also to contribute to the ease and dignity with which the individual confronts death. In this vein, the recent expansion of hospice care warrants continuing evaluation to determine its potential for easing the difficulties that patients and their families experience when recovery is no longer possible.

Although the demonstrations of community-based care for the elderly have not yet yielded positive results—at least not in terms of total dollar savings—they must be continued in the anticipation that cost-effective models will emerge that will enable more of the frail elderly to continue to live at home. On a related front, research into the causes and the treatment of incontinence and senility among the elderly should be intensified. These two conditions contribute greatly to the demand for nursing home care.

After long delays, it appears that as of the end of 1989 private insurance companies, sometimes with state assistance, are beginning to look more seriously at writing coverage for long-term care. It will probably require considerable experimentation before reliable results emerge, and it may turn out that private companies will never write policies for individuals and families of modest incomes and assets, but the result should not be prejudged.

For a long time there was much discussion but little action on permitting Medicare beneficiaries to convert their entitlements into vouchers that would enable them to enroll in an HMO and thus secure comprehensive health-care coverage. The federal government moved slowly and few HMOs were interested in opening enrollments to the elderly until they could get a better fix on the unknown risks. More recently, each of the parties has been somewhat more venturesome, but it will take several years before evidence accumulates about the interest of beneficiaries in joining and the willingness of HMOs to accept them. What is clear is that the federal government is willing to move ahead and reimburse HMOs at 95% of average adjusted costs for Medicare beneficiaries. What remains unclear is whether the government will benefit. It could suffer financially from adverse selection if the healthier elderly should opt disproportionately for HMOs, thereby increasing total Medicare expenditures.[8]

Recent efforts by the financial community to develop new ways whereby the elderly may turn their ownership of a home into an income stream for use during their last years can turn out to be an important factor in narrowing the gap between income and need. About 70% of all Americans own their homes, and most of the elderly no longer carry a mortgage. Hence they can look forward to significant increases in their annual incomes through a reverse annuity mortgage.

The continuation of present inpatient hospital benefits, together with greater opportunity for the elderly to join HMOs or to be treated in hospices in the event that they become terminally ill, seem, at least for the near term, to be ensured. On the other hand, there will be at most only modest government initiatives to enlarge nursing home capacity and home health care other than through "savings" realized by cutting back further on the current scale of inpatient care. In the presence of advancing technology, the potential of such savings is, of necessity, limited.

The standoff between additional governmental resources and unmet, growing needs of the elderly brings us face to face with the central theme formulated at the outset of this chapter: the necessity of combining new knowledge with humane societal values for the task of selecting among competing policy goals and alternative methods of implementation. The last years have witnessed moves in many different arenas—federal, state, and local—directed toward reducing the gap between the needs of the elderly for more and better health-care services and the inability and/or unwillingness of most governmental units to increase their appropriations for this purpose. In this condensed overview of policy alternatives, I will comment on the actions that have been contemplated or initiated and then outline other considerations that should inform policy in the years ahead.

President Reagan's successful effort in 1981 to reduce federal expenditures for domestic programs, coupled with his willingness to permit the states greater discretion in determining the specifics of their Medicaid programs, led many states to reassess their nursing home programs, with the result that they acted to slow nursing home growth. This measure of economy coincided with growing opposition from many groups of elderly persons to being shunted into nursing homes as the only means of receiving support services. The elderly much prefer to remain in their own homes and communities. It is essential, therefore, to continue the experimental programs that are now in progress to assess the feasibility and the costs of maintaining more of the sick and frail elderly in noninstitutional settings.

Under the best of circumstances some of the sick elderly will need institutional care, and therefore the states must ensure adequate capacity. Two radical proposals also merit attention and study. First, the federal government, in association with a representative group of states, should explore whether any significant gains can be achieved by prospective merging of Social Security, Medicaid, and other governmental programs as a means of enlarging the resources available for expanded institutional care.

Second, and even more important because of its scale and potential, private carriers, employer groups, and nonprofit organizations, such as the American Association of Retired Persons and foundations, should explore programs and mechanisms whereby middle-class families and individuals might be able to insure themselves for extended nursing home and home health care.

The last years have seen an ongoing series of measures by the federal government aimed at constraining its outlays for Medicare, including the introduction of DRGs, physician fee controls, cutbacks in funding for capital and graduate medical education, and the establishment of Peer Review Organization-designated restrictions aimed at reducing unnecessary admissions and lengths of stay. The most recent has been the introduction under the Medicare Catastrophic Coverage Act (signed into law in July, 1988) of income-conditioned cost-sharing by the beneficiaries in order to pay for expanded benefits. The provision has evoked opposition from advocates for the elderly and there are incipient moves in Congress for its modification. Moreover, the president requested, but was unable to elicit, Congressional support for substantial copayments by Medicare beneficiaries for the second to the sixtieth day of hospitalization.

Although the early results of many of these initiatives, particularly prospective hospital reimbursement, appear to be favorable, the long-term effectiveness of the new cost controls remains moot. Even if the DRG system falters, however, it is unlikely that cost-based reimbursement will be reinstated. We are much more likely to establish a new system of budgetary controls.

The last few years have called attention to the tenuousness of all long-term forecasts. In the early 1980s a potential deficit in the Medicare Trust Fund of $300 to $400 billion was widely posited. Today this prediction is no longer heard. Even in the face of continuing large deficits, Congress will avoid a radical reduction in Medicare benefits that would force the low-income elderly to contribute much more toward the cost of their hospitalization. It has moved to impose tax surcharges on the more affluent elderly, particularly for SMI coverage. If the federal budget goes totally out of control, it may be necessary to restructure Medicare into an essentially means-tested program.

Finally, the elderly must be more actively involved in decision making affecting their health care and life decisions. Many states have acted, and others are likely to follow, to give the elderly or their responsible agents a larger role in deciding about life-support systems. The prolongation of life without independent function is not necessarily a boon. Death is not always the worse alternative.

Aging, and its concomitants, is a process that can prove unduly burdensome in an era in which many lack faith and others have little appreciation of fate. The elderly have need for understanding, reassurance, and support to help them bear the many infirmities for which there are no cures and at best only modest alleviation. A simple, straightforward book written for the elderly to help them through their declining years could be an invaluable resource, much as Dr. Spock's volumes on infant and child care proved for the postwar generation of young mothers.

Concluding Observations

The extant system of funding health care for the elderly is fragile, and there is little or no prospect that the quantity and quality of care will be improved through substantially enlarged public expenditures in the near future. On the contrary, the current trend is toward constraints in both federal and state expenditures. However, in seeking to constrain public expenditures, care must be taken not to place excessive burdens on those least able to cope, namely, that half of the elderly population living on an annual income no greater than twice the poverty level. It should be a national imperative not to impose heavier burdens on those least able to bear them.

Some opportunities exist to reallocate resources. For example, reducing the quantity and intensity of acute hospital care utilized by the elderly (and others) would help finance the expansion of more appropriate and preferred services, such as home health care. It would be naive, however, to assume that such redirection of resources will come easily or quickly, given the power of the institutions and goals whose interest is to protect the status quo.

There is also little likelihood that potential improvements in the delivery of health-care services to the elderly will be realized unless the rapid inflation of health-care costs that has characterized the system during the past several decades can be slowed. The best prospect for moderating the anticipated steep increases in health-care services for the old-old, whose numbers are growing rapidly, rests with improvements in their health status through reduced morbidity, improved standards of living, and healthier lifestyles. If these improvements are reflected in fewer and lesser impairments in old age and if research and technology can modify the disabilities that are associated with dementia, incontinence, and immobility, our society will be better positioned to deal effectively and humanely with the health-care needs of the elderly.

Renewed economic growth would surely facilitate the allocation of additional resources to meeting health-care needs, but the long-term solution lies elsewhere—in a general improvement in the health status of the population at large, including the elderly; in advances in medical research and development that will reduce and eliminate many conditions afflicting

Eli Ginzberg

the elderly; and in a strengthening of family and community bonds to ensure that the elderly are not left to confront illness and death alone.

Acknowledgment

The author is indebted to Mrs. Miriam Ostow, Senior Research Scholar of the Conservation of Human Resources, for assistance in preparing this chapter.

References

1. United States Department of Commerce. 1987. *Statistical Abstract of the United States, 1987,* 446. Washington, D.C.: Government Printing Office.
2. See Ref. 1, p. 444.
3. See Ref. 1, pp. 95, 98.
4. United States General Accounting Office. 1982. Report to the Chairman of the Committee on Labor and Human Resources. United States Senate. *The Elderly Should Benefit from Expanded Home Health Care but Increasing These Services Will Not Insure Cost Reductions,* 26–31. GAO/IPE-83-1. Washington, D.C.
5. United States Department of Commerce. 1987. Statistical Abstract of the United States, 1987, 99. Washington, D.C.: Government Printing Office.
6. Lubitz, J., Prihoda, R. 1984. The use and costs of Medicare services in the last 2 years of life. *Health Care Financing Ref* 5(3):117–131.
7. Waldo, D., Lazenby, H. C. 1984. Demographic characteristics and health care use and expenditures by the aged in the United States, 1977–1984. *Health Care Financing Rev* 6(1):1–34.
8. Thomas, J. W., Lichtenstein, R., Wyszewianski, L., Berki, S. E. 1983. Increasing medicare enrollment in HMOs: The need for capitation rates adjusted for health status. *Inquiry* 20 (Fall):227–239.

Twenty-six

Is Comprehensive Care for the Elderly Fiscally Viable?

Anne R. Somers

At the time of its passage, Medicare was seen as a national commitment to adequate health care for most of the elderly. Its companion program, Medicaid, was intended to provide an additional safety net to those elders who were clearly indigent or whose medical expenses so exceeded their Medicare benefits that they became indigent in the process. Continued public commitment to this general concept has persisted through the years since Medicare became law. However, what seemed like a fairly simple, straightforward commitment two decades ago, has turned out to be extraordinarily costly, still incomplete, and generally unsatisfactory.

There are those who say that we simply cannot afford to provide the elderly with all the health care they need or think they need—certainly not anything like "comprehensive" care. In this view, any organization or nation that attempts to provide such care will find that it is not fiscally viable, that rationing is inevitable, and that the only question is how to ration. Others argue in response that the issue is not rationing, but rational management of existing resources, including transfer of substantial funds from other areas, such as the military, to the health-care economy, and some transfers within the health-care economy itself.

To evaluate these conflicting views and to provide some guidance to those responsible for designing, developing, and administering health programs for the elderly, it is essential to reexamine the original commitment in some detail. In this examination, we must ask: Who are the elderly? How long are they likely to be "elderly"? What are their major health needs? What do we mean by "comprehensive" health care? Should it be defined quantitatively, in terms of benefit / expenditure ratios or expenditure / income ratios? Or qualitatively, in terms of specific services? How do we define "affordability"? "Fiscal viability" in relation to what? What magnitude of expenditure are we talking about?

Complete answers are obviously far beyond the limits of this brief discussion. Other authors in this volume address the same issues from different perspectives. Definitive answers may never be available. Certainly, no answers will be permanent. The health-care field is dynamic; as needs change, so should professional and organizational responses.

Fortunately, however, we are not completely in the dark. We have accumulated a great deal of information about demographics, epidemiology, health care, and health-care economics during the past few decades. Even a cursory examination of these data yields two tentative conclusions: 1) With currently dominant assumptions, approaches and programs, it is probably *not* fiscally feasible to provide comprehensive care to the elderly. 2) Comprehensive health care for the elderly *is* possible if we are willing to make some reasonable adjustments to bring our assumptions, approaches, and programs into line with new realities. This chapter offers a defense of these two assertions by reviewing briefly each of the three major areas involved—the demographics of aging, the major health-care needs of the elderly, and the feasibility of providing this care. (See also other chapters in this volume.)

Who Are the "Elderly"?

Designation of 65 as the mandatory retirement age is a historical accident that should be, and is now gradually being, replaced by more flexible policies.[1] Social Security beneficiaries can now retire, on reduced pensions, at age 62, and the majority do retire before 65. Public Law 98-21, passed in 1983, raised the normal retirement age to 66 as of 2009, and to 67 as of 2027. This policy is sensible in view of our nation's increased life expectancy.

However, it does not follow that the age of eligibility for Medicare should be raised, as was recommended by the 1982 Advisory Council on Social Security.[2] It would be counterproductive to encourage older people to remain at work as long as their health permits, while denying them the health services that often spell the difference between ability to continue work or not. In the absence of universal national health insurance (which would be desirable for many reasons) I shall assume that in terms of eligibility for age-related health benefits, the 65-year threshold will be retained and that the elderly will continue to be defined as those 65 and over. However, I shall also assume that recent efforts on the part of leading gerontologists and geriatricians to emphasize health promotion and disease prevention for the elderly, through new concepts and programs, such as "preventive gerontology,"[3] "productive aging,"[4] and "successful aging,"[5] will gradually lead to a later average age of incidence or onset of chronic disease and/or disability even for those over 65. There is already some preliminary evidence of this effect.[6,7]

What of the other end of the old-age spectrum? How long can we expect to live on as "elderly"? Dramatic improvements in life expectancy in the course of the twentieth century have led to some speculation that the "natural life span" of human kind may be 100 years or even more.[8] The effect of such a development, not only on the viability of health and pension programs, but also on the entire economic, social, and political fabric of the nation, would be incalculable.

An opposing view holds that the recent increase in average life expectancy is by no means synonymous with an increase in the "normal" human life span, which is biologically determined and has remained virtually unchanged since Biblical times.[9] On the contrary, the rise in average life expectancy represents primarily progress toward the "normal" life span of the human species, which remains finite or close to it.

Recent figures from the National Center for Health Statistics suggest a slowing down in this rise, compared to the early 1970s, both at birth and at age 65. During the 5 years from 1971 to 1976, life expectancy at birth rose 1.8 years.[10] Between 1981 and 1986, it rose only 0.7 years, less than half as fast.[10,11] At 65, life expectancy rose 0.9 years during the early 1970s; only 0.2 years during the early 1980s. The figure is now 16.9.

James Fries of Stanford Medical School suggests that the "average" human life span is about 85–86 years, plus or minus 7–9 years.[12] The implications of this hypothesis, expressed in such concepts as "compression of morbidity,"[9] "active life expectancy,"[13] or "disability-free life expectancy"[8] are as great for our ability to pay for comprehensive health care for the elderly as for individual health. If the period of "old age" (the traditional term) can be compressed into a decade or so, rather than extended over an indefinite period, the costs of health care for the elderly—both to society and to the individual—could be reduced or at least contained. Very importantly, the cost of long-term care for the chronically ill—now frequently dismissed as prohibitive—could become supportable. Also, if it is understood that there is something like a "normal" life span, "heroic" efforts to prolong life—even in the presence of imminent death or extreme disability—would be seen more as a violation of the laws of nature than as an effort to help nature.

What Is "Comprehensive Care"?

Experts have debated the meaning of the term "comprehensive care" for years. Does it mean everything that anybody needs or wants? Clearly, this is impossible and probably even undesirable, since there are no limits to the applications and costs of modern medical technology.

But if not all health care is to be included, how much should be? The answer can be approached either quantitatively, in terms of dollars expended, or qualitatively, as services covered. Quantitatively, what would be a reasonable definition of "comprehensive"—90% of average expenditures? 75%? 50%? Qualitatively, should some categories of health care be emphasized more than others? Should some be excluded altogether? The implications of different options are at least as great for the health professionals and programs involved as for the elderly.

A Quantitative Approach

The average 1984 per capita expenditure for personal health services for the elderly was about $4200.[14] Assuming continuation of the 13% annual growth in per capita expenditures that prevailed for the previous 7 years, the figure for 1987 would be over $6000. This analysis, however, uses the 1984 "hard" figure. Few health-care authorities would maintain that even $4200 is truly needed to ensure comprehensiveness. Some portion is redundant or wasteful, some must be considered a luxury, some represents unjustified inflation, and some is dangerous.

Mental health care provides an instructive example. (This topic is explored in depth in Cohen and Hastings, Chapter 20.) There is a major discrepancy between the needs of the elderly and the type of mental health services they actually use. Their use of outpatient mental health clinics is very low. Cohen, citing National Institute of Mental Health figures, found that less than 1% of total mental health care time given to patients is provided to older people.[15] Only 4% of patients seen in outpatient mental health clinics were 65 or older; only 2% of those seen at private psychiatric clinics were in this age group. Yet the number of elderly in public mental hospitals is very high; they represent 30% of the total patient population. Furthermore, over 70% of the institutionalized elderly—some 5% of all those over 65—are reported to have mental disorders. In other words, few elderly receive relatively inexpensive outpatient mental health services, while most elderly mental health patients receive a disproportionate amount of the more expensive inpatient care.

Is it reasonable to assume that only half of the $4200, about $2100, was really essential? Given the prohospitalization climate within which doctors and patients have to function today, this is obviously too low. However, to say that 90%, about $3780, was essential strains credibility. But it is also unreasonable to assume that elderly individuals should be expected to bear anything like the full costs of unnecessary or overinflated care. The optimal degree of coverage must take into account the median income of the elderly, about $7500 in 1984,[16] as well as the essentiality of the services.

A conservative compromise would be to define "comprehensive" coverage for the elderly as that providing at least 75% of their average annual expenditures. In 1984, this would have meant that the average elderly individual would not have incurred out-of-pocket expenses of more than $1050. Given the median income of $7500 that year, it would also be in line with a 1985 recommendation of the House Select Committee on Aging: out-of-pocket health-care costs of the elderly should not be permitted to rise above 15% of income.[17]

A Qualitative Approach

The difficulty of defining "comprehensiveness" in dollar terms alone suggests that the definition must also take into account what the dollars are spent for. A thousand dollars might buy one night in an intensive care unit, or two weeks in a nursing home for a stroke patient, or two years of outpatient maintenance for a diabetic. Each may be justified under certain conditions. In order to ensure that each type is available when needed, but not to excess, so that other equally essential modalities can also be made available, it is necessary to spell out the essential services that make up the spectrum of comprehensive care.

Obviously, essential services should be defined in relation to the major health needs of the elderly, which today are related primarily to chronic disease and disability. Here is a suggested definition: *the prevention, early detection, treatment, and long-term management of patients with heart disease, cancer, stroke, alcoholism, Alzheimer's, and other chronic diseases of advancing age, as well as injuries, infectious diseases, and acute exacerbations of chronic conditions.* Unfortunately, the traditional definition of "essential" or "basic" services, embodied in most of our health-care financing programs, public and private, is just the opposite of this common-sense definition. In order to understand this apparent absurdity, it may be helpful to review briefly the historical evolution of policy in this area.

The modern concept of health insurance emerged in Europe in the early years of the twentieth century, when the major health problems of most people involved acute illness, childbirth, and trauma. In the United States, the "basic" coverages, developed and sold by the Blues, and later written into legislative concrete in the Medicare law, were also oriented toward acute care, emphasizing hospitalization and inpatient medical and surgical care, and almost totally ignoring the special problems of chronic disease—the importance of prevention and early detection and the frequent necessity of nonhospital long-term care. As has been frequently pointed out, although Medicare was created for the elderly, its benefits package, including the specific ban on "custodial care," was designed as if it were intended for the young. The same is true of most private Medigap or supplementary insurance policies. The likelihood of unnecessarily high costs was built into this approach, along with serious gaps in covered services. Recent efforts to fill the long-term care gap through traditional private insurance approaches, although well-intentioned, have thus far failed to meet the need. [18,19]

The first partial departure from this acute-care model was "major medical" coverage, developed by the insurance companies. While acknowledging the primacy of the "basic" coverages, major medical tried to fill some of the obvious gaps—office visits, long-term drug therapy, and "catastrophic" inpatient expenses beyond the usual basic limits. However, catastrophic was defined to exclude most long-term care—that is, care of patients with serious chronic illness or disability lasting six months or more. While it is extremely helpful in many individual cases, major medical still does not, and was not intended to, address the primary problems of chronic illness and disability. In fact, most major medical policies follow Medicare in ruling out reimbursement for preventive services and long-term nursing home or home care. Ironically, the Medicare Catastrophic Coverage Act of 1988 also excludes most long-term care expenses.

The next significant departure from the original acute-care model was the health maintenance organization (HMO). Not only does the HMO make primary care available on a fully insured basis (a nominal payment of a few dollars per visit is rarely a significant deterrent), but also each HMO member is usually required to designate one physician as his or her primary practitioner, and the latter then becomes the "gatekeeper" for all specialized services, including hospitalization. Although the HMO has been promoted primarily in terms of the capitation method of paying physicians as opposed to the fee-for-service method, potentially its most positive characteristic is the emphasis placed on primary care, with corollary controls on specialist care. [20] Equally important, the HMO structure, at least in its traditional group-practice model, makes it easier for the average primary physician to prescribe and follow through with preventive services.

Application of the HMO concept to the elderly came slowly but has increased since 1982 with the inauguration of "risk contracts" between Medicare and a number of HMOs. Preliminary evaluation of this experience suggests a mixed picture: Benefits have been "much more generous than standard Medicare benefits," cost-sharing requirements lower, and most reported hospital use-rates lower than average for Medicare beneficiaries. On the other hand, financial performance was mixed and there was a fairly high disenrollment rate—an average of 15.6% annually.[21] In 1986, 29 out of a total of 158 risk-contract HMOs terminated their Medicare contracts (K. Langwell, Mathematica Policy Research, Inc., telephone communication, December 28, 1987). Most of the terminators were of the independent practice variety and some clearly suffered from poor management.

Long-term care was traditionally neglected by HMOs, just as it was by most other carriers and plans. The social health maintenance organization (SHMO)—a concept aimed at adding long-term care benefits to the risk-contract HMO model and currently being tested in a four-site, multiyear demonstration funded by the Health Care Financing Administration—is discussed in Chapter 11.

Another nontraditional approach to health care for the elderly is potentially even more important than the HMO. The continuing care retirement community (CCRC), also known as the life-care community, is "an organization that provides housing, residential services, and health care to people of retirement age . . . the full continuum of housing and care, from independent living through nursing care, in order to meet the aging person's growing need for supportive services and care."[22–24]

The CCRC "offers a contract that is intended to remain in effect for the balance of the resident's lifetime. At a minimum, it guarantees shelter and access to various health care services. . . . A lump-sum entrance fee, paid upon moving into the community, and monthly payments thereafter, are typically required."[24]

According to the American Association of Homes for the Aging, principal trade association for CCRCs, 683 CCRCs met this definition in 1987. Analysis of 394 revealed three major types of contracts:

- *All-inclusive*, offering long-term care for little or no increase in regular monthly payments—33%;
- *Modified* contracts, offering only a limited amount of long-term care—31%;
- *Fee-for-service*, with guaranteed access to long-term care but at full per diem rates—28%;
- *Unclassified*—8%.

Probably the closest approximation to comprehensive care for the elderly available today, the CCRC faces a major obstacle to more rapid growth in its relatively high costs. As of 1987, entry fees ranged from $40,000 to over $150,000 (depending on type of contract, geographic location, size of residential unit, and number of occupants), and monthly fees from $500 to over $2000.[25]

A less expensive version of the CCRC model—the life care at home

(LCAH) concept—is currently being developed near Philadelphia and explored in a Robert Wood Johnson Foundation project.[26] LCAH omits the housing unit but provides equal access to long-term care. Entry fees at the first site, for a single person, range from $6500 to $12,500; monthly fees range from $210 to $260.[27] Several students of the LCAH concept believe it has a market potential of 10% to 25% of the elderly[26] and that 50% to 80% could afford to purchase one of the various emerging forms of long-term care insurance.[28]

However it is provided—by Medicare, CCRC, LCAH, HMO, or traditional insurance—if it is to recognize the centrality of chronic disease and functional disability in the elderly, comprehensive care should include the following categories of services:

- Primary prevention—immunization, counseling, etc., as part of ongoing primary care;

- Secondary prevention—periodic screening, physical and psychological exams facilitating early diagnosis;

- Definitive diagnosis, including functional assessment where relevant;

- Appropriate therapy—cure where possible, rehabilitation where necessary and possible, and stabilization, management, and long-term care of incurable conditions;

- Humane terminal care with maximum feasible patient autonomy.

Obviously, the procedures on this list could be categorized differently, but the point to emphasize is the broad spectrum of essential services. Still, the list leaves open the relative weight to be given to the different categories within the hypothetical commitment to meet at least 75% of the overall expenditures of the average elderly individual. Determination of these weights will require skillful reconciliation of utilization patterns under current benefit coverages, with estimates of unmet needs under the same coverages.

In view of the grossly skewed distribution of expenditures under most existing insurance programs, including Medicare, some resources will have to be transferred from the categories of definitive diagnosis and cure of reversible illness, where the lion's share is now concentrated, to prevention and primary and long-term care. In the case of mental illness, there is an obvious need to invest more resources in outpatient or community services.

What Is "Fiscal Viability"?

Fiscal viability can be defined in terms of an individual health-care plan or carrier or in relation to the national economy or gross national product.

Fiscal viability for a plan or carrier serving the elderly means the ability to generate adequate income to provide its older members or subscribers with the spectrum of services listed on page 474 in an amount sufficient to meet roughly 75% of their expenditures plus essential administrative and other overhead costs, including reasonable profits if it is a for-profit organization. As a practical matter, the question of fiscal viability today primarily concerns Medicare, not only because it is the principal source of third-party support for the elderly but also because it embodies national health policy and thus serves as pattern-setter for most other health insurers.

Could Medicare meet this test? On the basis of actual experience, the answer today has to be No. Despite its many accomplishments, Medicare fails to meet even minimal tests for comprehensive care. It specifically prohibits payment for most preventive services and for custodial or long-term care (Social Security Act, Sec. 1862). Instead, it emphasizes inpatient acute care, where it has been generous. Since inpatient acute care is the most expensive modality, it is not surprising that Medicare expenditures have spiraled upward dramatically, periodically endangering the Hospital Insurance Trust Fund, even with its currently restricted benefits.[2] Clearly if the Medicare benefit package were to be extended tomorrow to cover preventive services and long-term care, without any other changes, the program could not survive.

At the same time, the financial burden of illness falling on the elderly has increased. According to the House Select Committee on Aging, the elderly's out-of-pocket costs in 1984 represented a higher percentage of income than when Medicare began.[17] At that time, the committee estimated that the average older person was spending just over 15% of income for health care—an average of $1660 per person—and projected that, unless remedial action were taken, such payments would rise, from 1984 to 1990, about twice as fast as income, to nearly 20%.

Three years later, the same committee published an even harsher indictment of the financial plight of older Americans faced with the problem of paying for long-term nursing home or home health care.

> For those of you who are over the age of 65 living alone and have an annual income between $9,700 and $15,000 (between 200 and 300 percent of the poverty level), you would be impoverished after only **17 weeks,** on average, in a nursing home. However, if your annual income is between $6,000 and $10,000 (between 125 and 200 percent of the poverty level), it would take only **6 weeks,** on average, in a nursing home before you would be impoverished. Even if you have the average amount of financial assets for this latter income group, your income coupled with your financial assets will last only 32 weeks, on average, after you enter a nursing home.
>
> The sorry state of affairs can be traced to the almost complete absence of long-term care insurance protection in America.[29]

Obviously, for Medicare to achieve both comprehensive coverage and fiscal viability, some very significant changes will have to be explored, including:

- Serious emphasis on the prevention or postponement, early detection, and effective management of chronic illness;

- Some transfer of resources from inpatient acute care to primary and long-term care;

- Control over the excessive inflation in provider charges and costs, especially through fixed or prospective rates;

- Certain administrative reforms conducive to greater overall efficiency, for example, merger of Parts A and B and use of a community-based care coordinator or case manager to control the costs of long-term care;

- Enhancement of existing revenues through higher payroll taxes, special excise taxes on health-threatening products, such as alcohol and cigarettes, higher premiums, and more use of general revenues;

- More patient cost sharing;

- Greater emphasis on patient autonomy and responsibility for treatment decisions, including for terminal illness;

- Limitations on professional liability to minimize the counterproductive effects of defensive medicine;

- A greater role for states and private-sector bodies that meet public standards.

Some of these changes are already under way—most conspicuously the move to fixed provider rates through the diagnosis-related group payment system for hospitals. The reduction in Medicare payment for twelve procedures assumed to be overpriced, including coronary artery bypass surgery, total hip replacement, and cataract surgery, signed into law December 1987,[30] along with growing Congressional pressure for higher reimbursement for primary care[31] and for long-term care insurance,[32] may signal the beginning of some transfer of resources from acute to more comprehensive care.

All of the suggested changes involved some disadvantages as well as advantages, but overall they would probably facilitate achievement of fiscal viability for something approaching comprehensive care. Merger of Parts A and B could lead not only to greater administrative efficiency but also to the commingling of payroll taxes and general revenues, a development that would be furthered through transfer of Medicaid long-term care funds to Medicare. Inclusion of preventive and long-term services in Medicare would make the adoption of more substantial patient cost sharing more acceptable to consumers. Since 51% of all nursing home costs are now (1987) being paid for directly by patients or their families,[33] the substitution of a reasonable, income-related cost-sharing schedule as the price of Medicare coverage could help to redistribute this existing burden more equitably.

There is no question that even an expanded Medicare could be made fiscally viable if the political will were there to put through the necessary reforms. Similarly, HMOs and other private carriers could develop comprehensive programs in line with a revised Medicare benefit schedule if it were made clear through national policy that this is what the nation wants. But is it? Can the nation afford it? In other words, is comprehensive care for the elderly fiscally viable in relation to national income? In relation to other demands on the gross national product (GNP)? Does the nation gain enough from the productive efforts of its senior citizens to justify the inevitably high costs of their health care? Are we financially able to offer decent and humane care even to those who can no longer be productive but who are condemned—often through the success of the acute care that we so strongly encourage—to long periods of disability without adequate financial or other supports?

There are no easy answers. Those who say, "Let the proportion of GNP going to health care continue to rise indefinitely, reflecting the increase in the elderly in the population," evade the most difficult issues—how fast to let it rise, and how much. Clearly, some limits have to be imposed.

Others say, "The inevitable rise in health-care expenditures could easily be met simply through transfer of funds now being spent on unnecessary armaments, many of which pose more of a threat than a reassurance to national security." However, regardless of the obvious and urgent need for arms control, there is little evidence that any resultant savings would be made available to the health field when other international and domestic problems are so pressing.

However, those who say we cannot afford the "luxury" of caring for our "nonproductive" elders are similarly unpersuasive. To help put this into perspective, consider the magnitude of our current expenditures for the elderly—about $6000 per capita, as already noted. Consider, moreover, that we spend a higher percentage of the GNP on health care than any other nation. For example, the Health Care Financing Administration reports comparative 1983 percentages for ten nations as follows:

United Kingdom	6.2	West Germany	8.2 (1982)
Belgium	6.5	Canada	8.5
Denmark	6.6	France	9.3
Norway	6.9	Sweden	9.6
Australia	7.5	United States	10.8[34]

Consider, also, comparative life expectancy. Japan, with a 1985 figure of 77.1 years at birth, now has the highest life expectancy in the world.[35] Figures from 1985 for the same nations listed above[35] were:

United Kingdom	74.1	West Germany	74.1
Belgium	73.9	Canada	76.0
Denmark	74.8	France	74.8
Norway	76.2	Sweden	76.6
Australia	75.4	United States	74.6

Obviously, many factors other than health care enter into a nation's mortality rates and life expectancy. Explanations for international varia- tions in health-care costs are also complex and defy single-factor com- parisons. Nevertheless, the experience of so many other countries in equal- ing or surpassing our life expectancy, while spending a smaller proportion of GNP on health care, appears to refute the argument that advanced nations cannot afford adequate or comprehensive care for their elders.

The costs of health care for our elderly will, of course, continue to rise as their proportion of the population increases, but not without limits, assum- ing a reasonably finite human life span and some reins on medical tech- nology.[36-39] The challenge is to keep people relatively healthy, working (or at least able to care for themselves), and paying taxes as long as possible. When this is no longer possible and they need prolonged health care, we can and should help them secure the least expensive, most appropriate care, and we should make sure that it is conducive to maintaining their independence. This is the opposite of our present policy, which rewards acute illness and socioeconomic dependence.

There are some older people who would like to continue working—or not, as they prefer—while also enjoying the right to tax-exempt income, subsidized housing, transportation, health care, and other attractive "perks" designed to assuage the pangs of growing old. However, this will probably not be possible, even in our affluent society. Older people are going to have to keep on working as long as their health permits, to keep on paying taxes, and to continue accepting considerable responsibility for their own health or pay a price for irresponsibility. The elderly will also need more health care as they get older, and it is going to cost an increasing percentage of their shrinking income. Few, if any, will be able to command, at any price, all the care they would like.

Having said all that, it is still inconceivable that our nation cannot devise a viable health policy that ensures that all persons over 65 will receive, through a combination of public and private efforts—involving taxation, premiums, provider incentives and controls, and direct patient payments—the full spectrum of needed health services that constitute comprehensive care. The implementation of such a policy, requiring as it would some basic changes in the distribution of health personnel, capital investment, facilities, professional education, and other resources, is a different and primarily political matter.

References

1. Somers, A. R. 1981. Social, economic, and health aspects of mandatory retirement. *Health Politics Policy Law* 6:544–557.
2. Advisory Council on Social Security. 1983. *Medicare Benefits and Financing.* 1982 Report. Washington, D.C.: Government Printing Office.
3. Hazzard, W. R. 1983. Preventive gerontology: Strategies for healthy aging. *Postgrad Med* 74(2):279–287.
4. Butler, R. N., Gleason, H. P., (eds.) 1985. *Productive Aging: Enhancing Vitality in Later Life.* New York: Springer-Verlag.
5. Rowe, J. W., Kahn, R. L. 1987. Human aging: Usual and successful. *Science* 237:143–149.
6. Fries, J. F. 1988. Aging, illness, and health policy: Implications of the compression of morbidity. *Perspec Biol Med* 31 (3):407–428, Spring 1988.
7. Pell, S., Fayerweather, W. E. 1985. Trends in the incidence of myocardial infarction and in associated mortality and morbidity in a large employed population, 1957–1983. *N Engl J Med* 312:1005–1011.
8. Butler, R. N. 1987. The longevity revolution. *Mt Sinai J Med* 54:5–8.
9. Fries, J. F. 1980. Aging, natural death, and the compression of morbidity. *N Engl J Med* 303:130–135.
10. National Center for Health Statistics. 1986. *Health, United States, 1986.* DHHS Pub. No. (PHS) 87-1232. Washington, D.C.: Government Printing Office.
11. U.S. fertility at low and life expectancy at high. 1987. *New York Times,* September 8.
12. Fries, J. F. 1987. Reduction of the national morbidity. *Gerontologica Perspecta* (Montreal) 1:54–65.
13. Katz, S., Branch, L. G., Branson, M., Papsidero, J. A., Beck, J. C., Greer, D. S. 1983. Active life expectancy. *N Engl J Med* 309:1218–1224.
14. Waldo, D. R., Lazenby, H. C. 1984. Demographic characteristics and health care use and expenditures by the aged in the U.S.: 1977–1984. *Health Care Financing Rev* 6:1–29.
15. Cohen, G. D. 1980. Prospects for mental health and aging. In *Handbook of Mental Health and Aging,* ed. J. Birren and R. B. Sloane. New York: Prentice Hall.
16. United States Bureau of the Census. 1986. Money income of households, families, and persons in the U.S., 1984. *Current Population Reports,* Series P-60, No. 151, Table 31.
17. United States House of Representatives, Select Committee on Aging. 1985. *America's Elderly at Risk: A Report Presented by the Chairman.* Pub. No. 99-508. Washington, D.C.: Government Printing Office.

18. Wiener, J. M., Ehrenworth, D. A., Spense, D. A. 1987. Private long-term care insurance: Cost, coverage, and restrictions. *Gerontologist* 27(4):487–493.

19. Rivlin, A. M., Wiener, J. M. 1988. *Caring for the Disabled Elderly: Who Will Pay?* Washington, D.C.: Brookings Institution.

20. Somers, A. R. 1983. And who shall be the gatekeeper? The role of the primary physician in the health care delivery system. *Inquiry* 20:301–313.

21. Brown, R., Nelson, L., Langwell, K., Rossiter, L., Allen, P., Harkins, E., Tucker, A. 1987. *Second Annual Report: National Medicare Competition Evaluation.* Prepared for Health Care Financing Administration, Contract 500-83-0047. Princeton, N. J.: Mathematica Policy Research.

22. Somers, A. R. 1988. The continuing care retirement community (CCRC): One viable option for long-term care (LTC) insurance. *The DRG Monitor* 6(4):1–12.

23. Winklevoss, H. E., Powell, A. V. 1984. *Continuing Care Retirement Communities: An Empirical, Financial and Legal Analysis.* Homewood, Ill.: R. D. Irwin, Inc.

24. American Association of Homes for the Aging and Ernst and Whinney. 1987. *Continuing Care Retirement Communities: An Industry in Action: Analysis and Developing Trends 1987.* Washington, D.C.: The American Association of Homes for the Aging.

25. Tell, E. J., Cohen, M. A., Larson, M., Batten, H. 1987. Assessing the elderly's preferences for lifecare retirement options. *Gerontologist* 27(4):503–509.

26. Tell, E. J., Cohen, M. A., Wallack, S. S. 1987. Life care at home: A new long term care finance and delivery option. *Inquiry* 24(3):245–252.

27. *Jeanes/Foulkeways Life Care at Home.* 1986. Brochure. Gwynedd, Pa.: Jeanes Health System.

28. Cohen, M. A., Tell, E. J., Greenberg, J., Wallack, S. 1987. The financial capacity of the elderly to insure for long-term care. *Gerontologist* 27(4):494–502.

29. United States House of Representatives, Select Committee on Aging. 1987. *Long-Term Care and Personal Impoverishment: Seven in Ten Living Alone are at Risk.* Pub. No. 100-631. Washington, D.C.: Government Printing Office.

30. Pear, R. 1987. Physicians contend systems of payment have eroded status. *New York Times,* December 26.

31. Rovner, J. 1987. Disputes over health issues prove difficult to resolve. *Congressional Quarterly Weekly Report* 45(Dec. 19):3128.

32. Rovner, J. 1987. Pepper wins a round on long-term care bill. *Congressional Quarterly Weekly Report* 45(Nov. 21):2874–2875.

33. United States Health Care Financing Administration, Office of the Actuary, Division of National Cost Estimates. 1987. National health expenditures, 1986–2000. *Health Care Financing Rev* 8(4):1–36.

34. Waldo, D. R., Levit, K. R., Lazenby, H. 1986. National health expenditures, 1985. *Health Care Financing Rev* 8(1):1–21.

35. United States Bureau of the Census. 1987. An aging world. *International Population Reports,* Series P-95, No. 78. Washington, D.C.: Government Printing Office.

36. Somers, A. R. 1984. Why not try preventing illness as a way of controlling Medicare costs? *N Engl J Med* 311:853–856.

37. Somers, A. R. 1987. Insurance for long-term care: Some definitions, problems, and guidelines for action. *N Engl J Med* 317(July 2):23–29.
38. Somers, A. R. 1988. Aging in the 21st century: Projections, personal preferences, public policies—A consumer view. *Health Policy* 9(1):49–58.
39. Somers, A. R. 1986. The changing demand for health services: A historical perspective and some thoughts for the future. *Inquiry* 23:395–402.

Twenty-seven

Approaches to Health

T. Franklin Williams

Approaches to health maintenance and long-term care for older people have, as their overall goal, the maintenance of life styles, social independence, and dignity.[1-4] Included in this goal are following the older persons' preferences for living settings, maintenance of maximal health and functioning, restoration of lost function, and, when needed, appropriate supportive long-term care that also encourages as much independence as possible.

Table 27.1 summarizes the services needed to ensure the accomplishment of these aims. *Health maintenance* may be considered to include health promotion and disease-prevention activities, and primary, consultative, and rehabilitative care when needed. Long-term care (LTC) includes geriatric evaluation, and the management of LTC services, home-support services, and LTC in institutions.

The importance of rehabilitation in the care of older persons, including the use of the full spectrum of formal rehabilitative services where appropriate, cannot be overemphasized. Thus, in every health-care interaction with an older patient, physicians and other health professionals should keep in mind the functional status of the patient and take steps to restore or to maintain physical and mental abilities.

The full range of rehabilitative services is often needed to address the multiple, simultaneous medical, behavioral, and social disabilities of older

Table 27.1. Components of Health Maintenance and Long-Term Care Services for Older People

Health Maintenance
  Health promotion and disease prevention
    Consumer information
    Preventive practices
      Nutritional support
      Social opportunities
      Preventive check-ups
      Visual and hearing aids; other devices
  Ready access to primary and consultative care
    Care for acute problems, when needed, in office, home, or hospital; including consultative services
    Rehabilitative services—in day hospital, home, hospital, or nursing home
    Continuity of professional care
    Hospice care when needed
Long-Term Care
  Geriatric evaluation and care management
    Comprehensive multidisciplinary evaluation
    Care management
  Home support services
    Personal, social, and nursing care. Environmental modifications
    Counseling services for family
    Respite services
    Special services for special groups, i.e., Alzheimer's patients
  Long-term care in institutions
    Variety of options
    Rehabilitation orientation

patients. Comprehensive care can require not only the expert guidance of the physiatrist but also the contributions of physical, occupational, and speech therapists, social workers, rehabilitation psychologists, and other consultative specialists (for example, in rheumatic diseases and in neurology). In the United States, the development of rehabilitation has emphasized this team approach. Furthermore, rehabilitation services should be available on a consultative basis for older people in every care setting and in every community.

Health Maintenance

Demonstration Projects

Informed self-care is the foundation of health maintenance for everyone, including older people. Therefore, as recommended by Somers[5] and Ball (unpublished data), a health-maintenance program should provide information on self-care, symptom recognition, and when to see the doctor. It should provide social activities (e.g., day programs), nutritional guidance, periodic preventive examinations, and medical devices needed to maintain vision, hearing, and mobility. "One of the best ways to treat the problems of vulnerable and disabled older people is to provide appropriate services to them while they are still well."[6] The health-maintenance framework should also incorporate rehabilitative services, as already emphasized, in acute and continuing care settings, such as the day hospital approach so well developed in the United Kingdom.

There are many approaches to providing health-maintenance services, and all of them are useful as long as emphasis is placed on achieving and maintaining high-quality services—through professional education that deals adequately with gerontology and geriatrics and through incentives and standards for high-quality care. One approach emphasizes the individual primary-care physician, who oversees patient care and makes use of consultative and supportive services as necessary. Group practices are an excellent application of this approach. Particularly with regard to the complex, multifactorial needs of older people, health maintenance organizations (HMOs) are also unusually well suited to providing the comprehensive services needed. In addition, the typical HMO incorporates incentives, such as capitation payment for comprehensive care, that help favor the promotion and maintenance of health and the avoidance of unnecessary hospitalization.

Recent demonstration projects employing Medicare capitation payment to HMOs have documented the promise of this prepaid approach to comprehensive care for older people. The participating HMOs, which were located in varied geographic and urban/rural environments, undertook these demonstrations with funding by the Health Care Financing Administration (HCFA).[7] They found that older Medicare recipients were eager to enroll. Furthermore, the elderly clients were highly pleased with the simplicity of using one setting for multiple care needs and of avoiding Medicare forms or unpredictable copayments. Once enrolled, the Medicare recipient simply presented his or her card for services and paid a set monthly copayment that was often less than prior add-on charges to what Medicare paid. Also, to promote their services, the HMOs elected to provide some services not usually covered by Medicare, such as optician services and drug discounts.

The demonstration projects were also successful in significantly lowering hospital use by the enrolled Medicare recipients. The accompanying savings in costs in all but one of the participating HMOs resulted in a favorable financial balance at a capitation rate set by the HCFA that was 95% of the average Medicare costs for the region in which the HMO was located. The single exception was the Marshfield Clinic, in Wisconsin, where Medicare average costs are already considerably lower than those in comparable areas—due, it was thought, to the already established favorable effect of the Marshfield Clinic, the predominant source of care in that area.

The Department of Health and Human Services has made the option of capitation arrangements for comprehensive care for Medicare recipients more widely available. This approach seems certain to spread through HMOs, independent practice associations (IPAs), preferred provider organizations (PPOs), and similar practice arrangements. To ensure access for persons with greater care burdens, as well as soundness of reimbursement arrangements, it will be important to have adequate open-enrollment policies and allowance for rate adjustments in each practice organization.

Social Health Maintenance Organizations

The social health maintenance organization (SHMO) is another step toward health maintenance, providing social as well as health-care services aimed at minimizing the loss of function or independence.[8-10] (See also Greenberg et al., Chapter 11.) Demonstration projects to test the viability and value of SHMOs, funded through Medicare and Medicaid, are in progress.

Future Prospects

It is very likely that the organized-practice approach will be tested most extensively, and intensively, through Medicare financing of capitation payment for health maintenance and acute care. In the demonstration projects already referred to, this approach appeared to be excellent,[7] but there is a danger that, unless there is careful planning and appropriate regulation, including guarantees of financial soundness, some aspiring HMOs or similar groups might promise to provide care that they find they cannot deliver.

Long-Term Care

When an elderly person's health begins to fail significantly and/or the social support arrangements for a frail older person collapse, a thorough assessment is urgently needed to determine an appropriate plan for long-term care (LTC). (Techniques of case management and assessment have already been discussed elsewhere in this book.) In most instances the assessment is best accomplished in the setting of a comprehensive, multidisciplinary geriatric evaluation clinic or hospital service.[11-16] A consensus development conference on geriatric assessment at the National Institutes of Health endorsed this approach for selected older patients.

An unresolved issue is how these comprehensive clinics and services will be paid for. Evidence to date indicates that the use of such services decreases hospitalization rates and, at least in some settings, the use of nursing home care, and that the increases in home-care services that may accompany this approach are less costly than institutional care. A special reimbursement rate for such inpatient units and outpatient consultative clinics seems as advisable, surely, as having special rates for other specialty consultative clinics and services. In practices operating under prepaid, capitation arrangements, it would be wise to provide for such comprehensive assessment and LTC services as an integral part of the overall system, so that the organization not only would provide appropriate care but also would benefit financially by decreasing the overall cost.

To help ensure that care arrangements recommended by comprehensive geriatric assessments are accomplished, it is important to involve a professional person—the physician, or visiting nurse, or social worker—in ongoing case management.

Worldwide Innovations

We still have much to learn about providing continuing, appropriate, and dependable care in the home and in institutions. The range of home support services and institutional services that should be available across our nation is indicated in Table 27.1. In other countries (for example, in South Australia and in Kent, England), a "catchment area" approach to providing home support services has been developed. In this arrangement a team of home-support personnel has responsibility for all of the clients needing home-care services. In each area, "domiciliary care services" operated by voluntary health agencies are responsible for providing the domiciliary (home) care ordered by physicians for all patients in their areas. In South Australia the service is supported primarily by a budget provided by the state, including some federal funds, with a variable, income-based contribution by service recipients. There is no fee for any individual service nor any fixed duration of a service, in contrast to the fee-for-service home-care services in this country, where it is impossible to purchase less than an hour's visiting nurse service or, often, less than 4 hours' aide services. Rather, the domiciliary care team is flexible, paying brief visits to some patients, sometimes more than once a day, and spending longer times with other patients as needed. Supervisory support, team meetings, and good personnel practice can be much better provided in this type of organization than in the separate client approach in this country.

In Kent, England, a similar approach has been taken, with additional emphasis on combining nursing and social support services.[17] This model has now been tested in Rochester, New York, in a randomized clinical trial operated by the ACCESS long-term care program, with support from the Robert Wood Johnson Foundation. In this demonstration, a community health (or visiting) nurse and a social worker share care-management responsibility for a panel of patients in a catchment area and arrange for and supervise other home-support services. The nurse–social worker shared leadership provides flexibility in meeting the varied and changing medical and social needs of those served; at one time the nurse may be in charge, at another, the social worker. Obviously, close and sustained communication is necessary. Results indicate high patient satisfaction and a modest but important 10–15% overall decrease in the total health-care costs in the experimental group compared to a control population, attributable largely to decreased hospitalizations.

Undeniably, people who require nursing home care are entitled to high-quality services. Sounder guidelines for the quality of care in nursing homes was the objective of a special study completed by the Institute of Medicine, National Academy of Sciences, at the request of the HCFA.[18] The results of this study should help guide national efforts to ensure the quality of care in nursing homes. The National Citizens' Coalition in Nursing Home Reform, as well as other groups, is actively pursuing steps to follow up on this study.

A somewhat different concept of LTC has been introduced (in Rochester, N.Y.,) that holds that costly services requiring high-intensity care should be considered a "catastrophic" situation and should be approached like any other catastrophe (unpublished data). Examples of catastrophic situations include extensive, often around-the-clock nursing services in the home, intensive nursing care in a nursing home or chronic-care hospital, and frequent readmissions to acute-care hospitals. Available data indicate that about 20% of long-term care patients account for about 80% of the long-term care costs. These catastrophic costs are very burdensome to patients and families as well as to third-party payers, including public sources (Medicaid and Medicare).

By focusing on the special needs of this minority and by attempting to provide needed services most cost-effectively, desirable care may be provided at less cost. An example of this approach is the special short-term, hospital-intensity care that the ACCESS program provides (in the patient's home or nursing home) for LTC patients who have a "sudden decline" due to some intercurrent illness or exacerbation. Such situations usually lead to acute hospitalizations, but instead the ACCESS program provides additional nursing services as well as payment for daily physician visits for the duration of the acute episode. Evaluation of this program has shown that about 50% of what would otherwise have been acute hospital admissions from home or nursing homes were avoided, with no evidence of disadvantage to the patient's status and in fact a real advantage in not moving the patient to the strange hospital environment.

At the other end of the spectrum of long-term care are the majority of older persons, who have less intensive service needs and whose families provide most of the needed services, at times with limited additional purchased help. Families' contributions are being more widely recognized, and incentives for such contributions are now being provided in some states, through tax rebates or credits.

In conclusion, promising approaches are already being tested or introduced that should help provide more comprehensive, more effective, and less costly health maintenance and LTC services for older persons. What still remains to be established is an approach that effectively combines both health-maintenance and LTC services.

Note: The opinions expressed here are those of the author and not intended to reflect the views of the National Institutes of Health.

References

1. Fahey, C. F. 1983. Some personal views on long-term care. In *Grantmakers in Health*. Proceedings of Fourth Annual Conference: Long-Term Care and Chronic Illness—The Elderly and the Children, 10–11. New York: Grantmakers in Health.
2. Feinstein, P. H. 1984. Epilogue: Themes and issues. In *Long-Term Care Financing and Delivery Systems: Exploring Some Alternatives*. Conference Proceedings, January 24, p. 129. Washington, D.C.: Government Printing Office.
3. Williams, T. F. 1983. The aging of the American population. *Grantmakers in Health*. Proceedings of Fourth Annual Conference: Long-Term Care and Chronic Illness—The Elderly and the Children, 1–3. New York: Grantmakers in Health.
4. Williams, T. F. 1984. Introduction. In *Rehabilitation in the Aging*, ed. T. F. Williams. New York: Raven Press.
5. Somers, A. R. 1984. Why not try preventing illness as a way of controlling Medicare costs? *N Engl J Med* 311(13):853–856.
6. Kodner, D. L. 1984. Elderplan. In *Long-Term Care Financing and Delivery Systems: Exploring Some Alternatives*, Conference Proceedings, January 24, p. 67. Washington, D.C.: Government Printing Office.
7. Lamb, S. J., Gassaway, C. H., Gallagher, E. K. (eds.) 1984. *A Symposium on Financing Medical Care for the Aged*. Claverack, N.Y.: Caldwell B. Esselstyn Foundation.
8. Greenberg, J., Leutz, W. N. 1984. The social health maintenance organization and its role in reforming the long-term care system. In *Long-Term Care Financing and Delivery Systems: Exploring Some Alternatives*, Conference Proceedings, January 24, pp. 57–65. Washington, D.C.: Government Printing Office.
9. Kodner, D. L. 1984. Discussion. In *Long-Term Care Financing and Delivery*

Systems: Exploring Some Alternatives, Conference Proceedings, January 24, pp. 66–68. Washington, D.C.: Government Printing Office.

10. Kodner, D. L. 1984. Elderplan: An emerging social/HMO. In *A Symposium on Financing Medical Care for the Aged*, 37–42. Claverack, N.Y.: Caldwell B. Esselstyn Foundation.

11. Williams, T. F. 1983. Comprehensive functional assessment: An overview. *J Am Geriatr Soc* 31(11-12): 637–641.

12. Martin, D. C., Moryaz, R. K., McDowell, J., Snustad, D., Karpf, M. Community-based geriatric assessment. *J Am Geriatr Soc* 33:602.

13. Williams, T. F., Hill, J. G., Fairbank, M. E., Knox, K. G. 1973. Appropriate placement of the chronically ill and aged: A successful approach. *JAMA* 226(11):1332–1335.

14. Rubenstein, L. 1983. The clinical effectiveness of multidimensional geriatric assessment. *J Am Geriatr Soc* 31(11-12):758–762.

15. Williams, T. F. 1984. Characteristics of the aged in geriatric medicine. In *A Symposium on Financing Medical Care for the Aged*, 13. Claverack, N.Y.: Caldwell B. Esselstyn Foundation.

16. Rubenstein, L., Josephson, K., Wieland, G., English, P., Sayre, J., Kane, R. 1984. Effectiveness of a geriatric evaluation unit. *N Engl J Med* 311:1664–1670.

17. Davies, B., Challis, D. 1980. Experimenting with new roles in domiciliary service: The Kent community care project. *Gerontologist* 20(3):288–299.

18. Institute of Medicine. 1986. *Improving the Quality of Care in Nursing Homes*. Washington, D.C.: National Academy Press.

Twenty-eight

Vacating the Premises: A Reevaluation of First Principles

Robert L. Kane and Rosalie A. Kane

Essential Elements

Medical and Social Care

If one had the opportunity to start fresh in developing a system of care for the elderly, certain elements would be essential. The components are philosophically compatible but not generally available, at least certainly not in one place at one time. A system of care for the elderly should: 1) determine functional problems and ensure that they are treated to maximize functional abilities, 2) include environmental approaches to the improvement of functioning, 3) incorporate the preferences of older people, and 4) be predicated on universal coverage of health-care costs. These elements apply to long-term care as well as to acute care, because arbitrary divisions serve the elderly poorly.

The multiple, simultaneous problems of the elderly—the hallmark of geriatrics—make traditional diagnoses insufficient. The caregiver must be capable of identifying functional problems and their etiologies. Since the care process should begin by remedying the remediable, the first essential step is to treat those conditions that will respond positively to treatment.

This chapter was originally written in 1984 and revised in 1987.

The goal of care of the elderly is to maximize functioning. Function depends on two critical, mutually dependent elements: maximizing the individual's innate capacity, and developing a supportive physical and social environment. Careful medical evaluation to identify correctable problems is essential. In addition, choosing treatment is complicated. Elderly patients have a high potential for adverse consequences. Only a caregiver with considerable skill and training can attend to problems while working within a constrained risk: benefit ratio and imposing minimal risk. Without this training, more conservative practice is probably warranted.

Once the treatable problems have been addressed, the next goal of care is to maximize the elderly person's functioning by manipulating the environment, including both the physical and the social supports appropriate to encourage autonomy. Here, too, significant iatrogenic risks demand skillful practice. The caregiver must foster independence while strengthening and supplementing, not supplanting, individual and family resources. Thus, care of the elderly requires both a medical and a social approach. The approaches may be sequential, but they are clearly synergistic.

Care of the elderly should also accommodate the value preferences of the recipient. Although formal knowledge in this important area is limited, some studies have demonstrated that different people hold very different views about the goals of their care. Some may be concerned primarily about short-term survival to reach an important milestone; others value longer-term survival.[1] Differences also exist in choosing between details of care and preferred lifestyle. One preference has been recorded with unusual unanimity: surveys show that the preponderance of older people prefer to remain at home and to avoid the nursing home. Fatalistically, they may add that they expect to be sent to a nursing home if they need care, but the nursing home as they know it is a dreaded fate.[2] Surely, society can do better for its older citizens than to provide them with care so incompatible with their taste.

Thus, health care for the elderly is neither medical nor social, but a combination, and the issue is not whether to exclude one component or the other, but which component will dominate, if indeed dominance is the key issue.

Coverage of Costs

Another essential component in health care of the elderly is some system of universal coverage for health costs. Without this, health care quickly becomes either a welfare program or an uncontrolled industry. The elderly are triply vulnerable: they have the greatest number of health problems, they are more likely to have limited financial means, and they are more likely to be shunned by health-care professionals. Universal coverage provides a mechanism for controlling the costs of care and for distributing that care according to principles of social equity. The universality of coverage does not imply a single mode of delivering care, nor does it mean that delivery need be a government function. It does, however, place the responsibility for care in the public domain. By making health care an entitlement rather than a welfare benefit, it preserves the social resources of the elderly person, thus increasing the probabilities of autonomy.

Integrating Acute and Long-Term Care

The present health-care system, which separates acute and long-term care (LTC), is artificial and inefficient. Although it is true that most elderly persons need little or no LTC, the elderly are the group most likely to need such care. For the approximately one-fifth of the elderly population who need LTC, the poor articulation between acute and LTC services is dysfunctional. For many of the rest, a broader definition of useful interventions to include social activities would probably improve the effectiveness of health care. It is unrealistic to view acute and LTC as separate entities. Many of those in the LTC system enter because of an acute-care crisis. Many come directly from a hospital. Conversely, LTC recipients tend to be heavy users of acute care because they have a variety of medical conditions that create acute crises directly or precipitate them as a result of treatment.

A study of nursing home discharges, for example, has pointed to the tight linkage between nursing home care and hospital care.[3] Persons leaving the nursing home are very likely to go to the hospital. Some individuals followed for a period of two years moved back and forth between the nursing home and the hospital as many as six times.

Conversely, the hospital is a major source of nursing home residents, but under appropriate conditions the crisis surrounding hospitalization can be addressed in a manner that forestalls the inevitability of nursing home placement. Units can be organized in hospitals to assess patients from a broad functional perspective and to work with patients and their families to facilitate return to the community.[4] A randomized controlled trial of a geriatric evaluation unit has shown that it improves patient functioning and saves money by reducing subsequent utilization of institutional care.[5]

The value of integrating acute and long-term care is clear, but how the integration can be most productively accomplished is not. One scenario is to expand the definition (or jurisdiction) of acute care to encompass long-term care. Proponents have suggested extending Medicare benefits to cover long-term care under a "Title XXI" of the Social Security Act.[6] By design or default, many of the current shifts in American health policy seem to be moving toward integration.

Recent changes in Medicare's hospital reimbursement mechanisms toward fixed prospective payments by diagnosis-related groups have spurred enormous hospital interest in LTC. While such concern may be laudatory, its motivations must be recognized. Under a fixed payment per admission system, the hospital has a powerful incentive to discharge patients. The primary goal is to move them out; the secondary question is where. Under this payment system, hospitals have developed a keen interest in encouraging the availability of LTC resources in the community and in other institutions. Indeed, hospitals may well find it economically advantageous to subsidize nursing homes and home care (at least over the short term), with the rationale that this care is cheaper than hospital use. Certainly, hospitals are actively pursuing various modes of vertical integration. In fact, if hospitals can transfer costs from acute-care to LTC categories under a system of fractionated funding, they may be able to generate new sources of revenue.

Social versus Medical Sponsorship

The opposite position favors a separate system for LTC, in which participation in LTC services would in no way alter a client's eligibility for standard medical care. The heart of the separationist argument is simply that LTC is a social, rather than a medical, matter. In this view, medical professionals have a contribution to make, but they are not equipped to manage the system. The National Study Group on State Medicaid Strategies has taken this position in recommending a division of the Medicaid program into two distinct components: a federally financed and administered National Primary Health Care Program and a state-administered Continuing Care System.[7]

The case for a separate, social LTC system has many positive points. At one level, it may contain costs, since health care has an admittedly expensive style of operation. Some forms of care, alcohol treatment for example, have become very expensive under medical sponsorship, with no obvious gain in efficacy.

Health care also tends to follow a highly professional, technological style, which may not suit the needs of the LTC clients or the goals of their care. Indeed, movements like hospice care developed as a rejection of medicine's sterile approach to highly emotional issues like the care of dying persons. If the goal of LTC is autonomous functioning, the traditional health-care system's emphasis on efficacy may prove counterproductive by encouraging dependence rather than independence.

Although adequate medical assessment and treatment of the remediable problems of the elderly are essential, care of the chronically disabled has not attracted the enthusiasm of the medical profession. Patterns of practice up to the present suggest that the medical profession undervalues care of the elderly. To consign their care to a niche where it will be accorded second-class status seems inappropriate.

Social sponsorship is more likely to lead to creativity in developing new approaches to LTC. It could provide a wider variety of interventions, consistent with the diverse etiologies of dysfunction, than the medical profession can. Such variation may, of course, become a mixed blessing. In the present system of fee-for-service care, medical orthodoxy has proven to be a useful means of controlling expenditures. It establishes the bounds of what will be covered under a medical program. (The unit costs are high, but the allowable units tend to be definable and subject to limitations.) A move to more social sponsorship might open the floodgates for proponents of diverse interventions. Because the elderly tend to respond positively to a variety of stimuli, few interventions could be declared illegitimate and the public could be asked to pay for almost anything.

Those critical of the narrow bounds of medical orthodoxy may welcome such a shift. Certainly, if it were coupled with a requirement for evidence of efficacy (currently reserved for only a minority of medical practices), a shift to diverse interventions might move the care of the elderly in a progressive direction. In any event, more attention would be paid to quality-of-life issues and a "holistic" approach to care. A wider variety of caregivers could be accommodated, probably at a lower unit cost than that of physicians. The client may be less awed and hence more prepared to play an active role in the care.

Social sponsorship does not necessarily imply social-work leadership of the health-care team, nor does it automatically endorse the concept of a team at all. In many instances it may be more efficient to use disciplines as needed rather than have them all converge on the client to push their areas of expertise. Some form of case coordination will be needed, but it is not at all clear which profession is best suited to provide it. Although physicians seem unlikely candidates, Some would argue that primary care is similar to case management. Certainly if physicians want to assume such a role, they will need different training. More likely candidates seem to be nursing and social work, either separately or together. At present there is considerable overlap in their skills and interests. Whoever takes on the role, it must be done in a way that maximizes independence and accountability. As discussed below, case managers working for provider corporations are likely to become entrapped in role conflicts. The case manager has a sufficiently difficult time serving the client and society without having to meet the needs of provider constituencies as well. Such persons will best be hired independently, either as part of a contracted service or as a public corporation empowered to authorize care and responsible to the results of its provision.

Social operation is not inconsistent with health sponsorship. LTC funds are most likely to be successfully obtained from a reallocation of health dollars, for several reasons. The health budget is already large, and investment in LTC seems to yield savings in acute care, especially hospital care. Furthermore, precedents already exist in areas like acute home care. However, these resource-allocation decisions must be recognized to be very different from decisions that can be made on the firing line. Aaron and Schwartz pointed to health-care rationing decisions in the United Kingdom that work only because those closest to the actual sources of care are protected from having to deny that care.[8] It is therefore critical that the allocation decision be made at a policy level rather than being left to practitioners, who face constant demands for service. The reallocation can be accomplished by program budgeting, but because budgeting requires an ability to set bounds to spending, the open-ended health spending approach will not work with allocation strategies.

The social LTC program would cover the costs of providing a mix of services to the elderly needing assistance in maintaining independence. If community-based care is viewed as the preferred mode of service, institutional care would then be treated as a secondary choice to be used when the preferred mode was not feasible. The housing component of institutional care could then be addressed as a housing cost, and personal funds could be used to support this component to the same extent that these funds could have paid for noninstitutional housing. When financial subsidies are required, they should be provided in the same manner that rent subsidies are offered.

If LTC is viewed as a social provision to compensate for functional impairment, it follows that those receiving LTC would get health care in the same manner as people of all ages in society; that is, from doctors, hospitals, public health nurses, and home-health agencies. Indeed, it is possible that persons living in residential facilities might also be visited by a homemaker or a physical therapist under certain circumstances. Their transportation needs could be met by the community system used to transport handicapped adults. Recreational programs could be the responsibility of the city, mental health programs of the community mental health center, and adult education of the community college system. Through these measures, social sponsorship would counter the current tendency to view people living in residential facilities as having no further need of social institutions because their lives are essentially over. Furthermore, in this best of all possible worlds, their health care would be subject to the same standards of accountability as the care received by any other citizen.

However, separating extended hospital care from social LTC creates a new need for communication between systems as individuals move from chronic medical care to LTC and vice versa. Moreover, the shift is not necessarily any greater than that faced by an individual entering the medical system from the general population.

Finally, developing a socially based program with universal entitlement would mean taking a giant stride. The United States does not even have a program of universal health insurance, and yet the proposal outlined here calls for a universal program of both health care and LTC. Happily, the concept is not without precedent, since for most of this century the United States has had a universal program for public education and at least a basic universal benefit for almost all elderly Americans through Social Security. A universal health-care program would mostly benefit the elderly, just as universal education most directly benefits children, although making health-care benefits universal not only helps control overall costs but also eliminates intergenerational conflict over what is done for the old and what is done for the young when they are sick.

Capitation

A compromise position that postpones the medical–social debate proposes the use of pooled resources and assumed responsibility through prepaid capitation, whereby an organized unit that assumes responsibility for the health of a defined group defers the final question of which route to emphasize. Capitation strategies have several appealing points for different factions. From the standpoint of payers, they offer a means of limiting risk, since as long as the service organization is solvent and responsible, the payer need not decide which services to pay for.

For consumers, prepaid programs represent a commitment to service, rather than an insurance company's promise to simply pay the bill (or part of it). A prepaid system usually presents few disincentives to access, although expensive care may be rationed. In many instances, the prepaid dollar seems to buy more, or at least the prepaid package offers broader benefits for the same cost of an indemnity plan.

Providers of prepaid services have the opportunity to use the most efficient means to deliver care. The trade-offs usually precluded by traditional fragmented funding are more likely to be in evidence. One form of care may be used to offset another. If enrollment is expected to be constant, an "investment" strategy of care may favor more complete early efforts to recoup savings later on. If the program has control of its institutional resources, it may opt to hold down growth in that area and substitute noninstitutional care wherever feasible. Proscriptions against use of certain types of personnel established by Medicare reimbursement regulations need not apply.

Certainly, safeguards need to be incorporated into any prepaid system.

Not only are prepaid groups going to seek the most attractive (i.e., least risky) clients, but also they may try to undo any enrollment mistakes they make by encouraging the heavy user to disenroll. Thus, the constant danger in any system of prepaid care is the propensity to underserve by withholding care or making it difficult to get through gatekeepers. The usual argument to counter this threat is the ability of the client to disenroll, but disenrollment may not be punitive to the group if the client is a heavy user of care. The principles of free-market competition may not suffice to protect consumers, especially elderly persons, who tend to be less aggressive shoppers for medical care.[9] (For a discussion of SHMOs, see Chapter 11.)

Lessons from Canada

Each Canadian province has a universal health insurance program that protects citizens of all ages from virtually all health costs at delivery. Most provinces have also moved to include nursing home care and some degree of home care as universal benefits with limited copayments. Therefore, the Canadian experience provides an opportunity to examine systemwide innovations. The care systems in three Canadian provinces, Manitoba, British Columbia, and Ontario, provide some good examples.[10]

Manitoba and British Columbia

Manitoba, which has one of the oldest records of LTC coverage, deliberately divides responsibility for LTC. Nursing homes, along with hospitals and physicians, are under the Manitoba Health Services Commission. Community care and the assessment of clients for LTC are the responsibility of a separate Office of Continuing Care, which authorizes admission to nursing homes. This office and the commission report to the Ministry of Health. Thus, funding decisions, based on the relative service intensity of these two sectors, are made at the ministerial level, and specific areas of activity are decided on at the program levels.

British Columbia has an Office of Long-Term Care in the Ministry of Health that is responsible for community and institutional services. Its director reports to the same assistant deputy minister as those responsible for hospital care. Here, too, allocation decisions are made at a ministerial level.

Both provinces use case management as a primary mechanism for assessing the need for LTC services and authorizing admission to nursing homes, and the decisions are made by nonphysicians, although information from physicians on the client's medical condition is used as part of the data.

Manitoba has developed a noteworthy coordinating procedure, referred to as paneling. Prior to approval for nursing home admission, each case must be presented to an interdisciplinary group that includes a physician, a geriatrician whenever possible. The panel reviews the data and the decision and may request further evaluation by a special geriatric evaluation unit when there is reason to question the completeness of the medical data.

Both Manitoba and British Columbia demonstrate the feasibility of providing LTC services that are not under direct medical control. Physicians and hospitals continue to provide care as required by the patient's condition, and participation in the LTC program does not in any way reduce eligibility for medical care. Furthermore, all adults with functional impairment are eligible for the LTC benefits, so no arbitrary distinctions are made based on age. These provinces (and the rest of Canada) have been able to provide a more comprehensive set of health services for the elderly by making health-care coverage (broadly defined) a universal entitlement for all. Moreover, the cost, whether measured in dollars per capita or as a percentage of gross national product, does not imperil their economies. In fact, Canada's health-care costs have lagged behind those in the United States since the imposition of universal health coverage. While debates about universal health coverage in the United States have been peppered with fears of unconstrained cost, the Canadian experience demonstrates that vesting control in a single payer controls costs by controlling the supply of resources. The monopsonistic* state offers a means to determine what will be paid for, but the decision applies to everyone. There are no alternative markets for expensive services.

For the elderly, the Canadian experience shows that it is possible to cover both acute and long-term services at an affordable price. The LTC can include institutional community care. In fact, a review of province-wide programs clarifies at least one theory of LTC. As the growing evidence from American demonstrations has suggested, the implementation of active programs of community care does not automatically lead to reduced use of nursing homes. Rather, community programs provide a social and political climate for restricting the growth of nursing homes while still providing adequate LTC services.

The Need for Decentralization

Another major lesson from Canada concerns program scale. Although Canada is geographically larger than the United States, its total population is less than that of California. Some Canadian provinces have populations similar to those of many American counties. In Canada, LTC is largely a provincial issue, and even then it is administered at more local levels of

---

*A monopsony is a system in which *payment* is concentrated in a single place, in contrast to a monopoly, where the *production* of goods or services is the concentrated area.

government. As is the case in Europe, policies can be made centrally in Canada, but the program's operation requires active local control.[11] Extrapolating to the United States, planners must build programs around manageable geopolitical units, generally smaller than a state. The federal role would be heavily weighted toward financing, probably in some sharing arrangement with the states, and toward providing minimal program guidelines and standards that ensure at least a basic equity for the program. This pattern has already been established for Medicaid.

Community Care

The Canadian experience also offers support to advocates of community care. Providing community care that includes broad coverage of home-maker services as well as nursing did not lead to runaway utilization. Relatively simple case management can control the use of these services, and control becomes easier as the shape of the program and concomitant public expectations become established.

Thus, community care emerges as a flexible component of LTC, but sometimes its flexibility is to its detriment. When budget restrictions are imposed, cutting back on community care by limiting resources to each case-management unit is easier than closing beds. (Ironically, when service dollars are thus reduced, case-management agencies sometimes reduce case-management activities, such as reassessments, thereby vitiating their assertions about the efficacy of case management.) However, optimistically, community services can be created more easily than some have suggested. The short lag time between the introduction of a community-care program in British Columbia and the response of community agencies ready to provide services suggests that such programs can be mounted with little delay where potential foci of organization exist already.

The heart of the community-care programs is homemaking services. A few people need hands-on nursing, but the overwhelming majority need only assistance with basic tasks. Nursing and other therapeutic needs are more likely to be episodic. In Manitoba, British Columbia, and Ontario, homemaking programs are operated as social agencies, rather than as health programs, and are maintained separately from home nursing services. In many instances, the amount of weekly care needed is modest, sometimes only a few hours, yet these limited services, often provided to supplement informal care, are viewed as critical to an individual's remaining at home. Although scientifically sound data to support these contentions are lacking, the strength of conviction of both providers and recipients is impressive. At the very least, these observations should serve as an important caution to those who urge restriction of services to clients who have great gaps between service needs and extant resources.

An American Tragedy

Any effort to bring models of care from other countries to the United States must recognize the elements of American life that make it unique. Two major, related issues dominate American medicine, although they derive from American culture in general. One is historical, the other is recent.

America has a historical tradition of entrepreneurship, and many argue that this trait, an outgrowth of the pioneer spirit, is responsible for making the country what it is today. In its contemporary version, this entrepreneurial ethic makes it difficult to plan rationally. Whatever rules are developed, the goal of a good player is to find a way around them, to turn the situation to advantage. A direct corollary is the willingness to sue. Litigiousness as an expression of individual freedom makes it difficult to establish and maintain regulations, although regulations are critical to pursuit of social goals like universal health coverage.

The second major issue, related to entrepreneurship, is the rise of corporate medicine in both proprietary and nonprofit forms.[12] The concentration of health care in the hands of a few large corporations is likely to have profound effects. Even at a modest level, the hospitals' interest in developing vertical integration of acute and long-term care will mean, at a minimum, that the latter will be operated in a medical mode. The new system for prospective reimbursement by diagnoses creates pressure to reduce patients' length of stay in hospitals and has stimulated great interest in having available a sufficient supply of LTC services to facilitate hospital discharge. This byproduct of hospital prospective payment can serve the important social goal of linking the acute and long-term care sectors more closely, but unfortunately, it places the incentives on precisely the wrong objectives. Under diagnosis-related groups (DRGs), the hospital's goals are to spend as little as possible and to transfer costs to the LTC sector. It is a bitter irony that, just as we have begun to establish the value of careful evaluation of geriatric patients, the payment system is shifted to make the evaluations infeasible. The incentives created by prospective payment actively discourage thorough attention to geriatric patients or efforts to attend function problems. Instead, the emphasis is on focused care and rapid production.

The Rise of Corporate Medicine

Starr has identified the last quarter of this century as the era of corporate medicine in America.[12] There is a clear pattern of consolidation within both the proprietary and nonprofit sectors. Prospective reimbursement of hospitals has stimulated their interest in acquiring control of LTC resources to alleviate inpatient use, but this tendency to vertical integration had already begun before the introduction of DRGs. The advantages of controlling various levels of care, in order to diversify investments, had already been recognized.

At the same time, for reasons of economy, there has been a horizontal integration as chains of facilities have come under single management, with joint purchasing and common procedures. As a few of these corporations grow to vast size, the LTC industry will become consolidated in the hands of a few powerful giants that will have great leverage. Certainly, corporate care conjures up an image of impersonal, inflexible care. Regulatory efforts are more likely to confront powerful political and economic opposition. The balance between system control and provider control will favor the latter.

Existing providers already represent an active and often effective lobby. At the individual professional level, they often represent forces to maintain the status quo, and any efforts to modify the system will have to contend with these influences. Moreover, the greater the extent of change proposed, the more intense the opposition will be. The coalescence of large corporations will thus produce a politically potent force opposed to any increased role for government, especially one that threatens to systematize care.

These formulations especially discourage those wishing to reform nursing home care. A feeling of the inevitability of present conditions seems to permeate policy discussions. However, the longer action is delayed, the harder it will be to take action. Government has some strong cards, particularly its position as a major purchaser, and, just as important, in the instinctive and natural alliance of large segments of the general public. Public discontent with the current state and policies of LTC could be a force for change, if channeled appropriately.

Role of Competition

America's entrepreneurial ethic has led to a strong faith in free competition as a means of ensuring quality and reducing cost. This confidence may be misdirected in the case of LTC. Competition in medical and social services is more likely to produce both duplication and gaps in service as various providers compete for the most lucrative markets and leave others uncovered. With a product as nonspecific as LTC, it is particularly unrealistic to expect consumers to fend for themselves. When they must make decisions in times of crisis, the likelihood of careful shopping is even more remote.

Although a simplistic reliance on competition is unworkable, the concept can have a role in providing LTC. With a general system in place to define its direction, competition can be used effectively to achieve desired social ends. Currently, the United States lacks this guidance system. To use competition productively, it must have organizations that can assume authority and responsibility for populations in defined geopolitical areas, to ensure coverage and to avoid selection bias. Within this framework, various competitive strategies can be employed. Some strategies may feature competition among different providers of the same service, while others could foster competition among various modalities of care to serve the same problems or clients.

Case Management

Public expenditures require some mechanism to control spending and to exercise responsibility for the most effective use of available resources. Case-management programs provide this mechanism. Two of the Canadian provinces studied developed extensive case-management programs; the third is moving to develop this capacity. Moreover, case management is a mainstay of LTC demonstrations in the United States[13–15] and several states have introduced or proposed a case-management function for Medicaid clients and users of in-home supportive services.[16,17] Canadian experience reinforces the importance of case management and suggests some characteristics to be cultivated (and others to be avoided). The criteria for a case-management system proposed here do not necessarily represent any one of the programs encountered, but rather are a composite of the best of several.

Independence from Providers

In order to provide an unbiased judgment about the extent and type of care needed, the case manager cannot have a vested interest in any modality of care. Thus, the same organization cannot both provide care and perform case management. One of the prime characteristics of case management is objectivity, and the more that decisions are left to professional judgment, the more critical is such objectivity.

Coverage of a Defined Population

The case-management program should be designed to cover a defined geopolitical region. First, this design provides a visible program with a mechanism for accountability. Second, it minimizes the capacity for selection bias and provides a stronger relationship with the various provider agencies in an area. Target groups must also be defined. The British Columbia and Manitoba programs easily incorporated almost all adults with functional needs into the same case-managed financing system. However, British Columbia's program has recognized that the skills and resources for assisting the mentally disabled and the mentally ill qualitatively differ from those needed for frail elders and the physically disabled. The program has changed several times in an effort to determine the best way to provide case management and program responsibility for those populations, but, in general, specialized personnel have carried the responsibility. Similarly, some Ontario home-care programs have developed specialized care coordination (e.g., for hospices). The key seems to be clearly defining target groups and making sure that nobody in need falls through the cracks.

Control over Resources

The "broker" model, in which the case manager can only suggest care, is impotent. To succeed, case management needs responsibility and authority over resources. With this control also comes another important component: accountability. The case managers must be responsible for the results of decisions they make. Summing up their activities will produce a tally on the effectiveness of the case-management program.

Sensitivity to Client Preferences

The recommendations for care should be based on client needs and preferences. Decision making should separately ascertain the level and type of care needed, and then client preferences should help determine the best source for that care.

Minimizing Hospital-Based Decisions

The hospital is not the place to make decisions about how much LTC is needed and where it should be delivered. The assessment of functioning tends to be inaccurate, and the patient has little chance for decision making. Hospital personnel are often under pressure to facilitate discharge as expeditiously as possible and are rarely in a position to make community arrangements. The Canadian case-managed systems try to minimize the decisions being made from the hospital and by hospital personnel. The case managers try to give priority for facility admission to persons at home, rather than to persons in hospitals, so that the latter will have an incentive "to go home and try it." Powerful as the hospital is, it should not hold the cards in LTC planning. Perhaps the perversity of the current situation can be best expressed by proposing to redraft the Medicare requirement for a minimum hospital stay of 3 days before nursing home care is covered to require that the patient go home for 3 days before nursing home care is considered.

Case management is currently popular in the United States. Indeed, it has assumed a trendy legitimacy as the mechanism of choice for managing Medicaid long-term expenditures. However, it is important to distinguish between a case-management program for a universal public benefit and a program for a residual means-tested benefit, such as Medicaid. If case managers must keep hands off until individuals have exhausted their resources in the private market, the effect of case management on the overall system is blunted, and it becomes too little, too late.

Because of the concern in the United States over the potential for litigation, there has been a tendency to rely on complex forms and elaborate decision models; completing the form is often more arduous than working on the decision. A format that emphasizes common language and definitions but avoids pseudoscientific decision algorithms is much more desirable. Fortunately, case management, as it evolved in Canada, is desirably noncomplex, although it is an inexact science that must rely on common sense, good will, and a responsive stance on the part of the case manager.

Creative Tinkering

Various pundits have described the evolution of American LTC as "creative tinkering." This term refers to individual development of various segments in response to particular deficiencies or crises. The result is a disjointed program in which each action exploits the new opportunity and often requires countermeasures to stem the zeal. An occasional byproduct of this approach is the spawning of yet another interest group determined to expand its holdings in LTC.

How is the United States to get from where it is now to a more desirable situation? Surely many would agree that LTC in the Canadian provinces has enviable features: It is balanced between community and institutional care, its costs are subsumed as part of health costs that remain less than those in the United States, and the real risk of financial disaster for individuals and families faced with LTC needs is averted by collective measures. In the United States, suggestions to expand Medicare benefits to include LTC or to conduct more active experimentation with programs like social health maintenance organizations represent tinkering in the right direction, but they are not likely to bring about the necessary reforms.

The best system at first appears paradoxical: LTC should be run as a social program, but should be funded with health-care dollars. To be meaningful and workable, an LTC program must be a universal entitlement for people of all ages, covering hospital and medical care as well as LTC. This broad base of coverage must be supplied in an entrepreneurial environment, to prevent segmented development of covered services or covered populations, disproportionate distribution of the burdens of financing, and uncontrolled costs.

References

1. McNeil, B., Weichselbaum, R., Pauker, S. 1978. Fallacy of five year survival in lung cancer. *N Engl J Med* 299:1397–1401.
2. Kulys, R. 1983. Future crises and the very old: Implications for discharge planning. *Health Soc Work* 8(3):182–202.
3. Lewis, M. A., Cretin, S., Kane, R. L. 1985. The natural history of nursing home patients. *Gerontologist* 25:382–388.
4. Rubenstein, L. Z., Rhee, L., Kane, R. L. 1982. The role of geriatric assessment units in caring for the elderly: An analytic review. *J Gerontol* 37(5):513–521.
5. Rubenstein, L. Z., Josephson, K., Wieland, G. D., English P. A., Sayre, J. A., Kane, R. L. 1984. Randomized controlled trial of a geriatric evaluation unit. *N Engl J Med* 311:1664–1670.
6. Somers, A. R. 1982. Long-term care for the elderly and disabled: A new health priority. *N Engl J Med* 307:221–226.
7. National Study Group on State Medicaid Strategies. 1983. *Restructuring Medicaid: An Agenda for Change.* Washington, D.C.: Center for the Study of Social Policy.
8. Aaron, H. J., Schwartz, W. B. 1984. *The Painful Prescription: Rationing Hospital Care.* Washington, D.C.: Brookings Institution.
9. Olsen, D. M., Kane, R. L., Kasteler, J. 1976. Medical care as a commodity: An exploration of the shopping behavior of patients. *J Community Health* 2:85–91.
10. Kane, R. L., Kane, R. A. 1985. *A Will and a Way: What Americans Can Learn about Long-Term Care from Canada.* New York: Columbia University Press.
11. Kane, R. L., Kane, R. A. 1976. *Long-Term Care in Six Countries: Implications for the United States.* HEW Pub. (NIH) 76-878. Washington, D.C.: Government Printing Office.
12. Starr, P. 1983. *The Social Transformation of American Medicine.* New York: Basic Books.
13. Baxter, R. J. 1983. *The Planning and Implementation of Channeling: Early Experiences of the National Long Term Care Demonstrations.* Mathematica Policy Research. (Mimeograph.)
14. Capitman, J. 1983. *Preliminary Report on Work in Progress: Evaluation of Coordinated Community-Oriented Long-Term Care Demonstration Projects.* Berkeley, Calif.: Berkeley Planning Associates. (Mimeograph.)
15. Greenberg, J. N., Doth, D., Austin, C. 1981. *Comparative Study of Long-Term Care Demonstration Projects: Lessons for Future Inquiry.* Minneapolis: University of Minnesota Center for Health Services Research. (Mimeograph.)
16. Kane, R. A. 1984. Long-term care under the Older Americans Act. In:

Reauthorization of Older Americans Act 1984. Hearing before the Subcommittee on Aging of the Committee on Labor and Human Resources, Part I, January 17, January 31, February 24 and 28, and March 31, 1984. Washington, D.C.: Government Printing Office.

17. Toff, G. E. 1981. *Alternatives to Institutional Care for the Elderly: An Analysis of State Initiatives*. Washington, D.C.: Intergovernmental Health Policy Project.

Twenty-nine

Policies for People: A Proposal for Redirection of Long-Term Care for the Elderly

Tom Joe

Until the sun heats up her house a bit—which is quite late in winter days—
Anna doesn't feel like eating breakfast. The stairs, she says, are hard on her
knees and cold weather makes that unbearable. In the morning, the kitchen
seems miles away.

Anna broke her hip in January 1985. She's been in and out of the hospital a
few times, but her doctor says she's in prime physical shape. For someone her
age, he adds quietly. But after almost three years, she still uses a walker and is
reluctant to venture far from her home.

Her arthritis, she believes, was aggravated by the injury. Anna takes her
arthritis pills four times a day. Or at least she's supposed to. The other day, she
couldn't remember if she'd taken them or not, so she took a half dose—reasoning better some than none or too much.

Anna has also been forgetful when it comes to bills. She missed three electricity bills and the utility company couldn't reach her (the phone had been
disconnected). If it hadn't been for the community representative of the electric
company who arranged for payment, Anna might still be without electricity.
Financially, Anna's condition is marginal. She now lives on her $500 monthly
Social Security check. This pays for her food, utilities, medication, and property taxes, with a little left over for clothing and personal necessities. Fortunately,
she and her late husband paid off their mortgage years ago, but the house needs a
lot of expensive repair and, in fact, it is much too large for her to manage.

The last time her son, Don, traveled the 300 miles from his home to visit, he
talked about trying to find someone to take care of her. He said she needed

someone to look after her on a full-time basis. But he knew she could not afford to pay someone, and he had his own retirement nearing for which he had to save. Don said that as soon as her small savings were used up, Medicaid would pay for Anna to live in a nursing home. At least then she would have other people to talk to and look after her.

But Anna won't hear of it. She still vividly remembers the day when she had to put her husband in Bethel Home. That was different, though; he could not get out of bed, and she can still walk around. No nursing home for her. Not while she still has anything to say about it.

Although there was a time when Anna happily spent hours in her kitchen, these days she rarely feels much like cooking. She's taken a liking to canned fruit and easy-to-make macaroni and cheese mix. She apologizes for the mess in the kitchen, noting that she just hasn't felt up to cleaning the past few weeks. The hospital staff laid out an intricate menu for her at the end of her last stay, but Anna has difficulty making sense of it, let alone following it.

Anna has friends, though she doesn't see them much. It seems that all her friends have gotten old overnight. The girls can't come over very often anymore, but when they do, they have a good time talking about the past, and about their grandchildren.

The daughters of two of Anna's friends helped settle their mothers in nursing homes and Anna knows that they are not happy there. She tries to visit them once in a while, but really doesn't have a way to get there unless another friend's daughter takes her. She tries to call them at least once a week, anyway.

Anna knows that there are some organizations in town that help out older people. The Lions Club provides eyeglasses for the elderly, and a member of the club—an old friend of her son—made sure she received a new pair recently. The city pays Mr. Winchester from two doors down to shovel snow for older people in the winter, and a visitor from the Lutheran Church she used to attend arranged for her to receive one hot meal a day from the local Meals on Wheels program. There are lots of other services she's heard about other people getting, but she isn't quite sure who provides them. So she knows there's help to be had, but she's not sure she needs it, and she doesn't really know how to get it if she wants it. Luckily, she has a good neighbor who takes her food shopping every week.

All in all, Anna is making do. She misses her husband and her full, busy life of days past and she is a little scared about the future. But when her mind is in the present, she is fiercely independent. Perhaps this is the legacy from her parents' determined struggle during the Depression; perhaps it is the fear that dependence is a slippery slope. Managing one's family for over three decades is a formidable task; but admitting that one needs help managing one's self is even more formidable. Anna swears she will do everything she can to avoid becoming "dependent" on others.

The Problem of Long-Term Care: A Perspective for Policymakers

Anna's story, a composite based on real cases, illustrates the dilemmas many elderly people and their families face today. Her situation is not a "worst case"; she has at least minimally adequate food, clothing, shelter, health care, some social contacts, and a smattering of formal and informal supports. However, she and millions like her will, sooner or later, need some form of more intensive, consistent, long-term care (LTC). No one can hope to avoid confronting this issue, in the form of obtaining care for an elderly relative who can no longer cope alone, or planning for one's own old age, or at least as a taxpayer.

Even so, the problem of LTC for the aging should be kept in perspective. Implicit in much of the discourse on LTC is the assumption that every person age 65 or older is sick, poor, incompetent, and in need of care in an expensive nursing home at vast public expense. The facts are otherwise. Rice and Feldman's[1] analysis of demographic changes and their implications for the needs of the elderly reveals that only 5% of the elderly are now in nursing homes, and the need for institutional care is concentrated among the "old-old"—the median age of nursing home residents was 81 years in 1977, and 35% were 85 years or older.[2]

If the mortality rate continues to decline and if current patterns of morbidity and nursing home use rates remain unchanged, the need for LTC will grow apace. The proportion of people age 75 or more who are unable to perform some of the activities of daily living (bathing, toileting, eating, etc.) unassisted may rise from 36% in 1980 to 58% by 2040. These people, like Anna, will require less than institutional care, but more community support services. By 2040, the total nursing home population will be 3.5 times larger than it is now (1980), and over half will be 85 or older.[3] However, the United States is not facing an inevitable social disaster; there are some compelling arguments that healthier lifestyles and increased knowledge of disease processes will result in much shorter periods of disability prior to death (although arguments predicting more protracted disability periods attendant on a longer life span have been made as well). In addition, although the proportion of older people in the population is certain to increase, the magnitude of this change may turn out to be less drastic than anticipated—demographic projection remains a risky enterprise.[4] In any case, changes in the financing and delivery of services to respond to this challenge are well within the power of policymakers to bring about. These changes are necessary and desirable now. The predicted future demand should be seen as a positive incentive to develop a more humane and affordable LTC system in the 1980s.

The Present System of Long-Term Care: A Simple Response to Complex Reality

Although research has significantly improved understanding of the aging process and the needs of the elderly, it has had minimal overall influence on public policy and practice. The research effort must continue, but the results must be translated into action, so that programs serving the elderly are better in line with individuals' real needs and life situations.

One of the most critical insights gained from recent research is the understanding that the LTC needs of the elderly, once assumed to be dominated by medical problems, extend far beyond medical and health-related services. While the elderly do use a much greater share of medical services than the rest of the population, health care is just one component of a broader need for ongoing assistance. As Anna's case demonstrates, at times it is very easy to confuse an older person's need for health care with his or her social, personal, economic, and housing problems. Where do Anna's medical needs end and her needs for companionship, income support, nutrition, and appropriate housing begin? And, more importantly, how are they interrelated?

Data on the health and social factors related to LTC needs have shown that most elderly and disabled persons are institutionalized not because of a dramatic change in their health status, but because of a change in their marital status or living arrangements.[5] It has been facetiously suggested that a sensible LTC policy would be a dating and marriage service for elderly widows, since events like the death of a spouse or a child's moving away are most often the precipitating factors in institutionalization.

With the exception of a few demonstration projects, publicly financed LTC has focused almost exclusively on medical care of the elderly in skilled nursing and intermediate-care facilities. The dominance of medical LTC financing has inhibited society's ability to meet a range of other non-medical needs equally important to the elderly. Table 29.1 lists the types of services that many elderly people require and the range of settings in which they should be made available. If LTC programs are to be fully responsive, they must offer a broad spectrum of health and nonmedical services, in a variety of settings, by an array of providers.

Anna, for example, falls in Level II of Table 29.1, *moderately disabled,* and could probably benefit from nonmedical services, including companionship, telephone reassurance, escorted transportation to senior activities and congregate meals, and, potentially, a congregate living arrangement that would provide many of these services. At present, in most communities, Anna would have a great deal of difficulty orchestrating the range of services that could improve the quality of her life and prolong her ability to function independently.

Table 29.1. Range of LTC Service by Level of Individual Disability

Level of Disability[a]	LTC Service					
	Medical	Social	Housing/Living Arrangement	Income	Nutrition	Mental Health
Level I: Independent, low income Does not require personal care or supervision	Routine physician care Medications	Senior-citizen activities	Independent housing Congregate housing Supervised apartments	Social Security SSI VA pensions	Congregate meals programs Medications	Socialization activities
Level II: Moderately disabled Requires some health supervision, personal care, or help with activities of daily living	Physician care Medications Health supervision Rehabilitation	Companionship Telephone reassurance Escorted transportation Senior activities Homemaker/chore	Independent housing with help Congregate housing Supervised apartments	Social Security SSI VA pensions	Congregate meals programs	Socialization activities Counseling
Level III: Seriously disabled Nonambulatory or incapable of self-direction; requires ongoing assistance with personal care or protective supervision	Physician care Home health care Medication management Rehabilitation	Companionship Telephone reassurance Homemaker/chore Escorted transportation Adult day care Respite care	Congregate housing Board-and-care home Domiciliary care Adult foster care Independent housing with supportive services	Social Security SSI and state supplements VA pensions plus aide and attendant allowance	Congregate meals programs Meals on Wheels	Socialization activities Counseling
Level IV: Chronically ill Health condition requires continuous professional care	Physician care Home health care Skilled or intermediate nursing care	Live-in attendant companion Homemaker/chore Adult day care Respite care	Intermediate care facilities Skilled nursing facilities Independent housing with full-time care	Social Security SSI and state supplements VA pensions plus aide and attendant allowance	Congregate meals programs Meals on Wheels	Socialization activities Counseling

[a]Derived from *Working Papers on Long-Term Care*, prepared for the 1980 Under-Secretary's Task Force on Long-Term Care, OASPE, U.S. Department of Health and Human Services, October, 1981.

The current LTC system provides care only on each end of the disability spectrum: an institutional-care benefit for the most severely disabled and a sprinkling of services, through private enterprise and the Older Americans Act, for the relatively independent elderly. However, like Anna, many elderly people do not easily fall into one of these categories. They have needs that are not fully met by the current independent-care system; yet they do not require and do not want the confinement of institutional care. The elderly should have alternative middle-level models of care that provide a continuum of appropriate health and nonhealth services at all levels of disability.

Toward a New System of Care

Making LTC services more responsive to the needs of the elderly demands nothing less than a revolution in the way LTC services are financed and provided. Minor tinkering with current programs and policies will not suffice; rather, a fundamental restructuring is needed, and the task is not small. Any attempt to make LTC more effective, efficient, and acceptable to recipients must include both a service and a financing strategy. Specifically, "demedicalizing" the LTC system to respond to the social and economic problems of the elderly, improved coordination of existing services and financing mechanisms, and diversifying sources of financial support for LTC must all be addressed to achieve a system that is responsive to individuals—and affordable to the nation as well.

"Demedicalized" Alternatives for LTC

Proposals to demedicalize LTC focus on expanding personal care and other support services to individuals living in their own homes and on providing alternative community living arrangements for elderly people who cannot or choose not to live alone. Unfortunately, the real merits of such changes in the LTC service system are frequently confused with wishful thinking about what can be expected of them.

It is not uncommon to find home-based services and alternative living arrangements described as "alternatives to institutionalization," which in turn will "reduce the nation's mounting LTC costs." For some elderly people who become incapable of living in the community without assistance, however, the "alternatives" may prolong the period in which they can remain outside an institution but cannot substitute for nursing home care for the duration of the individual's life—as in the case of a person with a degenerative physical or mental condition that ultimately renders him or her incapable of any self-care or one in need of ongoing, sophisticated medical intervention. (Of course, even in such a case, noninstitutional care might continue to be provided if the individual or society were willing to bear the cost.)

The essential point is that demedicalizing the LTC system can be counted on to improve the quality of life, for at least some period of time, of a substantial number of elderly citizens. It can expand the range of choices open to older people and may preclude or postpone the need for institutional care—but the development of alternative services will not signal the demise of the nursing home.

Community-based alternatives may or may not be less costly, on the whole, than nursing home care. Institutional economies of scale often result in lower unit costs of care for severely ill or disabled individuals; on the other hand, institutional capital and operating costs require charges that would seem to be excessive for someone like Anna, whose current requirements are much less than the basic intermediate care facility (ICF) package. However, an alternative living arrangement in combination with all the support services Anna needs could still be as expensive as or more expensive than nursing home care. In fact, experience with the community-based components of the LTC system has been too limited in scope and duration to produce clear comparative cost data. Even if it were established that caring for someone with Anna's level of disability in a nursing home would be less expensive than meeting her needs in the community, would this justify her total loss of independence?

All in all, the relationship between costs of different forms of care and total system outlays is factually and ethically murky. Certainly, more data on the costs of community-based services in different combinations for people with different levels of disability are needed. Current state efforts under the Section 2176 Home and Community-Based waiver projects will hopefully provide data useful for assessing the relative cost-effectiveness of community-based versus institutional care and for identifying clients for whom home care is most appropriate. Whatever the findings of such efforts, the development of alternative services and settings will not alone provide a "quick fix" for runaway LTC costs.

Expectations for demedicalizing LTC must also take into account the willingness of the elderly person to acknowledge the need for help and to accept it. Relatives of elderly people frequently find that their aged family members—much like Anna—resist all suggestions that they might need homemaker or meal-preparation assistance, for example. They often refuse to move from an unmanageable home to a congregate living arrangement, and may insist on maintaining their independence long past the time that they have the ability to do so. In these cases, individual deterioration is fueled by poor nutrition, misuse of medications, household accidents, chaotic money management, and so on, until voluntary or involuntary admission to a nursing home becomes truly necessary. Changes in the LTC service system cannot solve this problem. What can be hoped is that the new cultural climate that has enabled younger generations to seek psychiatric help, demand special education for their disabled children, change residence frequently, and form self-help groups to cope with personal and social problems will also result in a greater willingness to seek help as they move toward old age.

In any event, there is little danger that immediate expansion of nonmedical alternatives to institutional care will outstrip demand. The burgeoning private sector home-health and full-service retirement housing industries attest to the willingness and desire of great numbers of today's more affluent elderly to use assistance to maintain their independence and quality of life. The vitality of this private market gives rise to the question of whether public LTC strategy should simply focus on income transfers to enable lower-income people to purchase their own care. This idea is appealing in principle, but its applicability to the elderly population raises many thorny questions of equity and practicality. For example, would Anna, forgetful and uncertain as she is, be able to set priorities for services to purchase? Would she be able to identify the best provider among several? Would income transfers be made available only to those who could demonstrate their capacity to be prudent consumers? Would the amount of income transfer be the same for all, or rise with changing needs? Who would determine when additional funds for services were needed, and in what amount? An income-transfer approach may have a role to play in the continuum of LTC for the elderly, but those who would rely primarily on this strategy have a large conceptual and experimental task ahead of them.

Regardless of financing strategy, an expanded system of in-home services should be developed in each locality and should include at a minimum homemaker/chore, home-health, personal care, and nutrition services for elderly individuals, along with respite care for those whose families have accepted the role of caregivers. Many states are now moving to develop these systems, but all confront needs that outstrip available financial resources.

The expansion of residential alternatives for the elderly should also be given high priority. A variety of models exist, offering different lifestyles and amounts of services. One of these is homesharing, in which the "homegiver" who owns or rents a dwelling unit and wishes to share expenses, or needs companionship and security, is matched by a responsible agency with a "homeseeker." In the few states where such a program exists, matches between unimpaired or moderately disabled elderly and younger people have been frequent and successful.[6]

Somewhat more common are semi-independent living arrangements for elderly people who can function fairly well with regular support services and minimal general supervision. Congregate housing projects, for example, typically provide residents with private space, including kitchen facilities, and one or more congregate meals a day. Core services, such as homemaker and health aides, are available to all residents, and the facility may organize additional activities and services. Supervised apartments, in which a resident manager or counselor provides general supervision to elderly occupants of a unit, are a variation on this theme. Housekeeping assistance and other support services are also provided.[6] Either of these settings would probably be appropriate for Anna, especially in view of her need for medication supervision and her increasing social isolation.

Sheltered living arrangements, appropriate for more seriously disabled elderly people, are exemplified by the board-and-care home, also known as a domiciliary home. As of 1987, approximately 41,000 of these facilities existed nationwide, housing 563,000 aged and disabled people.[7] In the best of these settings, the resident manager, often with staff assistance, provides a small group of elderly people with meals, personal care, unskilled health care, and recreation, and assists as needed with medical appointments and the like. Regulation of board-and-care homes has long been problematic, but many states are beginning to recognize these facilities as an important LTC resource and are developing strategies for improving their quality and for linking them with a network of supportive services in the community.[6]

Better Coordination of Services

Not only must a broader spectrum of LTC services be developed, but also the lack of coordination in the existing service system must be addressed. At present, each separate program operates in virtual isolation from others, and there are few successful models of service integration. In fact, clients or those acting on behalf of an elderly relative can rarely package the disparate community services available. Typically, each service arrangement must be identified and negotiated separately, sometimes with six or eight different service providers. It is no wonder that Anna's son sees a nursing home as the only answer to her problems.

Although it may seem minor from a policymaker's perspective, one of Anna's biggest concerns is the absence of a single contact person she can rely on when she needs assistance. Presently, Anna sees at least two or three different individuals in her home each week: one man delivers her Meals on Wheels, another woman comes to take her grocery shopping, and another man shovels her snow in the winter. Yet none of these people can help her identify her total needs or answer her questions about where she might get certain other types of assistance. The lack of a single contact also heightens Anna's sense of uncertainty about the future, because she does not know where to turn in case her situation deteriorates and she needs help quickly.

A new delivery system should be built around the clients, rather than around discrete service programs. Anna would like to have one person she can get to know and with whom she can feel comfortable and maintain steady contact. This person, a caseworker or case manager, would visit Anna regularly and locate any services that Anna may need. This ongoing contact person would give Anna and her family a much greater sense of security and would allow her to maintain an independent living situation as long as possible. This sense of security becomes even more critical when family members are not in the same city as the elderly individual. Unless they feel there is continuous and reliable ongoing monitoring of the situation, families often will decide to institutionalize the elderly person for his or her own "protection and comfort."

Although the use of case managers to arrange LTC services has become a widely accepted notion, case-management systems are not routinely available and exist in only a handful of innovative LTC programs around the country.[8] For several years, the U.S. Department of Health and Human Services investigated case management as part of the National Long Term Care Channeling Demonstration projects. Operating in ten sites, the channeling project employed two methods of case management. The first, basic model superimposed a coordination and accountability mechanism on the existing array of services and eligibility criteria. The case manager in the basic model helped clients gain access to the services they needed and could qualify for to remain at home in the community. The second, more flexible model provided a fixed budget for a demonstration site that could be used for a wider range of services under less restrictive eligibility criteria. Both models were tested by a rigorous experimental evaluation.

Overall, the project evaluation produced volumes of information and several significant findings. Under both case-management models, channeling led to an increase in total costs for clients. The increased costs, however, did produce benefits in terms of reduced unmet client needs and increased levels of life satisfaction by clients and primary caregivers.[9] The project did not produce conclusive evidence of the effects of different models of case management but it has given us invaluable experiential data on how to run a community-based model of LTC services effectively. The challenge for the future is to translate and amplify the positive findings into public policies and practices that go beyond the demonstration sites and experimental time frames.

More Coherent Financing

Many of the obvious coordination problems in the delivery of services reflect the fragmentation of LTC financing. A host of categorical programs exists at the federal, state, and local levels of government and in the private sector. On the federal level alone, they include Medicaid, Medicare, Supplemental Security Income, The Older Americans Act, Title XX Social Services, and the Veterans Administration. The funds for these programs flow from federal agencies to several state agencies or local governments, or directly to fiscal intermediaries, private facilities, or, occasionally, to the consumer. The fragmented financing at the federal level is mirrored at the state and local levels and is even further complicated by unique relationships between state and local governments and by state and county laws and regulations. In sum, there is little if any logical connection between funders or among levels of government.

Only major realignment of intergovernmental responsibilities can bring some coherence to public LTC financing and service delivery. A more integrated service system requires breaking down the categorical barriers. This formidable task has stymied well-intentioned planners for the past decade.

One starting point is a recommendation made by the National Study Group of State Medicaid Strategies,[10] which found no logical justification for maintaining the current combination of primary, acute-care and LTC services in one federal–state Medicaid program. The study group instead recommended that about one-half of the Medicaid program be allocated to a Primary Care System, with the remainder devoted to a state-administered continuing-care service system* that would provide a full range of health and social LTC services to elderly and other dependent individuals with demonstrated functional impairments. Federal funds for continuing-care services would be made available to states through an indexed capitation payment to provide services within broad federal guidelines. States would design and administer continuing-care service systems through designated local agencies. A critical component of the service system would be the development of local access agencies, which would have responsibility for:

- Assessing individual and family needs based on the presence of a functional limitation and taking into account the availability of social supports

- Recommending needed services

---

*"Continuing-care services" replaces the term "long-term care" and includes a broader range of in-home and community support services as well as long-term institutional care in a nursing home or other health-related domiciliary facility.

- Providing information and referral on available services, especially alternatives to institutional care

- Providing preadmission screening for institutional care and functioning as a gatekeeper for entrance into institutional care

- Determining financial liability for services on a case-by-case basis, based on established income eligibility standards

- Arranging for the provision of services through vouchers, purchase of service contracts, capitation arrangements, family subsidies or other arrangements developed by states and localities

- Monitoring the provision and quality of care.[10]

Giving financial and service-delivery authority to the states has a significant advantage over discretionary federal demonstration projects as a means for developing, testing, and incorporating changes into the LTC system. Although federal demonstration projects provide the flexibility to test new approaches, they often fall victim to bureaucratic and political whim. It is increasingly difficult to get an experimental effort off the drawing board, and even successful approaches may not be adopted if the political climate has changed since their initiation. An example of the political vulnerability of demonstration projects can be seen in the struggle of a proposed experimental program that would offer elderly people in four locations the choice of enrolling in social health maintenance organizations (SHMOs). SHMOs, which would provide a wide range of preventive, home-health, and social work services and limited nursing home care, were long delayed clearance by the Office of Management and Budget, evidently because the Reagan Administration feared the experiment would lead to increases in services and cost pressures on the federal budget.[11] Although the political battle over this issue was finally resolved in favor of the experiment, the implications of this example for timely federal LTC policy research are not encouraging.

Diversifying LTC Financing

It is unrealistic to think that government appropriations and the Social Security Trust Funds will be adequate to finance improvement and expansion of the LTC system either soon or in the long term. Additional financial strategies must be developed, including greater use of the private sector and the tax system.

Greater private-sector involvement has been the subject of much talk and little action during the past several years. The Health Insurance Association of America had a task force studying the feasibility of private LTC insurance, and individual insurance companies have begun to offer products on the market.[12] Research conducted by the National Center for Health Services Research suggests that private insurance may be financially feasible,[13] and we will learn much in the near future from how the elderly respond to the policies now being developed and offered. Utilization of LTC insurance would, of course, be encouraged by tax deductions for individual premiums and employer contributions.

Another proposed private-sector strategy is to stimulate individual savings for LTC through the creation of tax-free accounts that resemble individual retirement accounts.[14]

A third idea that has gained some legislative interest at the federal and state levels is to provide greater tax incentives for families to care for an elderly or disabled person. Oregon, Idaho, and Arizona have already passed such tax-subsidy laws, and at least a dozen more states are considering them. Although the full effect of this approach is hard to predict, an analysis by the Center for the Study of Social Policy concluded that a properly structured subsidy would reinforce desirable informal caregiving and, in conjunction with available community services, could prevent at least some premature and unnecessary institutionalization.[15]

The growing consensus in favor of strategies to stimulate private responsibility for financing LTC inevitably collides with concern over the federal deficit. This is indeed an awkward point at which to propose new tax expenditures, but hard choices must be made between existing subsidies for specific economic activities and control of public outlays for services that will be required in ever greater quantity with the aging of the American population.

Conclusion

None of the changes discussed here can stand alone. Demedicalizing care for the elderly and developing a humane and sensitive continuing-care service system to meet individual human needs will require a creative combination of public and private finances and services in conjunction with new federal, state, local, and family initiatives.

Too often, policymakers forget the Annas they are trying to help. As a result, they establish programs and policies in a vacuum. The resulting mosaic of scarce, confusing, and uncoordinated services can overwhelm elderly persons and their families. The story of Anna is a reminder that LTC is for real people with real needs. If policy planners will only keep Anna and the many others like her in mind in the coming years, perhaps she will be able to live her last decades as fully as her first.

References

1. Rice, D., Feldman, J. 1983. Living longer in the United States: Demographic changes and health needs of the elderly. *Milbank Memorial Fund Q* 61(3):362–396.
2. See Ref. 1, p. 364.
3. See Ref. 1, pp. 377–380.
4. See Ref. 1, p. 392.
5. Butler, L., Newacheck, P. 1981. Health and social factors relevant to long-term-care policy. In *Policy Options in Long-Term Care*, ed. J. Meltzer, F. Farrow, and H. Richman, 38–77. Chicago, Ill.: University of Chicago Press.
6. Harmon, C. 1982. *Board and Care: An Old Problem, a New Resource for Long Term Care*. Washington, D.C.: Center for the Study of Social Policy.
7. National Association of Residential Care Facilities. 1987. *1987 Directory of Residential Care Facilities*. Richmond, Va.: National Association of Residential Care Facilities.
8. Simpson, D. 1984. *Case Management in Long Term Care Programs*. Washington, D.C.: Center for the Study of Social Policy.
9. Mathematica Policy Research. 1986. *Evaluation of the National Long-Term Care Demonstration. Final Summary Report*. Princeton, N.J.: Mathematica Policy Research.
10. National Study Group on State Medicaid Strategies. 1984. *Restructuring Medicaid: An Agenda for Change*. Washington, D.C.: Center for the Study of Social Policy.
11. Fear of knowing. 1984. *Washington Post* March 31.
12. Lane, L. 1984. *AHCA Initiative on Long Term Care Insurance*. Washington, D.C.: American Health Care Association.
13. Meiners, M. 1982. *Private Coverage of Services Not Covered by Medicare: The Case of Long Term Care Insurance*. Washington, D.C.: National Center for Health Services Research.
14. Fullerton, W. 1981. Finding the money and paying for long-term care services. In *Policy Options in Long-Term Care*, ed. J. Melzter, F. Farrow and H. Richman, 182–208. Chicago, Ill.: University of Chicago Press.
15. *Tax Subsidies for Long Term Care of the Elderly.* 1982. Report on U.S. Administration on Aging Grant 0090-AR-0033. Washington, D.C.: Center for the Study of Social Policy.

Thirty

Using Field Data to Shape New Policies

Paul M. Densen, Ellen W. Jones, and Sidney Katz

Much of this volume is devoted to consideration of structural and/or fiscal policy changes designed to bring about a better match between the needs of the elderly and the resources available to meet those needs. In theory, at least, this match presupposes a direct relationship between changes in policy and desired outcomes of practice. Evidence of this relationship, however, has been incomplete. Many reasons for this state of affairs have been cited, along with calls for better data for policy and planning.[1-13] Although answers to policy questions often require well-designed and carefully controlled research, a source of information that is presently underdeveloped is the body of information collected, or potentially collectible, from the agencies in the community dealing directly with the elderly population. Several kinds of data, if systematically collected from the day-to-day operations of service providers, could improve policy and delivery and coordination of services in care of the elderly.

A Framework

Planning for change in the service system and then judging the effects of change on the elderly require baseline information about how the present

Supported in part by the Robert Wood Johnson Foundation (Grant 6845) and the Administration on Aging (Older Americans Act, Title IV-E, 90 AT-2164).

service system is working for the elderly population. Broadly speaking, there are three questions to be asked, and their answers should be retrievable from the service system itself: Who among the elderly are being served? What services do they receive? What effect does the receipt of services produce on the elderly? Information in these areas is currently incomplete because the system for financing and delivering services is disconnected. Many different agencies in the community, each of which may respond to a different mandate for collecting and reporting information, provide services to the elderly. This diversity has made it impossible, except under research or other special circumstances, to aggregate data on a population or community basis. However, in 1980 the Robert Wood Johnson Foundation funded eight projects* "to demonstrate the effectiveness of integrating and coordinating at a community level the diverse array of services needed by elderly citizens with health problems."[14] Two of the foundation's requirements signified the need for the projects to develop community-based information systems. The first requirement was use of a uniform assessment mechanism by all participating service agencies to determine each client's needs for service, and the second was the development, by the project staff, of a mechanism for systematic follow-up of all assessed clients to ensure their linkage with the appropriate services. The information systems being developed by the projects in response to these requirements provide much of the data used to illustrate the approach to answering the three broad questions outlined above.

Who Is Served?

Demographic Characteristics

All service agencies collect and maintain descriptive data about their clients, ranging from minimal name and demographic identifiers to detailed case histories. The ability to aggregate the information on demographic characteristics—age, sex, race, residence, and living arrangements—for the long-term care service network *as a whole* makes it possible to address issues related to targeting of services and access to care. For example, several projects on the health-impaired elderly are now able to compare the demographic characteristics of elders in any one (or more) of the participating service agencies with the characteristics of the total elderly population (see Table 30.1). In all three project areas shown in Table 30.1, the percentages of selected demographic characteristics are higher in

---

*These projects are located in Richland and Lexington Counties, South Carolina; eight counties in East Tennessee; Baltimore County, Maryland; Philadelphia, Pennsylvania; Erie County, New York; Summit County, Ohio; Northwest Cook County, Illinois; and Lincoln, Nebraska.

Table 30.1. Selected Demographic Characteristics, Expressed as Percentage of Clients[a] in Three Health-Impaired Elderly Projects, Compared with 1980 Census Data (in parentheses)

Demographic Characteristics	Project Area		
	East Tennessee[b]	Baltimore County[c]	South Carolina[d]
Age 75 and over	58.2 (36.1)	64.7 (36.3)	50.3 (34.0)
Female	78.1 (59.4)	73.8 (60.3)	70.1 (61.7)
Black	4.5 (1.8)	6.9 (3.2)	36.3 (22.8)
Living Alone	47.3 (25.6)	39.4 (21.8)	46.8 (24.6)
At or Below Poverty Level	27.2[e] (24.1)		

[a]Clients 65 and over, at initial assessment.
[b]Carter, Greene, Hancock, Hawkins, Johnson, Sullivan, Unicoi, and Washington Counties. Clients on file as of 2/1/84, N = 3765.
[c]Exclusive of Baltimore City. Clients on file as of 7/31/84, N = 870.
[d]Richland and Lexington Counties. Clients on file as of 8/21/84, N = 3116.
[e]Includes a small number of individuals below 65 years of age in both numerator and denominator.

clients than in the general population. This accords with the project objective of targeting those groups presumed to be at higher risk of needing service. If the comparison had been reversed, one might question the performance of the service network.

In another example, not shown in the table, the project in Baltimore County found that the census tract distribution of its clientele roughly paralleled the census tract distribution of the elderly population. Had there been a wide discrepancy between the two sets of figures, it might have signaled the need for a shift in the allocation of local resources.

It should be emphasized that the projects furnishing the data are in an early operational stage. The major service providers, but not all service providers, in the area are participating in the coordination effort. If participation were 100%, the proportion of each population subgroup that received service in particular time periods could be calculated directly. At present, the data in the project information systems only *begin* to give an overall view of who is served by the community's service system.

When data are collected periodically, changes in the distribution of persons being served can be analyzed in relation to changes in policy, particularly policy decisions affecting eligibility and/or coverage under public programs. The importance of system monitoring at the local level to determine the effect of policy shifts has been emphasized by Estes and Lee.[15]

Functioning Status Characteristics: The Basic Activities of Daily Living

In addition to knowing the demographic indicators of who receive services, program managers, planners, and policy evaluators must know the nature and extent of disability of those served. This knowledge is central to management concerns because of the need to make efficient use of agency resources, particularly when resources are shrinking or limited.

It is now generally recognized that functioning status assessment is an appropriate means of determining the nature and degree of disability in elderly people, not only for initial care planning but also, through sequential assessments, for identifying changes in disability and needs for care.[3,4,16–18] Although specific measures of functioning status have not been standardized to the extent that certain demographic indicators have, there is considerable agreement about measures characterized as the basic activities of daily living.[16] Once these measures are documented uniformly by service agencies in the community, the aggregate data can be used to determine whether community resources are being directed toward the most appropriate target population and to examine the effect of policy decisions on the actual delivery of service.

Development of a common assessment process among participating service agencies was a condition of the grant made by the Robert Wood Johnson Foundation to the eight demonstration projects for the health-impaired elderly. In addition, the projects were required to include in their assessment instruments information about the basic activities of daily living (ADL; see Table 30.2) that constitute the Katz Index of ADL.[19]

The distribution of Tennessee ACCESS project clients according to their functioning status in ADL (Katz Index) at their first assessment is shown in Table 30.3 for 3 consecutive project years. The percentage of clients with one or more disabilities increased consistently over the 3 years and the percentage without disability in any one of the basic activities decreased correspondingly. There are several possible reasons for the change, but the point is that the data collected show that change has occurred. Additional details, such as source of referral, services requested and provided, and demographic characteristics, will identify changes in associated indicators and yield insight into causes.

The importance of information about the functioning status of clients seen by community agencies is underscored by the possibility that Medicare reimbursements to acute-care hospitals based on diagnostic category classifications will result in earlier and more frequent discharges of severely disabled elders to the community.[20,21] This development requires data to identify the effect of the policy on practice and on the outcomes of the elderly affected by it.

Table 30.2. Items of Information Included in Assessment Instruments Used in Health-Impaired Elderly Projects[a]

Core Items Required	
Functioning Status	Demographic Information
Mobility	Date of birth
Walking	Sex
Transferring	Race/ethnic group
Bathing	Client's location
Dressing	Usual living arrangements (type of place and
Toileting	with whom)
Bowel and bladder continence	Other
Feeding	Date of assessment
Orientation	Type of assessment (initial or reassessment)
	Source of referral for initial assessment
Sensory Impairments	Services needed by client
Sight	Services requested for client
Hearing	Agency to provide service(s)
Speech	Assessor/service planner

**Other Functioning Status Items Commonly Obtained
(with number of projects obtaining each)**

Transportation use (8)
Housekeeping, housecleaning (8)
Meal preparation (8)
Shopping (7)
Telephone use (6)
Laundry (5)
Medication, self-administration (5)
Money management (5)

[a]Core items required of all projects as well as certain other items commonly obtained. Definitions of items are as in Ref. 52. Basic ADL activities are classified as: performing without help, performing with help, or not performing the activity.

Functioning Status: The Instrumental Activities of Daily Living

Another measure of functioning status commonly used by community service agencies is the client's ability to carry out the instrumental activities of daily living (the IADL), a term introduced by Lawton and Brody.[22] The IADL are shown in Table 30.4. Information about an older person's performance of the activities indicates what specific services must be arranged if the person is to maintain an otherwise independent living status.

Table 30.5 shows the importance of measuring IADL separately for males and females. Many more females than males are able to carry out the activities of cooking, housecleaning, and shopping. Whether these differences will continue in the future as changes take place in sex-role

Table 30.3. Distribution of Tennessee ACCESS Clients According to Their ADL at Initial Assessment[a] for Three Time Periods

ADL Status	Year Ending 2/1/82		Year Ending 2/1/83		Year Ending 2/1/84	
(Katz Index)	N	Percent	N	Percent	N	Percent
A	1104	81.8	897	71.7	999	66.1
B	96	7.1	145	11.6	199	13.2
C	50	3.7	65	5.2	94	6.2
D	31	2.3	43	3.4	47	3.1
E	47	3.5	58	4.6	97	6.4
F	14	1.0	35	2.8	59	3.9
G	8	0.6	8	0.6	17	1.1
Total	1350	100.0	1251	100.0	1512	100.0

[a]ADL status refers to function in six areas: bathing, dressing, toileting, transferring, continence, and feeding. A = no dependency, B = 1 dependency, C = 2 dependencies, D = 3 dependencies, E = 4 dependencies, F = 5 dependencies, G = 6 dependencies.

Table 30.4. Percentage Distribution of Clients in the Baltimore County (exclusive of Baltimore City) Coordinated Services for the Elderly Project, According to Level of Function in the Instrumental Activites of Daily Living (IADL)[a]

	Level of Function		
Activity	Performs Without Help	Performs With Help	Does Not Perform
Housekeeping	16.4	17.2	66.4
Laundry	18.6	11.6	69.7
Meal Preparation	27.2	15.6	57.2
Shopping	10.8	20.9	68.3
Medication Administration[b]	54.6	11.8	33.6
Money Management	45.5	19.6	34.8
Telephone Use	66.0	9.6	24.5
Transportation Use	15.8	50.2	33.9

[a]Total of 1063 clients with initial assessments as of 2/10/84. Clients were screened for potential need of multiple services. Small numbers of clients with unreported levels of function were excluded from some of the individual calculations.
[b]Percentage based on 929 clients taking medications.

definitions remains to be seen. In any event, the data suggest a direction for community educational efforts designed to help people to help themselves.

The Relationship Between ADL and IADL

When elderly clients seen by community service agencies are described in terms of their ability to perform both ADL and IADL activities, there is a marked relationship between performance of the ADL and IADL activities. Individuals with one or more impairments of function in the basic

Table 30.5. Housekeeping, Cooking, and Shopping Activity of Male and Female Clients of Tennessee ACCESS Project[a]

	Both Sexes		Males		Females	
Level of Function	N	Percent	N	Percent	N	Percent
Performs All Activities Without Help	788	20.0	125	10.9	663	23.8
Has Help in Some But Not All	2188	55.7	630	54.7	1558	56.0
Has Help in All Three Activities	955	24.3	396	34.4	559	20.1
TOTAL	3931	100.0	1151	100.0	2780	99.9

[a]All clients with an initial assessment as of 10/25/83.

ADL are at very high risk of needing help with one or more of three home-maintenance activities. This fact has implications for the training of service providers, which should focus attention on the individual's *total* functioning and needs rather than "health-care needs" or "social service needs" alone. It also argues for policies and practices that strengthen communication between those agencies whose primary concern is with medically oriented care and those that provide other services necessary for maintenance in the community setting.

The relationship between the basic ADL and IADL has significance also for the classification of population groups on a scale of ADL functioning. Although the individual items that make up the Katz Index are commonly used by workers in the field, the Index per se has not come into general use outside of the research environment. The Index has been thought by some to be insufficiently revealing of client needs for community social services, since a large proportion of the noninstitutionalized elderly will be classified in the single category A, independent in all six basic activities. If the A clients are further classified as those with and without IADL dependencies, however, one gets an expanded, more sensitive scale of eight classes as follows:

A without IADL dependency

A with IADL dependency

B with IADL dependency

.

.

.

G with IADL dependency

When the assessment data from the Tennessee ACCESS project were looked at in this way, 99.6% of the clients could be described by one or the other categories of the expanded scale. Only 0.4%, those with ADL status of B or worse who said they were independent in the listed IADL functions, did not fit into one of the descriptive categories.

Population-Based Estimates of Functioning Status

Unlike demographic data, data on the distribution of the elderly population by functioning status are not available from the U.S. Census. Reports issued by the National Center for Health Statistics contain national estimates, by age, of persons needing help with basic physical activities and with home-management activities.[23] Several special community surveys, such as those of Branch in Massachusetts[24] and the Government Accounting Office in Cleveland,[25] provide similar figures. With appropriate adjustments for age and sex it is possible to estimate from these data the prevalence of individuals in any community needing help with ADL or IADL activities—providing one understands that such estimates assume the rates in the community are the same as those in the country as a whole or in the special survey.

When the aggregate data from service agencies are compared with the prevalence estimates, the proportion of the total community problem being addressed by the service network can be examined. The difference may be large; it has been shown repeatedly that a large proportion of the help received by elders is help from family and friends.[26–28] Comparison over time, however, would reveal whether the difference changes. The change, or lack of it, could then be reviewed for its policy implications.

Services Provided

The services being provided in the community and the length of time between the request for and receipt of service concern individual clients and their families as well as those responsible for providing services effectively.

Table 30.6 illustrates that data on these concerns can become available through area-wide uniform assessment and a centralized information-management system. The data in Table 30.6 refer to reports of services provided by agencies whose clientele, for the most part, reside in the community, that is, in noninstitutional settings. Data about hospital and nursing home resources are discussed in a later section.

As might be expected, the time between request for and receipt of service varies among the types of services in Table 30.6. For example, in the Tennessee project, 95% of clients with referrals for home health care received the service within one week, while only 29% with referrals for

Table 30.6. Time Between Referral and Start of Service[a]

Service for Which Referral was Made	Total Referrals	Distribution of Referrals by Time to Start of Service					
		0–7 days		8 days or more		Not started	
		N	Percent	N	Percent	N	Percent
Home Health Care	38	36	94.7	1	2.6	1	2.6
Hearing Evaluation and Service	48	22	45.8	13	27.1	13	27.1
Other Medical Evaluation and/or Therapy	24	17	70.8	2	8.3	5	20.8
Home Medical Equipment, Supplies	7	5	71.4	2	28.6		
Home-delivered Meals	187	77	41.2	36	19.3	74	39.6
Homemaker Service	137	39	28.5	91	66.4	7	5.1
Chore Services	133	16	12.0	114	85.7	3	2.3
Transportation	14	5	35.7	6	42.9	3	21.4
Congregate Meals	13	13	100.0				
Food Stamps	14	2	14.3	3	21.4	9	64.3
Energy Assistance	364	60	16.5	25	6.9	279	76.6
Emergency Assistance	28	24	85.7			4	14.3
Legal and Protective Services	17	4	23.5	8	47.1	5	29.4
All Other Referrals	15	4	26.7	3	20.0	8	53.3

[a]Quarterly report of selected referrals for Tennessee ACCESS clients, October–December 1983.

homemaker services and 41% with referrals for home-delivered meals received those services as promptly.

Review of information like that in Table 30.6 can stimulate a program manager to initiate some inquiries. The rate of completion of referrals may indicate the need for better communication between agencies at one or both ends of the referral process, for repeated or better staff education and supervision somewhere along the line, or for increased resources. Used in this way, the information-management system becomes a tool for monitoring the performance of the service network in the community as a whole, just as the case-management function is designed to monitor care of the individual client.

People and Services

Most service agencies in the community have data on the number and variety of services they provide in terms of volume (or units) of service or agency activity. Many also count the numbers of clients for whom they provide a particular service. These data can be aggregated for the service network as a whole, or at least for that part contributing to a central information system (see Table 30.6). Data have not been available, however, on the *unduplicated* count of individuals to whom these services or combinations of services are provided. Table 30.7, an example of an analysis of data for the Baltimore County project area, shows the clients for whom a service plan was developed based on a comprehensive assessment of their functioning status and need for care. Of the total 838 clients with a service plan, 40.1% were said to need only one type of service, but over half, 59.9%, were said to need two or more types. In particular, although a total of 169 clients, or 20% of the total, needed transportation services (data not shown in the table), only 7 of the 169 (4%) needed transportation services alone. Thus, 96% of clients needing help with transportation also needed other types of community service. In this context it should be recalled that individuals with one or more disabilities in ADL almost always need help with one or more IADL associated with maintaining a noninstitutional living situation.

Should these relationships prove to be generalizable, their implications must be considered in developing policy about health care for the elderly. Since policy is directed at meeting needs as they occur among the elderly, addressing health needs or social service needs alone, as if they were

Table 30.7. Services Recommended for Clients in the Baltimore County (Exclusive of Baltimore City) Coordinated Services for the Elderly Project[a]

| Number and Type of Service | Clients with Specified Number and Types of Services Recommended | | | |
| | N | Percent | Cumulative | |
			N	Percent
One Type Only	336	40.1	838	100.0
Transportation[b]	7	0.8		
Housekeeping and other homemaker services[c]	69	8.2		
Social support services[d]	164	19.6		
Personal care services[e]	38	4.5		
Continuing medical/nursing services[f]	58	6.9		
Two Types of Services	244	29.1	502	59.9
Three Types of Services	161	19.2	258	30.8
Four Types of Services	79	9.4	97	11.6
Five Types of Services	18	2.1	18	2.1
Total	838	100.0		

[a]Clients with initial assessments and service plans as of 8/15/84.
[b]Includes all types of transportation and escort services.
[c]Including light housecleaning, chore services, minor house repairs, and meal services.
[d]Including administrative and legal services, leisure socialization services, material aid, and placement services (both housing and institutional).
[e]Assistance with ADL (bathing, dressing, etc.).
[f]Including specialized therapies and mental health services.

independent of each other, will present barriers to maintaining individuals in the community at their highest possible level of functioning.

The Need for a Common Service Terminology

One of the problems in comparing service data over time or between programs is the lack of agreement on definitions or classification of services, that is, the specific tasks included in a given service title or the grouping of services into broader categories. The problem is illustrated in Table 30.8.[29,30] The congruence and incongruence among the three classifica-

Table 30.8. Comparison of Three Classifications of Selected Services[a]

CSE Project	National Long-Term Care Channeling Demonstration	NASUA, N4A, and TSDI
Personal care	Home health aide Homemaker, personal care	Personal care Homemaking Shopping Chore Escort
Homemaker	Homemaker, personal care Housekeeping	Personal care Homemaking Housekeeping Shopping Chore
Chore	Housekeeping Chore	Homemaking Housekeeping Shopping Chore Repairs, maintenance, renovation
Home Repairs, Maintenance	Chore	Chore Repairs, maintenance, renovation
Meals (home-delivered and congregate)	Home-delivered meals	Meals (homedelivered and congregate)
Transportation	Transportation Companion	Transportation
Supervision	Companion	Shopping Escort Supervision Visiting Telephoning Recreation

[a]Comparison was made on the basis of specific inclusions in definitions of service categories. Congruence (i.e., overlapping definitions) is indicated by the repetition of terms. CSE Project (Baltimore Co.) definitions as of 1/17/83. Channeling Demonstration (NY State) definitions are from Ref. 32. NASUA definitions are from Ref. 30.

tions shown in the figure were determined by comparison of inclusions in the service categories and their definitions. Clearly, some inclusions are congruent with one category and others with a different category, and the lack of overall congruence among the three classifications is apparent. However, judgments about the efficiency or effectiveness of different eligibility and coverage combinations in terms of cost rely on comparisons based on a uniform terminology for the classification of services. What is one to make of unit costs, for example, that differ as much as tenfold (from $0.61 to $6.78) among five agencies within the same community?[31] The first question to ask about such variation (beyond checking the arithmetic) concerns the nature of the product being purchased: Are the tasks paid for with $0.61 the same as those paid for with $6.78? In what respect do they differ? The National Association of State Units on Aging (NASUA) has published a classification of services contracted for by Area Agencies on Aging and a proposed classification scheme.[30] This scheme has been the basis for the expanded categories of services used by several projects for the health-impaired elderly. An agreed-upon nomenclature and classification of services would be useful to all agencies concerned with care of the elderly at local, state, and national levels. An authoritative body should take on the task of developing and promoting such a classification.

Tracking Changes in the Functional Status of Elders

It is natural that concern for meeting the long-term care needs of elderly individuals should focus on the process, that is, the efficiency, of providing service. Yet, whatever the immediate focus of social policy, legislation, or regulation intended to translate policy into practice, the ultimate goal is to enable individuals to maintain or improve their ability to function in their chosen environment. Data on changes in functional status, therefore, are necessary to examine effectiveness as well as efficiency. These measures of change represent one aspect of the *outcome* of the process of care.

Reports of longitudinal studies showing change in time in the individual's ability to function have begun to appear in the literature.[33,34] These studies, based upon successive observations of representative samples of the elderly in the general population, provide a picture of the natural history of the aging process as reflected in functional status.

Changes in functioning status of patients in nursing homes have also been reported. One approach to the measurement of quality of care in such settings is a comparison of progress in functioning of patients in different nursing homes related to their functional status at time of admission.[35,36] Widespread adoption of uniform assessment procedures would make these comparisons possible.

The use of a common assessment instrument by community service agencies participating in the health-impaired elderly projects now makes it possible for the project information systems to provide data on functioning status change among elderly people receiving service from the community service network as a whole.

Table 30.9 shows functioning ADL status change, as expressed by the Katz Index, among Tennessee ACCESS clients who were reassessed 6 months (plus or minus 2 weeks) after their initial assessment. The horizontal axis shows status at initial assessment and the vertical axis status at 6-month reassessment. For those with a reassessment, the numbers on the diagonal represent individuals whose functioning status was the same at first assessment and at 6-month follow-up. Numbers above the diagonal show persons whose status improved; numbers below the diagonal, those whose status deteriorated. The types of change are summarized for two functioning status groups in Table 30.10.

Of the 1609 clients reassessed at 6 months, 87.1% were functioning at the same level on follow-up as at initial assessment, but 5.1% had improved and 7.8% were worse. Because individuals in the A category were functioning independently in all six of the basic activities, they could not be shown to have improved within the range of classes of the ADL scale. Improvement was revealed, however, for 21.3% of the individuals with one or more dependencies at the time of their initial assessment.

The data in the tables also show that people without ADL dependencies at first assessment had better outcomes than those with one or more dependencies: fewer deteriorated and fewer died. The small group with dependencies in all six activities (the G group) had very poor outcomes. Seven of the eighteen (38.9%) had died within 6 months, and none of the four who were reassessed had improved (Table 30.9). These data on the relationship between dependency in function in the basic ADL and the risk of deterioration or death are consistent with past studies. They indicate that long-term care services should be evaluated in terms of maintenance of function, that is, avoidance of or delay in deterioration and death.

Tables 30.9 and 30.10 also provide information of value in considering ways of improving practice. Of the 3304 clients entered in the tables (all those with an initial assessment in the indicated period of time), 1365 were receiving service from a participating agency but did not have a reassessment reported to the central file during the 180 ± 14 days follow-up period. Yet the stated policy of the ACCESS project was to assess clients every 3 months. From the standpoint of continuity of care and coordination of services for the individual, and from the standpoint of monitoring the performance of the network as a whole, these 1365 cases warrant further inquiry. If, indeed, reassessments were not done on these individuals at this time, changes in their needs for care would have gone undetected. On the other hand, it is possible that reassessments were done but not reported to

Table 30.9. Changes in ADL Status 6 Months after Initial Assessment[a]

ADL Status at 6 Months (180 ± 14 days)	ADL Status at Initial Assessment							
	Total	A	B	C	D	E	F	G
A	1194	1145	33	7	1	5	3	—
B	162	37	108	7	3	5	2	—
C	73	11	6	47	5	2	2	—
D	52	12	3	7	26	2	2	—
E	77	12	5	4	7	46	3	—
F	42	6	1	1	—	9	25	—
G	9	1	1	—	1	—	2	4
Total with 6-month Reassessment	1609	1224	157	73	43	69	39	4
Total Not Reassessed but Receiving Services	1365	1054	143	57	29	53	25	4
Died During Period	165	76	19	22	12	18	11	7
Relocated During Period, Other Terminations	165	127	13	3	3	11	5	3
Total with Initial Assessment	3304	2481	332	155	87	151	80	18

[a]Tennessee ACCESS clients first assessed 4/1/81–6/30/83. ADL is expressed as the Katz Index and refers to function in six areas: bathing, dressing, toileting, transferring, continence, and feeding. A = no dependency, B = 1 dependency, C = 2 dependencies, D = 3 dependencies, E = 4 dependencies, F = 5 dependencies, G = 6 dependencies.

the information-management system. The situation needs to be clarified and the findings incorporated in ongoing training programs for staff and supervisors of community agencies in order to bring policy and practice together.

Tables 30.9 and 30.10 are examples of a class of information that a well-organized data-management system can be expected to produce. Obviously, other periods of observation can and should be looked at for determination of outcomes. As data production becomes more sophisticated, more variables, such as client's age and living arrangements, can be incorporated into the progress measures. Examination of trends over time will greatly enhance assessment of the effect of policy on practice in the community.

Comparison of different communities with different service structures or policies can also provide clues about which organizational arrangements or policies relate to improvement in functioning status outcomes. Routine administrative reporting systems seldom can answer the question of why differences occur, but they can reveal areas for further investigation through specific research.

Table 30.10. Reassessment Status and Change in ADL 6 Months after Initial Assessment[a]

Reassessment Status at 6-Month Follow-up and Change in ADL Status[b]	N	Percent of Clients with Initial Assessments	Percent of Clients with Reassessments	ADL Status at Initial Assessment					
				A (no ADL Dependency)			B–G (one or more dependencies)		
				N	Percent of Initial Assessments	Percent of Reassessments	N	Percent of Initial Assessments	Percent of Reassessments
Improved	82	2.5	5.1	—	—	—	82	10.0	21.3
Same	1401	42.4	87.1	1145	46.2	93.5	256	31.1	66.5
Worse	126	3.8	7.8	79	3.2	6.5	47	5.7	12.2
Total with 6-Month Reassessment	1609	48.7	100.0	1224	49.3	100.0	385	46.8	100.0
Total Not Reassessed But Receiving Services	1365	41.3		1054	42.5		311	37.8	
Died During Period	165	5.0		76	3.1		89	10.8	
Relocated or Other Termination During Period	165	5.0		127	5.1		38	4.6	
Total with Initial Assessment	3304	100.0		2481	100.0		123	100.0	

[a] Tennessee ACCESS clients first assessed 4/1/81–6/30/84. ADL is expressed as the Katz Index and refers to function in six areas: bathing, dressing, toileting, transferring, continence, and feeding.

[b] Change to a less-dependent status (to fewer dependencies, such as from D to C) is classified as improved; change to more-dependent status is classified as worse.

Hospitals and Nursing Homes

To bring about a better match between the needs of the elderly and the resources available to meet those needs, the parts of the service network— family, physician, hospital, nursing home, and community agency—must mesh smoothly. In other words, answers to the three broad questions— who among the elderly gets service, what services do they get and how does their status change over time—need to include the *entire* array of long-term care services in the community.

The increasing proportion of the elderly and chronically ill among the patients of acute-care hospitals has led to recognition of the significance of hospitals in long-term care.[37,38] Implementation of the prospective payment system regulation,[39,40] resulting in earlier discharge of elderly patients, increases the importance *to the hospital,* for financial as well as humanitarian reasons, of early identification of those patients who will need help after discharge. The sooner arrangements for posthospital care can be made, the more feasible the early discharge. Again, systematic assessment of elderly patients can identify individuals at high risk of needing long-term care and can contribute to discharge planning and to more effective communication with the other agencies that may be called upon to help meet the patient's needs.

If federal and state efforts to reduce inappropriate placement of long-term care patients are successful, the distribution of places to which hospitals discharge the elderly should change. Data on discharge destination of hospitalized patients are regularly available in a number of states. Table 30.11 shows the data for 1980–1982 for patients age 65 or older in two of the health-impaired elderly project areas and in their states as a whole. Similar data can be used to monitor trends in discharge dispositions. The data could also display institutional or noninstitutional residence of patients before admission. The percentage of elderly patients discharged to long-term care institutions *for the first time,* that is, the percentage of these discharges among those *not* admitted to the hospital from nursing homes or other long-term care residential facilities, would indicate the hospital's and community's success in promoting alternatives to institutional care.

One aspect of the dynamics of patient movement within the long-term care system is illustrated by the data in Table 30.11. In the geographic areas shown, between 4.5% and 7.1% of elderly persons discharged from the acute-care hospitals went to nursing homes. Knowledge of the interaction of nursing homes with other parts of the long-term care system is also important. There is a considerable body of information about the characteristics of individuals *in* nursing homes,[41–44] but much less is known about what happens to those leaving nursing homes. Contrary to the popular impression, not everyone who enters a nursing home stays for an

Table 30.11. Percent Distribution of Hospital Discharges by Place to Which Discharged

| | Maryland[a] | | South Carolina[b] | |
	Baltimore County (excluding Baltimore City)	State (excluding Baltimore County and City)	Richland and Lexington Counties	Entire State
Total Discharges 65 Years and Over: Number	108,192	200,272	44,723	284,606
Percent	100.0	100.0	100.0	100.0
Home Without Mention of Home Care	80.5	81.5	81.1	83.2
Home With Organized Home-Care Service	2.0	1.6	2.3	1.8
Nursing Homes, LTC Facilities	6.8	7.1	4.9	4.5
Other Hospitals	2.2	1.8	0.6	2.0
Against Medical Advice	0.3	0.3	0.1	0.2
Other Place and Unknown	0.2	0.3	4.4	1.3
Died	8.0	7.4	6.6	7.0

[a]Data are resident data. Source: Information Service Center, Baltimore, MD.
[b]Data are for hospitals in the specified areas. Source: Budget and Control Board, Division of Research and Statistical Services, State of South Carolina.

extended time period.[45] Liu and Manton, using data from the 1977 National Nursing Home Survey, found that one-third of an initial admission cohort had been discharged within 30 days or less.[46] Furthermore, in 1980, 27% of over 12,000 live discharges from long-term care facilities in one health-impaired elderly project area were discharged to their (or another's) private residence.[47] Tracking these individuals as they move back into the community is essential for continuity of care. Health-care planners should know what educational programs are needed to help families support these individuals, what services from other community agencies the discharges require, how many of these discharges remain at home or are readmitted to a nursing home, and their subsequent hospitalization. Determination of these intermediate and long-term outcomes is important for coordination of services to the individual, for improving communication among the various components of the service network, and for understanding the implications of different methods of financing long-term care. Lewis and her colleagues have made a start in this direction.[48]

As community-based data systems, such as those being developed by the health-impaired elderly projects, incorporate data on elderly patients in hospitals and nursing homes as well as from other sources, they move closer to making a continuum of care a reality.[49] A well-organized, community-based information system, including both service input and client outcomes, can be a catalyst that moves people and organizations closer to achieving their mutual goals for care of the elderly.

Discussion

"The great source of misery of mankind is not their numbers, but their imperfections, and the want of control over the conditions in which they live. . . . There is a definite task before us to determine from observation, the sources of health, in the two sexes under different conditions. The exact determination of evils is the first step toward their remedies."

Those words, written in the middle of the nineteenth century by William Farr,[50] are equally pertinent today to the task of reshaping health care for the elderly. We need to know both how well policy is being translated into practice and what practice tells us about which policy changes are required.

The answers to these questions can come from a systematic, well-organized information system based on the day-to-day operations of service agencies. The information system has two requirements: all providers of service must express the information in a common language, and some organizational body must collect and analyze this information on a communitywide basis.

The first of these requirements can be met through the use of a uniform assessment instrument. As Kane and Kane[51] point out, "Any strategy for altering the health status of the elderly population requires a technology for first assessing that health status and then detecting increments of progress." A common assessment instrument provides the *lingua franca* for describing long-term care problems and need of the elderly. The information derived from the instrument contributes to every operation of the long-term care service network, from the developing of individual care plans through planning programs and managing the service agencies, to monitoring systems and making policy for all the elderly in the community. The multiple uses of a uniform assessment mechanism have been well set forth by Jones et al.[52] and by Callahan and Wallach.[1]

As early as 1956, the Commission on Chronic Illness[53] called for the development of a terminology for use in evaluating the needs of patients in order to provide appropriate treatment and to make better use of resources. Since then, the population of elderly has increased and the need for systematic assessment is more widely recognized by service providers. A minimum data set has been recommended,[54] and many items from it are already in use. The field is also gaining experience in how to use assessment information in care planning, operations, and system management.

The time has come to take the next step toward translating policy intended to reshape health care for the elderly into efficient and effective practice. That step calls for official sponsorship of a uniform terminology for needs assessment by federal funding agencies and regulatory agencies at the state level in a manner similar to the sponsorship of the *International List of Diseases, Injuries and Causes of Death,* originally sponsored in the United States by the predecessor of the present National Center for Health Statistics.

Another common language needs to be developed to define and to classify services. Recognition of this need and support of efforts to develop a terminology by official and voluntary agencies would lay a solid groundwork for the future.

The second requirement of a well-organized information system is a centralized information-management unit responsible for monitoring the service network through analysis of the activities of the service agencies. The centralized state-level reporting systems now in operation are limited in scope and in their accessibility for analysis of the whole health-care system. Available health-care data are generally claims data, clinical data, or administrative data, such as admissions or discharges, and collection is uncoordinated.[55] As a result, there can be little analysis for long-range planning of a continuum of care for the elderly. This is not surprising. The pressures of day-to-day demands at the direct service level and at the systems level (the state) make management, (in the words of Iglehart, who was describing the problems of the British National Health Service) "oriented toward operations, not strategic thinking."[56]

Yet the problem has not gone unrecognized in the United States. For example, a report on long-term care system development in Washington State recommended that "the department (of Social and Health Services) should improve its long-term care data collection and retrieval capabilities . . . to augment its capability to generate useful information on clients characteristics, utilization and cost for management, planning and research purposes."[57]

The information described in this paper should provide the foundation for strategic thinking on data collection. The data can be produced on a regular basis in the same way that vital statistics on the general population are regularly produced. The findings, of course, can be elaborated in many ways by special analyses, but the primary function of the data compiled here is to provide an illustration of how the long-term care service network is actually operating and to reveal areas that require further investigation or re-examination of policy.

Furthermore, a centralized client information system facilitates a count of people as well as services or problems. Thus it permits an estimate of the number of elderly with multiple needs, the very individuals who generate the greatest pressures to coordinate and integrate services for long-term care. The ability to make these estimates will become increasingly important in the future as the numbers of elderly persons, particularly the old-old, continue to increase.

Moreover, if policy is to meet people's needs, treating the various needs as though they were independent of each other perpetuates problems in the efforts to match needs and resources. Focusing on the service rather than the person tends to result in financing efforts that contribute to fractionation of services, duplication of effort, and high costs.

The data given here indicate a high correlation between the needs for help with ADL and IADL. As a consequence, many different service organizations, including the hospital, the physician, the nursing home, the home-care program and others, may be involved in meeting the needs of the elderly individual. Efforts to coordinate this complex service structure have resulted in the introduction of the case manager. At the systems level, however, there has been very little analysis of how individuals move through the system. This analysis will require longitudinal observations and is a subject for research. The questions for research can and should arise from the ongoing information-management effort.

Public policy is largely dictated by politics. It is naive to expect policy to flow neatly from a data base to the passage of legislation, and then to development of a rational service structure. However, because policy and practice are intimately related, a well-conceived data system can unify the development of policy by identifying the options available and clarifying the advantages and disadvantages of each.

References

1. Callahan, J. J., Wallach, S. S. 1981. *Reforming the Long-Term Care System.* Lexington, Mass.: Lexington Books.
2. Congressional Budget Office. 1977. *Long Term Care for the Elderly and Disabled.* Washington, D.C.: Government Printing Office.
3. Katz, S., Hedrick, S. C., Henderson, N. S. 1979. The measurement of long term care needs and impact. *Health Med Care Serv Rev* 2(1):1–21.
4. McDermott, W. 1981. Absence of indicators of the influence of its physicians on a society's health. *Am J Med* 70(4):833–843.
5. New York State Coordinating Council. 1979. Long term care. In *Statewide Health Needs and Practices.* Albany, N.Y.: New York State Coordinating Council.
6. Gurland, B., Bennett, R., Wilder, D. 1981. Reevaluating the place of evaluation in planning for alternatives to institutional care for the elderly. *J Soc Issues* 37(1):51–70.
7. Vladeck, B. C. 1982. Understanding long term care. *N Engl J Med* 307(14):889–890.
8. United States Office of Management and Budget, Interagency Statistical Committee on Long-Term Care for the Elderly. 1980. *Data Coverage of the Functionally Limited Elderly.* Springfield, Va.: Department of Commerce, National Technical Information Service.
9. United States Office of Management and Budget, Interagency Statistical Committee on Long Term Care for the Elderly. 1980. *Inventory of Data Sources of the Functionally Limited Elderly.* Springfield, Va.: Department of Commerce, National Technical Information Service.
10. Kovar, M. G. 1977. The population 65 years and over. In *Health: United States, 1976–1977.* HEW Pub. No. (HRA) 77-1232. Washington, D.C.: Government Printing Office, 3–26.
11. Maddox, G. L. 1981. Alternative models for health care. In *Allocating Health Care Resources for the Aged and Disabled,* ed. R. Morris. Lexington, Mass.: Lexington Books.
12. United States General Accounting Office. 1981. Improved knowledge base would be helpful in reaching policy decisions on providing long term care. HRD-82-4. Gaithersburg, Md.: United States General Accounting Office.
13. Kamerman, S. B., Kahn, A. J. 1976. *Social Services in the United States: Policies and Programs.* Philadelphia, Pa.: Temple University Press.
14. The Robert Wood Johnson Foundation. 1979. *Program for the Health-Impaired Elderly.* Princeton, N.J.: The Robert Wood Johnson Foundation.

15. Estes, C. L., Lee, P. R. 1981. Policy shifts and their impact on health care for elderly persons. *West J Med* 135(6):511–518.
16. Hedrick, S. C., Katz, S., Stroud, M. W. 1980/1981. Patient assessment in long-term care: Is there a common language? *Aged Care Serv Rev* 2(4):13–19.
17. Duke University Center for the Study of Aging and Human Development. 1978. *Multidimensional Functional Assessment: The OARS Methodology. A Manual,* 2nd ed. Durham, N.C.: Duke University Center for the Study of Aging and Human Development.
18. American College of Physicians, Health and Public Policy Committee. 1984. Long-term care of the elderly. Position paper. *Ann Int Med* 100(5):760–763.
19. Katz, S., Akpom, C. A. 1976. A measure of primary sociobiological functions. *Int J Health Serv* 6(3):493–508.
20. Meiners, M. R., Coffey, R. M. 1983. Hospital DRGs and the need for long-term care services: An empirical analysis. Paper presented at the 111th Annual Meeting of the American Public Health Association, Dallas, Tx.
21. Estes, C. L. 1984. Fiscal crisis and public policy for the aging. Paper presented at the Annual Meeting of the American Association for the Advancement of Science, New York, N.Y.
22. Lawton, M. P., Brody, E. M. 1969. Assessment of older people: Self-maintaining and instrumental activities of daily living. *Gerontologist* 9(3):179–186.
23. National Center for Health Statistics. 1983. Americans needing help to function at home. *Advance Data from Vital and Health Statistics,* No. 92, DHHS Pub. No. (PHS) 83-1250. Hyattsville, Md.: Department of Health and Human Services.
24. Branch, L. G. 1977. *Understanding the Health and Social Needs of People Over Age 65.* Boston, Mass.: Center for Survey Research, University of Massachusetts and the Joint Center for Urban Studies of MIT and Harvard University.
25. Comptroller General of the United States. 1977. *The Well-Being of Older People in Cleveland, Ohio.* HRD-77-70. Washington, D.C.: Government Printing Office.
26. Branch, L. G., Jette, A. M. 1983. Elders' use of informal long-term care assistance. *Gerontologist* 23(1):51–56.
27. Cantor, M. H. 1979. Neighbors and friends: An overlooked resource in the informal support system. *Res Aging* 1:434–463.
28. Shanas, E. 1974. Health status of older people: Cross-national implications. *Am J Public Health* 64(3):261–264.
29. New York State Office for the Aging. 1982. *Long Term Care Channeling Demonstration Project, Annual Progress Report.* Albany, N.Y.: New York State Office for the Aging.
30. National Association of State Units on Aging. 1981. *Uniform Descriptions of Services for the Aging.* Washington, D.C.: National Association of State Units on Aging.
31. Erie County Department of Senior Services. 1981. Monthly Program—Fiscal Reports. Buffalo, N.Y.: Erie County Department of Senior Services.
32. New York State Office for the Aging. 1982. *Long-Term Care Channeling Demonstration Project, Annual Progress Report.* Albany, N.Y.: New York State Office for the Aging.

33. Katz, S., Branch, L. G., Branson, M. H., Papsidero, J. A., Beck, J. C., Greer, D. S. 1983. Active life expectancy. *N Engl J Med* 309(20):1218–1224.

34. Branch, L. G., Katz, S., Kniepmann, K., Papsidero, J. A. A prospective study of functional status among community elders. *Am J Public Health* 74(3):266–268.

35. Jones, E. W., Densen, P. M., McNitt, B. J. 1978. Assessing the quality of long-term care. Research Summary Series, HEW Pub. No. (PHS) 78-3192. Hyattsville, Md.: National Center for Health Services Research.

36. Linn, M. W., Gurel, L., Linn, B. S. 1977. Patient outcomes as a measure of quality of nursing home care. *Am J Public Health* 67(4):337–344.

37. Campion, E. W., Bang, A., May, M. I. 1983. Why acute-care hospitals must undertake long-term care. *N Engl J Med* 308(2):71–75.

38. Eisdorfer, C. 1981. Care of the aged: The barriers of traditions. *Ann Int Med* 94:256–260.

39. Medicare program. Prospective payments for Medicare inpatient hospital services. 1983. *Federal Register* 48(171):39752–39890.

40. Medicare program. Prospective payment for Medicare inpatient hospital services. 1984. *Federal Register* 49(1):234–334.

41. United States Senate, Special Committee on Aging. 1974. *Nursing Home Care in the United States: A Failure in Public Policy.* Washington, D.C.: Government Printing Office.

42. New York State Moreland Act Commission. 1976. *Long Term Care Regulation: Past Lapses, Future Prospects, a Summary Report.* Albany, N.Y.: New York State Moreland Act Commission.

43. United States General Accounting Office. 1979. Entering a nursing home: Costly implications for medicaid and the elderly. *Report to the Congress by the Comptroller General.* PAD-80-12. Washington, D.C.: Government Printing Office.

44. United States Department of Health, Education, and Welfare, Public Health Service, Office of Nursing Home Affairs. 1975. *Long Term Care Facility Improvement Study.* Washington, D.C.: Office of Nursing Home Affairs.

45. Liu, K., Palesch, Y. 1981. The nursing home population: Different perspectives and implications for policy. *Health Care Financing Rev* 3(2):15–23.

46. Liu, K., Manton, K. G. 1983. The length of stay pattern of nursing home admissions. *Med Care* 21(12):1211–1222.

47. Illinois Department of Public Health. 1980. *Annual Long Term Care Facility Questionnaire.* Springfield, Ill.: Illinois Department of Public Health.

48. Lewis, M. A., Kane, R. L., Cretin, S., Clark, V. 1985. The immediate and subsequent outcomes of nursing home care. *Am J Public Health* 75(7):758–761.

49. Ross, E. C. 1984. Programming for chronically disabled persons: The impact of federal financing policies in the political climate of the early 1980s. *J Health Hum Resources Administration* 6(4):425–449.

50. Eyler, J. M. 1979. *Victorian Social Medicine: The Ideas and Methods of William Farr.* Baltimore, Md.: Johns Hopkins University Press.

51. Kane, R. L., Kane, R. A. 1981. *Assessing the Elderly.* Lexington, Mass.: Lexington Books.

52. Jones, E. W., McNitt, B. J., McKnight, E. 1974. *Patient Classification for Long-*

Term Care: User's Manual. HEW Pub. No. 75-3017. Washington, D.C.: Government Printing Office.

53. Commission on Chronic Illness. 1956. *Chronic Illness in the United States,* Vol. 2, *Care of the Long Term Patient.* Cambridge, Mass.: Harvard University Press.

54. National Committee on Vital and Health Statistics. 1980. *Long Term Care: Minimum Data Set.* HHS Pub. No. (PHS) 80-1158. Washington, D.C.: Government Printing Office.

55. Birnbaum, H., Burke, R., Pratter, F. 1983. Managing programs for the elderly: Design of a social information system. *Health Care Financing Rev* 5(2):11–23.

56. Iglehart, J. K. 1984. The British National Health Service under the Conservatives, Part II. *N Engl J Med* 319(1):63–67.

57. Garrick, M. A., Rubin, D. D., Wilke, D. C. 1983. *Long-Term Care System Development Project, Final Report.* Olympia, Wash.: Washington State Department of Social and Health Services.

Index